Intelligent Interactive Multimedia Systems for e-Healthcare Applications

Amit Kumar Tyagi · Ajith Abraham ·
Arturas Kaklauskas
Editors

Intelligent Interactive Multimedia Systems for e-Healthcare Applications

Springer

Editors
Amit Kumar Tyagi
Vellore Institute of Technology
Chennai, Tamil Nadu, India

Centre for Advanced Data Science
Vellore Institute of Technology
Chennai, Tamil Nadu, India

Arturas Kaklauskas
Department of Civil Engineering
Vilnius Gediminas Technical University
Vilnius, Lithuania

Ajith Abraham
Machine Intelligence Research Labs (MIR Labs)
Auburn, WA, USA

ISBN 978-981-16-6541-7 ISBN 978-981-16-6542-4 (eBook)
https://doi.org/10.1007/978-981-16-6542-4

This Springer imprint is published by the registered company Springer Nature Singapore Pte Ltd.
The registered company address is: 152 Beach Road, #21-01/04 Gateway East, Singapore 189721, Singapore

Preface

In the recent decade, machine learning and learning and Internet of Things have been emerged at a very high rapid rate. Internets of Things are primary source to machine learning techniques. Machine learning techniques require raw data to analyse, which is provided by Internet of things. Today's IoTs or smart devices are being used by almost all sectors like manufacturing, transportation, agriculture, healthcare, etc., to provide automation (including intelligence) in respective sectors. Using IoTs by industry increase productivity and fulfil demands of many consumers at the same time. Data produced by IoT devices is at rest or in communication/flight. Machine learning help analyses produced data (by IoTs communications) and provide better decision to utilize available resources in a perfect way. For example, when IoT is used in health care (or e-health care), refereed as Internet of Medical Things (IoMT) and Machine Learning (also deep learning) can be used to refine or analyse data produced by a hospital. But, producing, analysing, or fulfilling consumer's demands are not the terms which complete this critical sector. Security of healthcare records is a primary concern in this sector. Security, privacy, trust, standardization of devices, and many stakeholders, battery limitation, etc., are few serious issues of IoTs. On the other side, not having modern tools for machine learning and skilled professional for analysing this large amount of data is also a big problem. Artificial intelligence (AI) which includes machine learning and deep learning as its subset will be in trend in next few decades and will be used at a larger scale by many sectors/applications.

Hence, this book starts with introduction of IoTs and machine learning and then discusses ever possible topics including possibilities of these technologies (IoMT and machine learning) with other technologies like cloud/edge computing, blockchain technology. Hence in last, several recent trends, future opportunities and open challenges in the machine learning/ deep learning techniques have been included in this book.

This book will be helpful to readers who are looking forward to find effective strategies, mechanisms for health care or intelligent and automated (interactive) systems. Undergraduate, postgraduate students, researchers, and scientists from industries can use this book to clear their doubts and find problems for their research work in near future.

In last, we want to thanks our God, family members, teachers, friends and in last but not the least to all our authors and their hard work from bottom of our heart for helping us in completing this book. Really, kudos to all.

Chennai, India	Amit Kumar Tyagi
Auburn, USA	Ajith Abraham
Vilnius, Lithuania	Arturas Kaklauskas

Contents

About the Editors

Amit Kumar Tyagi is Assistant Professor (Senior Grade) and Senior Researcher at Vellore Institute of Technology (VIT), Chennai, India. He received his Ph.D. Degree from Pondicherry Central University, India. He is a member of the IEEE society. His current research focuses on machine learning with big data, blockchain technology, data science, cyber-physical systems, smart & secure computing, and privacy. He has contributed to several projects such as "AARIN" and "P3-Block" to address some of the open issues related to the privacy breaches in vehicular applications (such as parking) and medical cyber-physical systems.

Ajith Abraham is the Director of Machine Intelligence Research Labs (MIR Labs), a Not-for-Profit Scientific Network for Innovation and Research Excellence connecting industry and academia. He received his Ph.D. Degree in Computer Science from Monash University, Melbourne, Australia. As an Investigator and Co-Investigator, he has won research grants worth over 100+ Million US$ from Australia, the USA, EU, Italy, Czech Republic, France, Malaysia, and China. His research focuses on real-world problems in the fields of machine intelligence, cyber-physical systems, Internet of things, network security, sensor networks, Web intelligence, Web services, and data mining. He is the Chair of the IEEE Systems Man and Cybernetics Society Technical Committee on Soft Computing. He is the editor-in-chief of *Engineering Applications of Artificial Intelligence* and serves on the editorial board of several international journals.

Arturas Kaklauskas is a Professor at Vilnius Gediminas Technical University, Lithuania. His areas of interest include affective computing, neuro-marketing, intelligent tutoring systems, effective intelligent tutoring systems, massive open online courses (MOOCS), affective Internet of Things (IoT), smartly built environment, intelligent event prediction, opinion mining, intelligent decision support systems, life cycle analyses of built environments, energy, climate change, resilience management, healthy houses, sustainable built environments, big data and text analytics, intelligent library, and IoT. He is the Editor in Chief of the *Journal of Civil Engineering and Management*, Editor of *Engineering Applications of Artificial Intelligence*, and

Associate Editor of the *Ecological Indicators Journal*. He has published nine books. The Belarusian State Technological University (Minsk, Belarus) has awarded him an Honorary Doctorate.

Introduction About Intelligent Systems and Multimedia Systems for Healthcare

Comparison, Analysis and Analogy of Biological and Computer Viruses

Sanskar Gupta, Aswani Kumar Cherukuri, Chandra Mouliswaran Subramanian, and Amir Ahmad

1 Introduction

Virus is an external entity or foreigner that has malicious intent to reside on its host, thereby disrupting the normal functioning of the host causing malfunction in the system and using the host resources to exist and thereby multiplying and propagating to other systems by connection making them the new host. This external agent is microscopic in size and infectious in nature. Viruses can be broadly categorized into two types, namely biological virus and computer virus. The association of viruses into an ordered structure is a significant method for researchers to have the option to contemplate and comprehend the biodiversity of infections. By and large, virus characterization is a concern as indicated by some given measures. The organization of natural life forms much complex processing, and they are found on phylogenetic (transformative) connections. In any case, there is no proof that virus have a typical precursor are in any means phylogenetically related. There are noticing similarities between natural infections and their digital counterparts. Similarly, as your resistant framework responds to infections by recognizing their genome code, conventional digital security guards rely upon their capacity to distinguish the structural codes of the malware [1].

Experts recommend that taking a look at how organic infections show and spread can illuminate our way to deal with shielding all the more successfully in the computerized world [2]. Infections do not have the hereditary material and biochemical hardware to recreate freely. In any case, after contaminating a cell, a virus can guide the cell's proliferation apparatus to create more virus. All the while, infections are fit for transforming and transforming at least one of their qualities during cell division as

S. Gupta · A. K. Cherukuri (✉) · C. M. Subramanian
Vellore Institute of Technology, Vellore, India
e-mail: cherukuri@acm.org

A. Ahmad
College of Information Technology, United Arab Emirates University, Abu Dhabi, UAE

A. K. Tyagi et al. (eds.), *Intelligent Interactive Multimedia Systems for e-Healthcare Applications*, https://doi.org/10.1007/978-981-16-6542-4_1

DNA is copied [1]. In its digital counterpart, at whatever point, a document or bit of code is created, changed or downloaded by anyone or any procedure in your system. It is executed against this tremendous and ever-developing malware database. In those events that a match with a known "terrible" mark is discovered and the document is distinguished as malware and subject to a type of remediation. The current trend in fighting against the computer security-related threats and malware is to develop the techniques based on machine learning and artificial intelligence. In principle, these techniques are inspired by the nature and human brain learning abilities. While combating against the malware, we can aim at developing techniques that model the human immune system. The rationality for choosing immune system is that biological immune systems automatically and proactively fight against the biological viruses. In this direction, we analyze the similarities, dissimilarities on how computer viruses and biological viruses originate, spread and damage that they causes. Further, we believe understanding this is essential in building artificial intelligence and machine learning-based techniques that fight against the malware.

2 Background

Biological viruses are one among the oldest and long living species which have undergone many genetic revolutions. Experts have estimated the existence of numerous and countless biological viruses, and if they were all lined up, they would stretch the entire galaxy. In a more advanced technological term, it can be thought that they are nature's self-build nanotechnology, small entities measurable on the scale with nanometer reading, possess alterations and processes to invade upon the host such as other living creatures to regenerate and reproduce. Although a vast variety of these viruses are not of any harm to humans, few of the types prove to be fatal [3]. They are sometimes referred to as non-living because they cannot function in open environment without any host body and also cannot store or build energy by their own [4].

2.1 Biological Virus

Termed as pathogen, they are infectious agents of sub-microscopic size responsible of causing various diseases and threat to human life by replicating inside the living cell of an organism. The effects of the virus depend on the severity of its composition and the immunity of the organism. These host are of all sizes of life forms from biggest of whales to the smallest microorganism including bacteria which are infected by them scaling according to the host vulnerability. On attacking the host, the virus injects its DNA into the cell and forces the cells of the host to supply enough of resources to help it produce several duplicates of the original in a rapid fashion [5]. By considering alive in nature because of long life, adapt and evolve through natural selection process, reproduce themselves by the formation of duplicates and multiplying possess genetic material.

2.2 Computer Virus

Computer virus are computer programs in actual which multiplies itself by modifications done to other system programs and pasting their code when executed in host system. These viruses are developed intentionally by adversaries [6]. They are triggered in many ways, either executing the applications or running demo files and many others. They are engineered by exploiting the necessary detailed knowledge of security vulnerabilities and process to reach denial of service intent mostly rather than the intention of breaching privacy on accessing data.

3 Biological Viruses

3.1 Origin

There is no proper evidence about the origin of virus [7]. The clear origination of these biological viruses is an ongoing debate as scientists have not been able to solidify the origin hypothesis. The history of discovery of virus dates back to late nineteenth century when Russian Scientist Dmitri Ivanovsky captured that certain pathogens can pass from filter which was meant to hold bacteria test on the sapling of infected tobacco plant. The origin of the viruses has been recalled under three main hypotheses such as progressive hypothesis, regressive hypothesis and virus-first hypothesis [7]. Finally, it is concluded that none of the hypothesis discussed is all true, but these are the possibilities that are considered today for their studies. Today, virus grows through multiple mechanisms and have many complex unknown traits.

3.2 Architecture

The specification of the architecture of the viruses is specified by the properties of its constituent and macromolecules. Mutual affinities, their population, surface properties of inclusive protein molecules highly influence the shapes and sizes of the viruses. Specific requirement of each type of virus have led to huge diversity and geometrical design. Apart from these vast diversities, the general architecture and certain common features apply to all viruses.

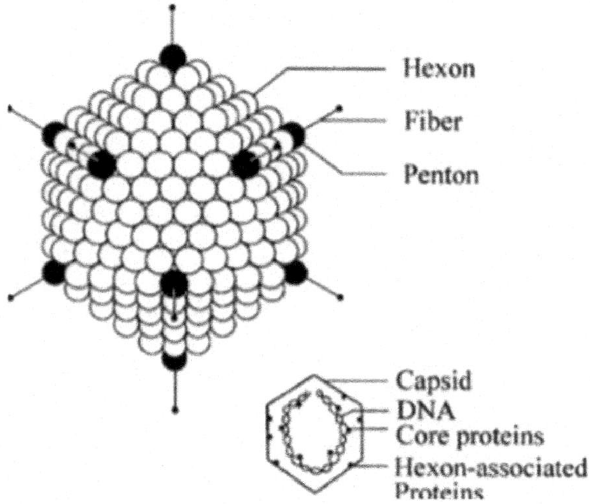

Fig. 1 Structure of icosahedral capsid

Based on architecture of their protein core or capsids, they can be defined under four types are enveloped viruses, icosahedral viruses, helical viruses and complex viruses. The enveloped viruses develop the coating or envelope through plasma membrane of the host which is a protective lipid. Since the budding process in not lethal to the host cell, thus, they do not kill their host cell but instead setup persistent functions to get released. These viruses are highly infectious only in the envelope is intact, for example HIV, influenza. Icosahedral capsids is the main characteristics of nucleocapsids of many spherical viruses. It mostly contains three types of different proteins and fibers. Most animal viruses are like this. Most of the proteins involved in the making of capsids and other are associated with viral DNA. Icosahedral capsids structure is shown in Fig. 1.

Helical capsid is mostly seen in virus with high variability and content in their protein core and nucleus (nucleocapsids). Length, width, pitch of helix and the number of protein subunit per helical turns are the parameters that characterizes the helical capsid structure. The structure of helical capsid is shown in Fig. 2.

3.3 Mutation

Viruses are undergoing constant changes because of genetic selection process. Genetic changes develop via mutation and through recombination. When error in the genome of virus is incorporated mutation occurs. Recombination is the result when genome information is switched between viruses co-infecting together. This leads to creation of novel virus.

For an organism, the mutation rate can be described down as the random experimental conclusion for difference in genetic information that is passed down to

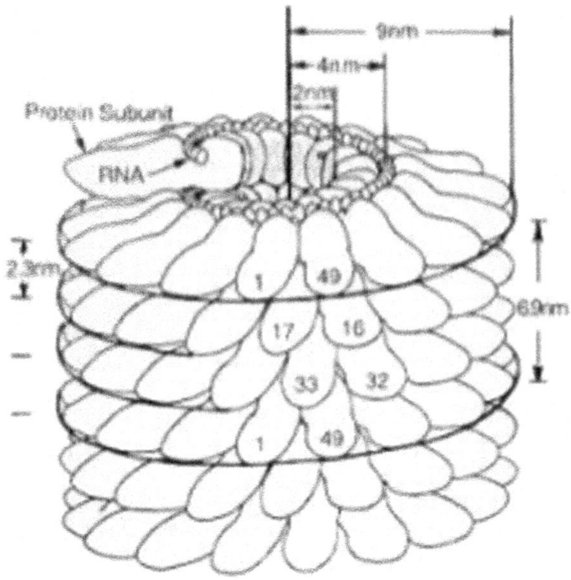

Fig. 2 Structure of helical capsid

upcoming generation. In viruses, the cycle of cell infection is a generation. This comprises of the attachments on the surface of cell, expansion of genes, entry and exit and producing particles causing severe infections. Damage of nucleic acid and genetic material being edited can also result in mutations. Studies show that viruses having DNA of single-strand generally have mutation at higher speed than viruses with double-strand DNA. Although the difference is dependent on work with only a particular bacteriophage, as for eukaryotic viruses of single-strand DNA, no estimates for mutation rate have been gained. The mutation rate shows up no obvious difference for the RNA viruses. One explanation given by scientists and biologists on comparing between viruses of single and double-strand is that nucleic acids of single-strand are more susceptible to deamination and other kinds of chemical damage. Higher levels of reactive oxygen species (ROS) and other cellular activities during viral infections can activate mutations. Also, viruses with genomes of small size moves to faster mutation, but there has been no quantitative universally accepted explanation for this.

Independent assortment shows up when viruses which possess segmented genomes exchange while replication. These genes have no linkage in them and are miscellaneous at random. The prevailing 6–20% rate of frequency of recombination is by independent assortment. Recombination likewise happens between genomes living on a similar bit of nucleic acid. Genes that by and large isolate together are called linked genes. On the off chance that recombination happens between them, the linkage is supposed to be deficient. Recombination of not completely connected genes happens in all DNA infections (virus) that have been examined and in a few RNA infections.

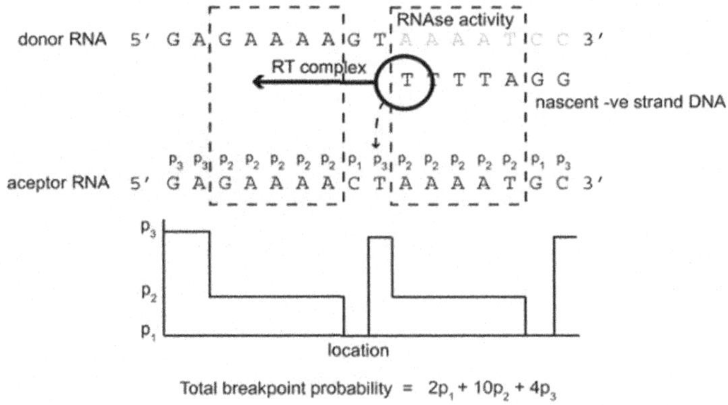

Fig. 3 Representation of copy-choice mechanism

In coronaviruses, recombination happens at the degree of the communication of the viral RNA genomes and is not accepted to happen by a break–rejoin mechanism. The system is right now accepted to be a duplicate decision mechanism. The image in Fig. 3 provides the copy-choice mechanism.

3.4 *Propagation*

The build-up of virus challenges its ability to spread. The main idea behind the existence of virus is to reproduce. As soon as the offspring develops or it multiplies, they spread to new cells making new host. The mediums through which they can spread are physical contact, sexual contact, air exchange, contaminated eatables, carriers like insects, indirect exchange like passing by exchanging infected object. The mechanism of propagation of virus happens in two stages [8].

While the primary stage consists of injection and residing in host to develop condition suitable for propagation, the secondary stage focuses on the virus multiplication and switching between cells by any process like budding and other. The primary stage propagation is shown in Fig. 4 and secondary stage propagation is shown in Fig. 5.

3.5 *Functioning and Impact*

The main component of a virus particle is its genome, which is the primary molecule either made of DNA or RNA, and it holds the necessary directions for reproduction. This is enveloped in a layer of proteins called a capsid, which provides protection to the genetic material. Generally, there is an external layer made of lipids, which are

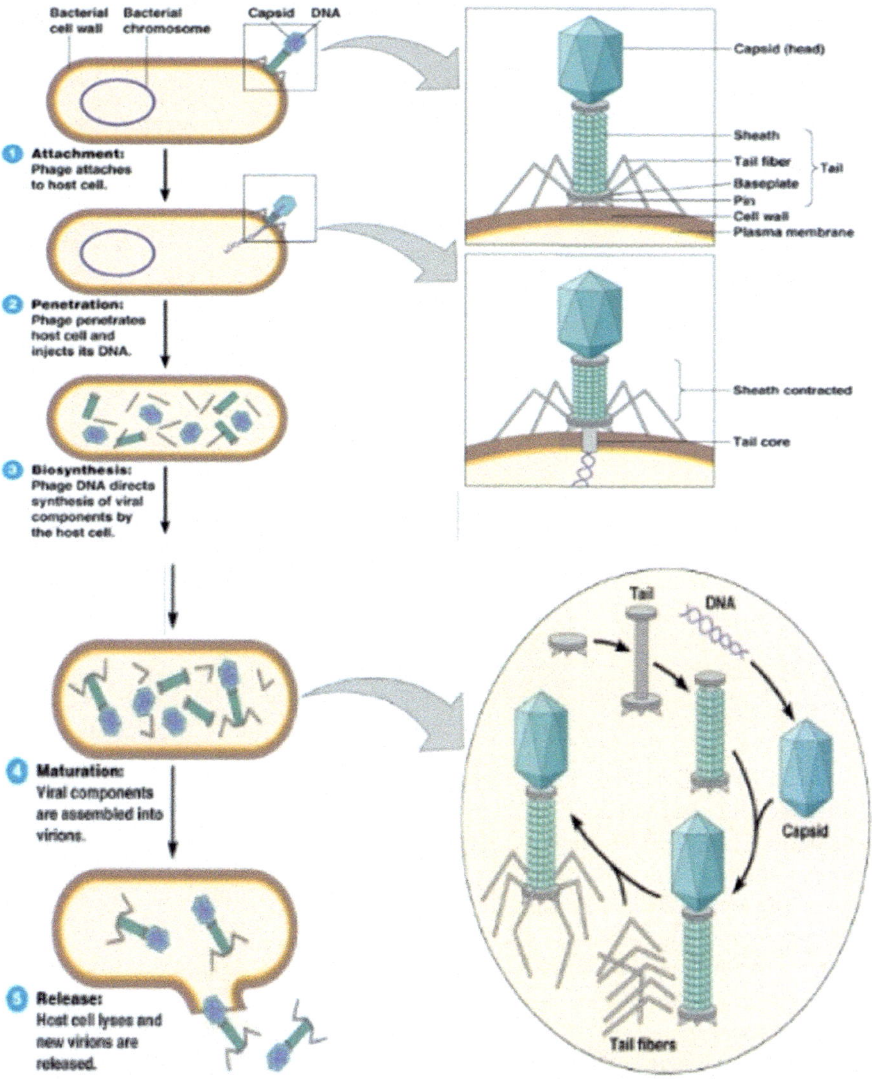

Fig. 4 Phases of virus in primary stage propagation

fatty natural molecules. The coronavirus that causes COVID-19 comprises this layer [9]. Cleanser like soap can break up this fatty enclosing, prompting the annihilation of the entire infection molecule and that is one explanation washing our hands with disinfectants and cleanser is important to keep ourselves fit.

Viruses have a specific target they can recognize and attack. The choice of organism a virus attacks depends on how well that particular virus can grow and reproduce in that virus. Depending upon the enzymes inside the structure of the

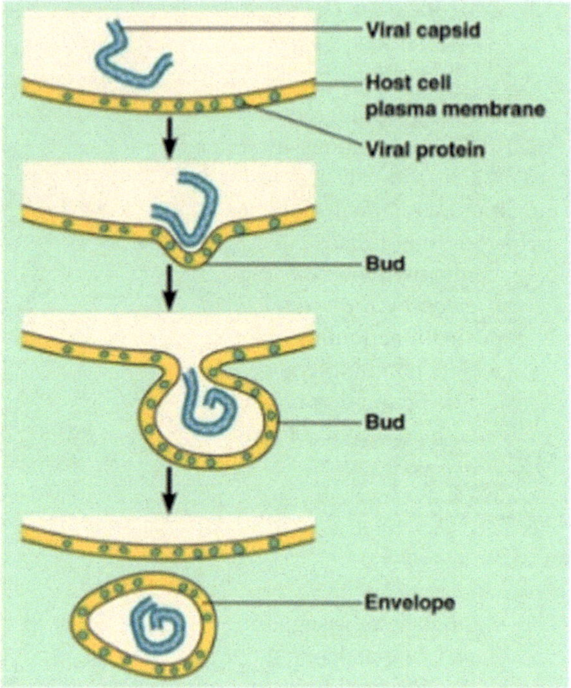

Fig. 5 Phases of virus in secondary stage propagation

virus, some organisms may not genetically be appropriate hosts for the virus. This is the reason why most viruses do not harm human beings, while some can exist in our cells but not have that severe of an impact. This also explains that how can several animal including plant species possess their own viruses. For instance, the HIV virus causes AIDS in humans. A similar kind of virus, FIV targets the cats' species.

When an individual is exposed to an infection, their body turns into a warehouse of infection particles which can be discharged in organic liquids, for example, by sniffling or by shedding skin or sometimes in any event which is contacting surfaces. The infection particles may then either wind up on another possible host or a lifeless thing. These polluted items are known as fomites and can have a significant job in the spread of infection.

Infections can be transmitted in miscellaneous ways. Some infections can spread through touch, spit, or even the air. Different infections can be transmitted through sexual contact or by sharing tainted needles. Fliers including ticks and mosquitoes can go about as "vectors" or "carriers" transmitting an infection starting with one host then onto the next. Spoiled food and water are other expected potentials of viral contamination.

3.6 Effect and Infect with Its Detection and Emergence

Viruses totally depends on their host because they are unable to make their own proteins hence cannot reproduce or multiply without acquiring the host. They capture upon the host functions by infecting it with its own genetic material. Viruses are omnipotent and call acquire by infecting all living organism's present from plant kingdom and animal kingdom to the smallest of bacteria and thus are potentially dangerous to life. They have an edge for the uninterrupted production since they can outpace the immune system evolving more quickly. Many parameters into the host gets affected by the virus having great effects like disrupting the immune collaboration, malfunctioning in antibodies production, fluctuation in immunoglobulin levels, induction in tolerance and rejection by host, delayed skin reactions, internal transformation at microbiological level.

People are continually encountering a variety of viruses. These infections are hereditarily differing and new varieties, strains and species advance quickly. A small amount of all these viruses infect people severely. It is not certain whether a portion of these human-infective viruses will be equipped for arriving at more elevated levels of the pathogen pyramid or whether ensuing development of their capacity to contaminate and transmit from people is normally required. The distinction is conceivably significant as it suggests various determinants of the pace of development of infections with pandemic potential.

The frontier line of barrier against developing infections from viruses is a viable inspection. This topic has been broadly talked about; however, we will repeat a couple of key focuses here. Number one, developing infections from upcoming viruses is everybody's concern: The simplicity with which viruses can scatter, conceivably worldwide in few days, combined with the extremely wide geological dispersion of emerging occasions, implies that a planned, worldwide observation network is basic on the off chance that we are to guarantee quick recognition of novel infections. This quickly highlights the tremendous national and territorial contrasts in the discovery limit, with by far most suitable facilities situated in Europe or North America.

Another, announcing of uncommon infection occasions is inconsistent; even once identified, it reflects both administration issues and the absence of incentives. We have to consider stretching out the inspection efforts to other warm-blooded animals just as people, in light of the fact that these are the most probable source of new human infections.

3.7 Prevention

As we have seen, infections from viruses can cause various ailments in our body, some of which can even lead to death. These illnesses can be treated by antiviral medications or by antibodies, yet some infections; for example, HIV have capabilities of both, keep away from the immune response and changing to get impervious to antiviral medications [10].

While we do have restricted quantities of viable antiviral medications, for example, those used to treat HIV and flu, the essential technique for controlling viral infection is by vaccination, which is proposed to prevent outbreaks by building resistance to an infection or virus family. Antibodies might be readied utilizing live viruses, executed infections or atomic sub-units of the pathogen.

The dead virus antibodies and subunit virus vaccines are both incapable of causing the ailment. A few vaccines are in growing advancement in light of the fact that certain infections, for example flu and HIV, have a high transformation rate contrasted with different viruses and cells of normal hosts. With flu, changes in the surface particles of the virus help the life form dodge the defensive resistance that may have been acquired in a past flu season, making it important for people to get inoculated each year.

Different viruses, for example, those that cause ailments in the young ones measles, mumps and rubella, transform so rarely that a similar vaccine is utilized quite often. At times, vaccines can be utilized to treat the functioning of active viral contamination. The concept driving this, is by giving the antibody, immunity is boosted without including more infection-causing viruses. In case of rabies, a deadly neurological sickness transmitted by means of the saliva of rabies-infected creatures, the movement of the infection from the hour of the animal bite to the time it enters the focal neuron system might be fourteen days or more. This is sufficient time to immunize a person who speculates that they have been bitten by an unknown creature, and their immune response is adequate to keep the infection from entering sensory tissue [10]. Along these lines, the possibly lethal neurological outcomes of the illness are deflected, and the individual just needs to recover from the infected bite. This methodology is additionally being utilized for the treatment of Ebola, one of the quickest and deadliest infections on earth.

3.8 Infection Encountered

The prevention of disease and handling infection caused by the virus include methods like active prophylaxis or vaccination which involves monitoring of the virus making in host which triggers the immune system of person to release its own specific combating bodies [11]. Vector controls and sanitization includes reduction of exposure to virus by improving cleanliness and eliminating non-living carriers around our surrounding. Certain chemical therapies follow procedure that involves producing agents that directly combat virus cells and inactive them, agents which boost the immunity response of host and some other that inhibits the replication of viruses. Practicing methods like avoiding grouping and social distancing help in significant way.

3.9 *Coronavirus (COVID-19)*

3.9.1 Origin of Coronavirus

On December 31, 2019, China's office of the World Health Organization (WHO) came across the news of a less explored and unaware virus behind most cases of pneumonia in Wuhan, a Chinese city with gross population exceeding 11 million. The new linking virus shown in Fig. 6. briefly named COVID-19 is believed likely to be originated from bats. The first ever trace of this virus was discovered in Wuhan province of China. The disease outbreak from a market of seafood in Wuhan. There wild creatures, including marmots, winged animals, hares, bats, and snakes, are additionally traded in illegal way. Coronavirus is observed to be transformed from animals to humans and is suspected that the people early diagnosed with this disease are of group consisting mostly seafood vendors who acquired it through contact with animals. Since, then via person-to-person contact the virus has spread globally.

The genetic makeup of the current coronaviruses is matching 96% to the coronavirus found with bats, although a report released on 26 March suggests that the hereditary groupings of coronavirus in pangolins are somewhere in the range of 88.5 and 92.4% like the human virus. In any case, some early instances of COVID-19 appear to have dispensed individuals with no connection at all to the market of Wuhan, recommending that the underlying course of human contamination may predate the counting of cases in market.

The virus can effect both animals and humans. It causes mild fever and respiratory problems because it is a virus that is responsible for harsh but short-termed breathing

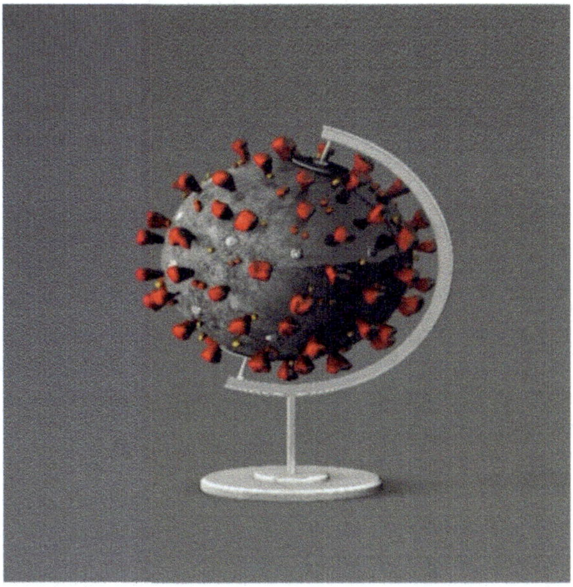

Fig. 6 Coronavirus across entire globe

and nasal problems (SARS-V) [12]. The virus has a tragic effect on the people suffering from more than one health problems or probably possess weak immunity. The worst part of the virus is that it is still under research and new traits related to it are getting discovered presenting its real characteristics.

3.9.2 Spread of Coronavirus

It spreads in close community from person-to-person via various forms of contact. People suffering from COVID-19 when cough or breathe out, they expose the surrounding with the small droplets containing virus. The people around them when inhale these droplets they cause infection and thus the virus spreads all around. Hence, because of all mentioned, it is mandatory to stay away from a sick person by more than 1 m (3 feet).

The virus droplets can also land on the objects of daily use. People can pick up virus from infected objects as after touching they unknowingly touch their faces then entering the body through nose, mouth or eyes.

3.9.3 Mutation of Coronavirus

Corona virus has been declared a novel virus. There are too many rapid mutations to map a family tree of COVID-19 cleanly. Two importance transformations in the bat coronavirus set us making progress toward pandemic COVID-19. The primary changed the course of action of the spike-like structures from which the virus extends. The modified spikes help the virus to hook on a protein called ACE2, which lines the flying route. The second key change permitted the coronavirus to build up a protein blade called a furin, which can cut through different proteins to tie the virus firmly to the throat and lung cells. The furin protein made the COVID-19 infection irresistible and dangerous to people. It is also probable that either of one or of present both mutations could have exploded in a human who had been diagnosed with an earlier form of the virus but who did not display any symptoms. The mutations which propagate as a virus are detrimental to the virus itself or do not affect how it operates.

Figure 7 provides the viral samples of a patient and visualizes the genome sequence along with its mutation. Samples A and B share the same variables. C and D have different versions, even though C has more versions corresponding to A and B than D. An analysis of these similarities allows scientists to build a genetic tree. The virus samples from A and B are closely related and both are more similar to C than D. Figure 8 describes it. Sorting the samples from the tree according to the date they are taken, Fig. 9 visualizes how the virus spreads over time.

The gene tree shown in Fig. 10 helps to visualize the transmission. The clusters due to genetic similarities belong to those patients within the same transmission chains. The confidence level of the transgenic tree improves as the number of virus samples increases.

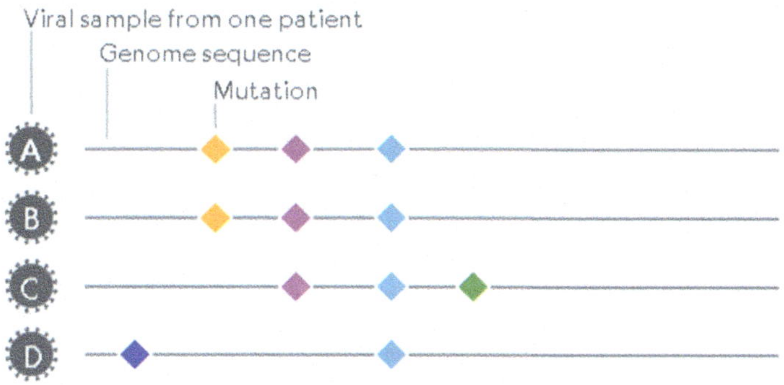

Fig. 7 Probability of mutation of genome—analysis

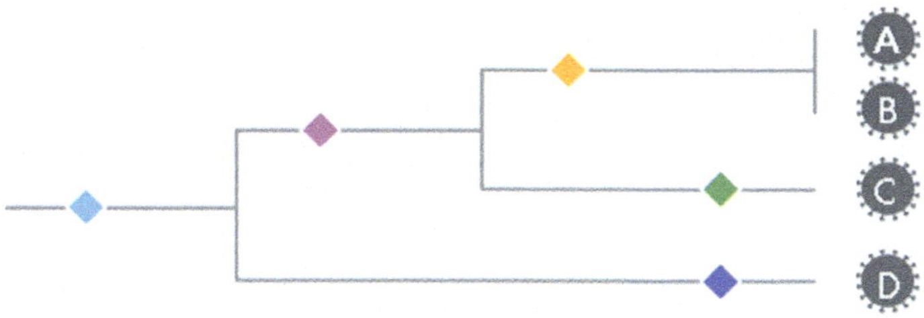

Fig. 8 Generic tree builds out of analysis from virus samples

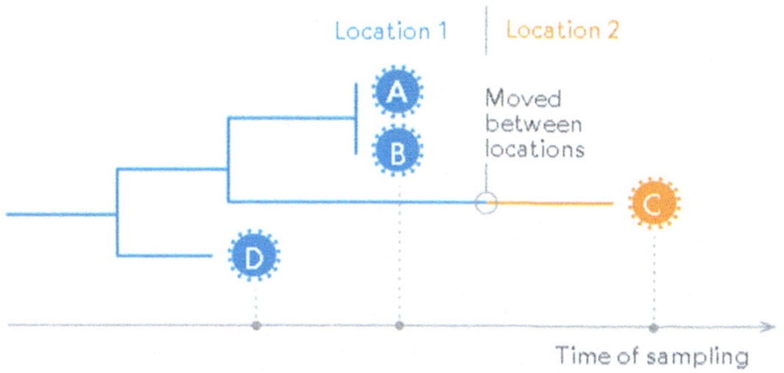

Fig. 9 Study of spreading of virus over time from generic tree

"These mutations are just as effective and useful as a puzzle piece to find out how the virus spreads," said Nextstrain cofounder and a biologist Trevor Bedford, of the Fred Hutchinson Cancer Research Center.

This genetic-tracking coronavirus has emerged as a bright spot amid the complexity of deadly epidemic topics. The same science helped record previous epidemics, such as Zika and Ebola [13]. But experts say that the decrease in costs and the rapid growth and efficiency of genetic sequencing tools have enabled a small

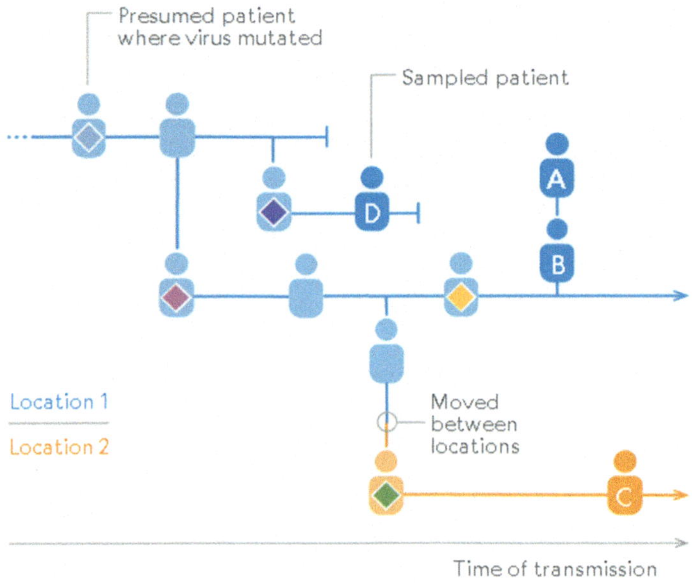

Fig. 10 Transmission of virus genome

army of researchers around the world to quickly document the deadly coronavirus [14]. That information can help officials decide whether to move from mitigation plans, especially in areas where testing is lagging.

"When we went back to the Ebola virus five years ago, it was a process that took a whole year from samples from which genomes were started and publicly shared," Bedford said. "Now the transition is very fast—from two days to a week—and that real ability to apply these strategies in a way that contributes to new outbreaks is new."

3.9.4 Working of Coronavirus

The new coronavirus hooks its proteins having spikes on solid cells to receptors, particularly the ones present in the lungs. The proteins of virus expressly blast off into cells through receptors of ACE2. The coronavirus seizes healthy cells and takes over the control once reported inside. In this process, a large portion of the good cells gets damaged. The virus descends down your breathing route. This route incorporates your mouth, your nose, your throat and your lungs. The lower part has a greater number of receptors for ACE2 than the remainder of the respiratory tract. Along these lines, COVID-19 is bound to go further than the normal cold infections.

The lungs get swollen, making breathing difficult for you. This tends forward to pneumonia, an inflammation of the small air sacs (alveoli) within your lungs, where the blood binds oxygen and carbon dioxide together and any, the infection gets worse.

They have shortness of breath (called dyspnea) about 5–8 days after symptoms begin. A few days later, acute respiratory distress syndrome (ARDS) starts up.

ARDS can cause rapid breath, fast pulse, dizziness, and perspiration. It harms your alveoli's tissues and veins, making flotsam and jetsam get together inside. This causes you rapid breath, or even incomprehensible. They carry less oxygen to your body, as liquid pools in your lungs. That implies that your blood may not convey enough oxygen to your organs for survival. This can cause your kidneys, lungs and liver to quit working and shut down. The brain will have a shortage of amounts of oxygen and eventually the person will collapse.

3.9.5 Difficulty in Detection

Major problem faced is that the virus is able to spread by someone not showing the symptoms of it. When symptoms are at peak, it is highly contagious. Due to sudden breakout of COVID-19, the estimation for the severity of disease is difficult. The cases may not seem serious at the first and then suddenly transforms to become severe leading to death. The main failure in detection is that the symptoms itself takes 14 days to show up after the exposure to virus, till then living normally affects man others in contact. Although some recognized common symptoms are fever, breathlessness, cough, body aches and pain, congested nose, sore throat, muscle pain and loss of taste.

A fast indicative test (RDT) dependent on antigen identification was additionally directed on COVID-19, which included taking examples of the nose, throat and lungs. RDT—rapid diagnostic tests for a sample of the human respiratory tract assists with distinguishing viral proteins (antigens) related to the COVID-19 infection. This guarantees quick and exact discovery and its utilization is endorsed by the CDC. RDT dependent on the accessibility of an immune response identifies the nearness of antibodies in the blood of individuals contaminated with COVID-19. The quality of the antibody agent reaction relies upon a few factors, for example age, drug, infection and seriousness of the disease and so on.

Using clinical models in patients with a high respiratory infection, we demonstrated that the repeat of trade transcript-polymerase chain reaction (80% of fecal models and 25% urine tests) was subsequently in large rate than that of polyclonal (half unit and 5%) and monoclonal (35% and 8%) nucleocapsid antigen capture-associated with the synthetic immunosorbent.

3.9.6 Prevention

Although pardoning to the exact effective ways to prevent the spread of the virus is a global challenge yet the best method to count is avoiding close contact with others and thus practicing social distancing. Prevention through antiviral vaccines is only way to battle, but it takes time to develop and distribute effective vaccines all around. Washing hands properly and maintaining personal hygiene. Use of soap and water to wash hands for 20 s minimum per time and sanitizers with at least 60% alcohol content. Avoid touching face and use of mask to properly cover the opening part of mouth.

If you ever feel that your symptoms have been described in coronaviruses, your healthcare provider can contact the CDC or your local health department for instructions on testing. There are a few laboratories build-up for coronavirus tests so that one can be coordinated to any one of the laboratories. There are various sorts of coronavirus tests that can be carried out. Swab testing—for this situation, a swab is utilized to gather a sample out of the patient's nose or throat. Nasal desire—for this case, solution saline in nature will be embedded into your nose and the sample is taken. Dermal goal—For this case, a little tube embedded with a light called a bronchoscope is inserted into the mouth to get to the lungs for the collection of samples. Sputum examination—sputum is a shallow knot that is found in the lungs and usually exits with the cough. For this test, a request for cough in a medical cup is utilized to take a sample of the respiratory section. Blood test—in this case, a sample of blood unit is collected via a vein. In the same way, the working, propagation, mutation, detection and prevention of Ebola and H1N1 virus can be analyzed.

4 Computer Virus

"Network virus" defines a fairly new form of malware that spreads from machine to machine without the need to drop a file-based copy of itself on any of the computers affected [15]. These viruses only exist as network packets when, and in memory, they travel from one device to another. Malware is any software or file that is harmful to a user's computer. Malware types can include computer viruses, worms, Trojan horses, as well as spyware. These programs may perform a number of functions, like hijacking or altering core computing functions, stealing, encrypting and deleting confidential data, monitoring user computing without permission.

Viruses are capable of damaging or destroying resources present on a system and exchanging via previously infected portable media, executing malicious attachments arriving on mails, and visiting web pages having malicious content [16]. Worms belong to the category of virus that propagates itself from one computer to other. Its function is to utilize every resources of the system so that your computer stops responding. Trojan horses are computer programs that hide viruses or malicious programs. It is too common for software available for free to have a Trojan horse, which makes the client feel that they are working with legitimate copy of software, although it carries of malicious work on your computer. Cybercriminals have kept on creating approaches to misuse PCs and gadgets for financial gain [17]. Most recently, the CryptoLocker group of ransomware has risen [18]. For the most part spread by means of email as a connection, the program can encode focused on documents, which hinders the particular clients from getting to them. The malware shows a message requesting payment by means of Bitcoin or Moneypak in return for the encryption key [19]. On the off chance that installment is not delivered by the cut-off time, the key would be erased, leaving the client without access to their information.

4.1 Origin

People write viruses on their computers. An individual is required to create and run the code, check it for ensuring that it spreads widely and afterward launch it. Often, an individual plot the attack process of the virus, it might be a dumb message or the corruption of storage memory. Released in 1971, it was an experimental self-replicating virus called Creeper System was the first computer virus [20]. The name itself describes it was meant to cover up the whole hard drive causing malfunctioning until a system could not further execute any operation. It was developed under the BBN technologies in USA. People have to write code and thus develop or produce a virus initially. Testing it before deploying to check spreading and severity and also has to define the attack phase then release it. Piggybacking on top of documents, files, programs and other executable application is the main need for a computer in order to launch itself.

There are four simple reasons coined for the programers to create viruses are psychological that drives out of curiosity, thrill to overcome rules, bragging the rights and challenging tasks, cash (legal or illegal) and ethical in terms to reach for new developments and procuring technological progress [21]. Identity theft/restricted data theft—the virus records data from your PC and transmits that data back to the host machine of virus creator. Much of the time, the virus does not really search out information on your PC but instead sits and screens your movement on the web and information you send to the web like for instance: Visa data, passwords or individual personality data. At that point, the virus sends that data to the host PC of the virus creator. Stealing rights—the more PCs that come into infection by the specific virus, the more feeling of achievement the virus creator can guarantee. To gain remote control of a PC—the virus captures your PC to the host machine of the attacker which may deliver your PC commands to undertake activities that advantage the virus engineer anyhow. To damage organizations or competing business entities—these kinds of viruses are normally made by a developer who has a contrary plan than the plan of the corporation on which the attacker has launched the virus [14].

4.2 Architecture

The three main component of computer viruses are infection mechanism, trigger and payload. As part of infection mechanism, the infection vector deals with the propagation of the virus [8]. This component comprises of the searching and routing routine that act as guide and radar to find the potential host [14]. Trigger is the compiled version of the executable file containing the virus code, which when run activates the virus that conditions to the malicious event which is to be delivered. Payload is the actual entity of the virus and have data for the malicious purpose of the virus to get launched. This harmful activity is noticeable as it causes changes in system performance and is thus distributable. Based on the feature of the virus, they can be classified in various forms. They are macro-viruses, logic bomb, boot sector virus, polymorphic virus, encrypted virus, stealth virus, etc.

4.3 Functioning and Propagation

The potential computer virus consists of a search routine that tracks down for new disks and new files that can actually prove to be a worth target for infection and thus copy itself into the program. Infected files can be downloaded from websites, by file sharing activities or as email attachments. Visiting infected Websites, downloads from online drive, viruses may be concealed in Javascript, thus installing itself while web page loads up.

Activation of the virus highly relies on the pattern of coding of the virus. They either require some specific event to be performed from user side or get triggered just by when the user open an effected file. The exposed program executes (at the demand of client), and the virus is stacked into the memory of CPU prior to any of the needed code executes.

Security breaching attacks including scams like phishing, tricking victims to obtain confidential data, or accessing your systems of the workplace via attacks that are customized to show itself as legal organizational proceedings that are further reported false as they force the victim to respond quickly without a chance for second thought. Smart devices, cloud services and other system peripherals act as access points that are hijacked by the attacker and controlled by him.

Viruses in the past were basically code snippets embedded in a bigger, functioning program, likewise a game or development tools. Upon execution, the legitimate code the virus runs itself within memory and searches for any other programs on the disk. If it comes across any one, the virus intents to modify the program to embed its code snippet into that program, sort of like how a biological virus uses the host organism to function. All this time, the client is completely oblivious to the functioning of the virus.

Unfortunately, the virus reproduces itself after capturing program, so two programs get infected. When user launches either of those programs the next time, the virus infects other present programs and the chain flows like a domino effect. This is very similar to how the biological viruses spread and propagate through the host body—exponential growth. But viruses would not be unwanted to such an extent if they did was replicate themselves.

Most viruses likewise have a destructive stage when they do real harm. The developer would have typed a trigger that can actuate the attack mode, and the virus at that point launches something destructive, for example eradicating your information. The trigger may be a particular date; on various occasions, the infection has been repeated or something comparative. One probable approach is the capacity to stack viruses into memory so they can continue running in the background as long as the PC stays on. This provides viruses a considerable successful approach to repeat themselves. Another approach is the capacity to damage the boot sector on storage drives. The boot sector is a snippet of a program which is the initial part of the OS that the PC loads. It contains a small program that advises the PC to stack the remaining working framework. By placing its code in the boot area, a virus can surely be executed. It can stack itself into memory quickly and run at whatever point the PC is on. These kinds of virus propagation are shown in Fig. 11.

Current infections are significantly more severe in their attacks. Files that are received as word records, excel spreadsheet and images can include viral connections. In any event, opening an infected site can download a program infected by virus. Documents having extensions, for example.exe or.vbs, are executable and can harm the user functions needs. Numerous virus camouflage by multiplying with the addition of the name of program, for example stuff.gif.vb. When the virus is active on the PC, it duplicates itself into records, files and projects when they are utilized by the PC.

The life cycle of computer virus involves various phases of virus such as dormant phase, propagation phase, triggering phase and execution phase. In order to start, a computer virus has to piggyback any other software or file in addition. A computer virus upon running can infect other documents or programs. Similar to its biological

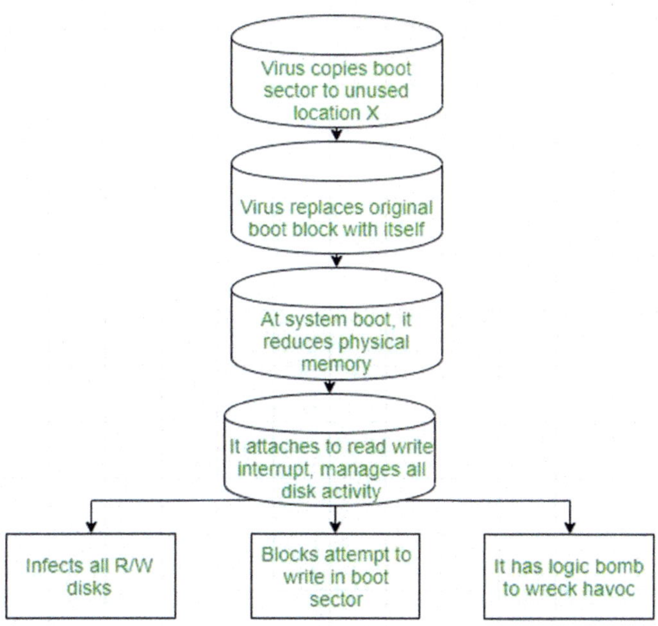

Fig. 11 Boot sector virus propagation

counterpart, viruses bind themselves to safe and uninfected files and infect them. They spread uncontrollably, damage core functionality of a device and remove or corrupt data. They normally appear as a file which can be executed (.exe). Trojans are the kind of malware pretends to be a legitimate software or is embedded in corrupted applications. It misleads to function discreetly along with build backdoors to let other malware inside your system. Spyware is a kind of malware specified to keep eye on movements. It slips behind the scenes and jot down about online activity, including passwords, ATM card details, net surfing and more. Worms attack whole computer network by using network interfaces, either locally or over the Internet. This uses any computer that has been infected consecutively to spread infection.

Ransomware locks down computer and files. It tries to delete anything until a ransom is paid [18]. Adware are not severely malicious in nature, and offensive advertisement programs will compromise system protection for showing advertisements—which pave way for other malware. Botnets are networks of systems infected and are designed to work together under attacker power.

4.4 Infects and Its Detection

The creators of the virus miss out the main point that their creation and testing leads to brutal consequences of causing real losses to common people. Damaging the hard disk of an individual which may contain his needful data or wasting of resources and time of tech giant or MNC in cleaning up their systems and servers causing trouble to many. Thus, the authorities and administration have to take severe steps and have to undergo harsh implementations with rigorous penalties for those dealing in hand with malicious virus. Viruses are also known to cause traffic in network by spreading, thereby suspending all the ongoing internet activities. Unexpected data losses, denial of service, breach of privacy by activating spying malwares, frequent crashes are some popular effects of the viruses executed on a system.

The types of detection are broadly classified into two categories: static and dynamic. By static investigation, a virus is identified by looking at records for the events of infection pattern without running any snippet of code. Static methods incorporate the following techniques such as string scanning method, wildcards method, bookmarks method and heuristic analysis. String scanning method looks for series of bytes that are pertaining to a specific virus but not likely present in other programs. Wildcards method permits to skip byte ranges. For instance, "?" characters are ignored and the % implies that the scanner will attempt to look for the following byte. Bookmarks method ascertains the separation between the beginning of the virus body and the recognition string. Heuristic analysis is a specialist recommended observation that determines the vulnerability of a framework toward specific danger utilizing different standards or techniques. One of the methods for weighing is multi-criteria analysis (MCA).

The dynamic detection strategy chooses if the code is contaminated or not by executing the code snippet and watching its output. The program screens the known strategies of virus action which consist of attempts to contaminate and evade detection. This may likewise incorporate entices to write on boot sectors, alter vectors, modify framework documents and so on. For instance, most virus movement needs to call some system functions similar to I/O activities—considering only these activities. Regardless of how jumbled are the static I/O calls, the calls will show up plainly when the code runs. Programing screens work best when the ordinary use attributes to the framework are boundlessly not quite the same as the movement profile of an infected framework. A virus may show a powerful signature like, opening a running file, having both read and write consent, reading the part of the file header containing the executable location and composing a similar file header and trying to limit the file by attaching to the document.

A behavior blocker is programing for an antivirus which screens a running system's conduct progressively, looking for unsure actions. On the chance, if such action is seen, the behavior blocker can keep the dubious tasks from succeeding, can end the task or can approach the client for the proper activity to perform. Behavior blocking permits code to run on the genuine machine. Interestingly, antivirus procedures utilizing the code being dissected in a copied domain. The expectation is that, under mirroring, a virus will uncover itself. Since any virus found would not be running on the genuine PC, no damage is finished [22].

Network quarantine disconnect the local network immediately from the Internet as a precautionary measure against further external source infection. This can also prevent malware from linking to external sites already present in the network for more mischief [16]. Quarantine occupies the middle ground, transferring the file to protected storage that is under the control of the antivirus program, so it cannot harm your device. This gives you the right to restore the file if you believe that the file was marked as harmful by mistake. Once the infection is detectable, it is easier to quarantine an infected device. Plan is only successful against worms and viruses which our safety products recognize, not against new and undetectable ones.

Anti-malware is one type of program that you install on your device with reference to protect the system from intrusion and contamination with malware [22]. Anti-malware applications can do so in following ways: they discover the presence of malware on the system, delete it with precaution, and clean up all the damage that has been done by malware to the device [23].

Likewise, some top notch programs, such as malware bytes, have blocking feature of malicious website and real-time protection. This means the programs block Websites that have been developed with the purpose of distributing malicious virus. It ensures that in the background this anti-malware runs continuously, so as to avoid any piece of malware that attempt to install itself on the system [22].

Antivirus program runs as background process on the user computer, scanning every document that is opened. This process is commonly called as on-access scanning, or similar to this, relying on the term user's antivirus program may use.

On the chance, if one executes a setup file, it might appear as though the program dispatches quickly—however, it does not. The antivirus programing scans the program first, contrasting it with known viruses, worms and different sorts of malware. The antivirus programing likewise does "heuristic" checking, logging programs for kinds of awkward conduct that may tell about another, new infection. Antivirus software likewise examines various sorts of documents that can contain infections. For instance, a compressed archived record may contain viruses in compressed format, or a Word file can contain a dangerous large scale virus. Documents are examined at whatever point they are utilized.

A full access scan is usually done when an antivirus software is installed for the first time. At this stage, it will check if the system already has any viruses lying dormant in the background. An essential part of the antivirus software is the definitions of virus. Antivirus programing depends on definitions of viruses to distinguish malware. That is the reason it consequently downloads new records. The definition documents contain identity marks for infections, viruses and other malware that have been experienced earlier. At the point when an antivirus program checks a document and notifies that the record coordinates a known bit of malware, the antivirus program prevents the document from running, placing it into isolation. Depending on the antivirus program's settings, it can directly delete the file or one can choose to allow the file to run anyway, on the chance of it being a false positive. False positives are when the antivirus software declares a file as a threat even though it does not contain any virus. Antivirus organizations need to constantly stay updated with the latest and most recent bits of malware, discharging definition updates that guarantee the malware has infected their projects.

An antivirus software is judged based upon its detection rate, which includes both the false positives and the virus definitions and heuristics. One may have a higher detection rate because of better, updated virus definitions provided by the software company, or maybe, it results in fewer false positives than its competitors. Upon the dawn of the open source era, many open source antivirus software has also been developed and is quite accurate. One of the leading open source antivirus software is the Avast Antivirus Software.

4.5 Infections Encountered

Use of a reliable antivirus software with updated patch of virus blocking can prove as a best shield against the attacking body [4]. This depends on the quality and services provided by the software. If the system still gets affected by the virus, then the program used is not reliable. Every then and now when you connect and surf through Internet a lot of cookies and cache also gets infected and may contain some threat. Dealing this has an easy option of regularly scanning the system. This helps in recognizing any unknown and malicious intent file which can be treated before causing any trouble. Many a times, the updates and patches of software you are using gets infected and act as carrier of viruses [24]. This common mistake can lead to downloading and activating of virus, thus scanning of files before downloading and uninstalling random apps and malware that come attached can help get rid of future risk.

4.6 Code Red

Code Red was discovered on the internet on July 15, 2001, as a computer worm. It targeted computers running the IIS web server at Microsoft. It was the first mixed threat-attack on a wide scale to effectively threaten business networks. Code Red resides in background disguised a request from GET/default. In this manner, the code is built to misuse a flaw within the Internet Information Server (IIS) of Microsoft's buffer overflow, which is the indexing program. That way, the code snippet executes in the IIS server. The virus is running entirely within the memory and is not present on the disk. This takes up approximately 3600 bits. It attempts to spread its contamination by discovering numerous IIS servers from starting day to 19th day on the Internet. Further, the device linked by unique addresses will become compromised by attacks like denial of service from 20th day to 27th day. After, there are no dynamic assaults since last day of the month. The worm did not verify whether the server running on a remote system was executing a powerless variant of IIS, or to even observe whether it was performing on IIS somehow while searching for vulnerable machines. Data logs for Apache. The working of Code Red is shown in Fig. 12.

Code Red infected more than 2 million machines, which forced companies to spend $2.75 billion to recover the lost output. Code Red propagates via Internet without user intervention and u updates the most recent security patch on Windows OS. (Microsoft issued an update to security patch to secure compromised systems against Code Red attacks). Actualize the utilization of a powerful web protection bundle that incorporates antivirus programing for testing, recognizing and evacuating unknown dangers, a firewall which interrupts dubious outbound information traffic from the web server of IIS to evade malware spreading and different sorts of attacks, and above all control innovation—that isolates suspicious dangers and executes them in a confined domain.

Similarly, there are other popular viruses such as ILOVEYOU [25] and Slammer which are sent through email and SQL server respectively.

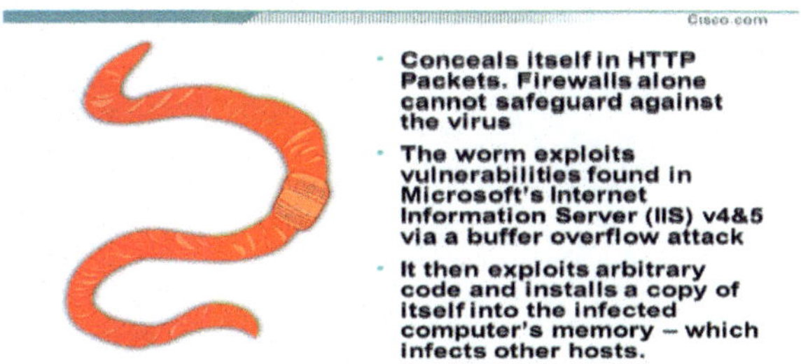

Fig. 12 Working of Code Red worm

4.7 MBR—Rewriting Malware (COVID-19 Virus)

The coronavirus pandemic (COVID-19) over the globe led to few ideas of developing a malware which completely destructs virus attacked computers, either by cleaning records or by revising the record of master boot record system (MBR) of a computer [9]. A security researcher discovered the first of the MBR rewriters. This malware infects a device using COVID-19.exe as the name. It is shown in Fig. 13. The malware has two phases of infection.

The first phase of the malware is it only shows an annoying window in the first phase which clients cannot shutdown since the adversary would have disengaged the Task Manager. When clients seek to tackle the current corrupted window, the infection secretly rewrites the master boot record in the background. It afterward reboots the system and kicks in latest MBR, trapping client in an earlier boot panel. It is shown in Fig. 13.

Clients can again have access to own devices, but recommended apps which are in need to construct and store MBR to work again will be required. Again, a second strain of coronavirus-based malware was present that rewrote the master boot record which is a higher complex operation of malware. It acted like the "ransomware coronavirus." The essential capacity of the malware was to take passwords from an infected system, and afterward mirror ransomware to deceive the client and cover their genuine reason. It was not ransomware in real, however, it simply acted like one [26]. Endless supply of the information by self-taking tasks, the malware entered a stage in which it revamped the MBR and blocked clients into a pre-boot message forestalling access to their PC. With clients seeing payment notes and afterward

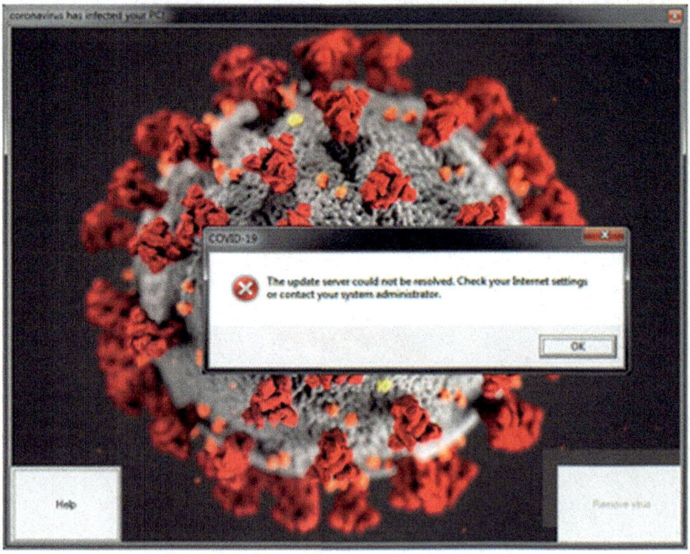

Fig. 13 MBR rewriting virus in action

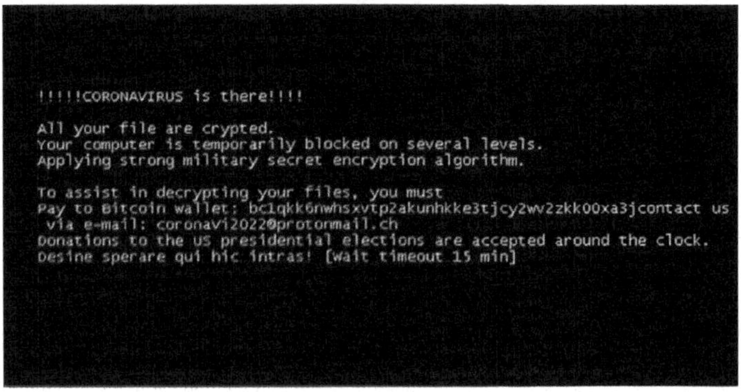

Fig. 14 Command prompt showing the presence of virus

being not able to get to their PCs, the exact opposite thing clients would need to do is check whether somebody has invaded passwords from their applications. The presence of malware is show in Fig. 14.

4.8 Ransomware

Ransomware attackers use a variety of strategies to activate malware, grant sophisticated privileges and submit demands to find its food. Available infection carriers for ransomware are phishing, exploitation package, downloads and botnets of Trojan, strategy of social engineering along with heavy load equivalence systems. Phishing is till now being practiced in preferred option, with a significant growth in utilization of predatory tools, which were utilized in 2015 to expand crypto walls along with Tesla cryptos. Main features include the way ransomware attacks client files by locating them. The files to be attacked are latest and are of much worth and significance, so ransomware do check at the history of earlier files accessed, and folders, likewise, Pictures, Downloads, My Documents and Other Simple Files in folders, such as Recycle Bin [18]. During mapping, a process maps, extends and calculates their position and delivers the result to the Command and Control (C&C server). To decide the significance of the records, the latest access time is noticed and the net time is calculated between the creation and last revision date, both indicating the amount of work done in a file and the level of user. To verify that documents are real and unaltered, ransomware assess information density, names of file and contents present in them. If the net work done is too high or too small, featuring random content, the ransomware will translate the document as auto-generated and remove it away from its directory. There are two types of ransomware such as encryption and lock screen. Encrypts individual files or documents and after encrypting, the file is deleted. Usually, there is only a text file after encryption, which is now not accessible with payment instructions. We can see the screen after phone is locked, but all available variants do not show one, until you have problems when you try to open those files. It is shown in Fig. 15.

Lock screen type of ransomware returns a full window picture which restricts all other screens. Single important documents are not encoded here. It is shown in Fig. 16.

Master Boot Record is the partition on the PC storage drive that permits the working OS to ensure for booting, yet the MBR ransomware changes the PC's MBR, consequently disturbing the typical processing of boot services. Obviously the payoff request is shown on the screen of user.

Generally, threatening messages indicate that it is imperative that the computer is not shut down, and stay aware of the requests, in any case, the decoding key, client records, or decoding system will be lost or the installment will increment. Possibly, malware which encrypts MFT, such as Petya, by corrupting the Master Boot Record, imposes ransom on the ransom note and blocks gain to the working OS. After deploying the Stalez group, the user is vulnerable to the environment. We suppose that all crypto-malware encrypts the targets to obtain files which require encryption, or to process the files and deliver it in the encrypted form. Therefore, remedial steps are more proven if it in course of the map phase.

While considering all unauthorized transaction operation for files, preventing ransomware in its path is genuinely straightforward. However, this creates a huge bias toward collectible tools, such as false-positive identification of applications, and thus reduces user experience and performance. Computer users should have a proper stability with a high incorrect assumption rate. Operating on an end-point machine is inappropriate, as it allows the model to continue the map phase.

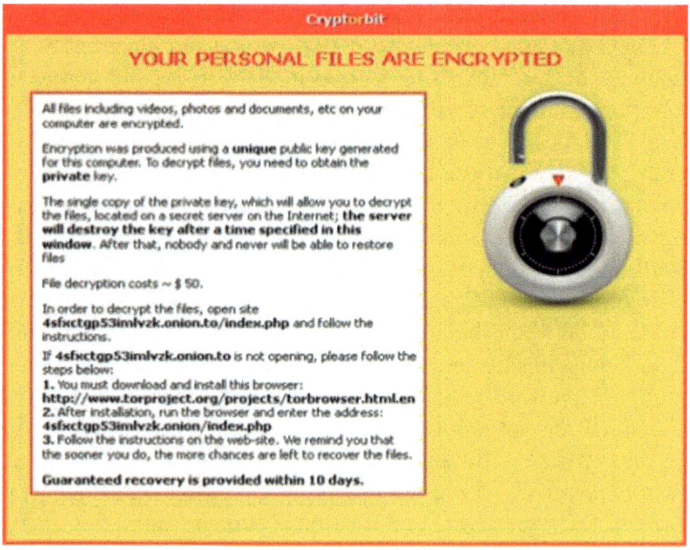

Fig. 15 Encryption type ransomware

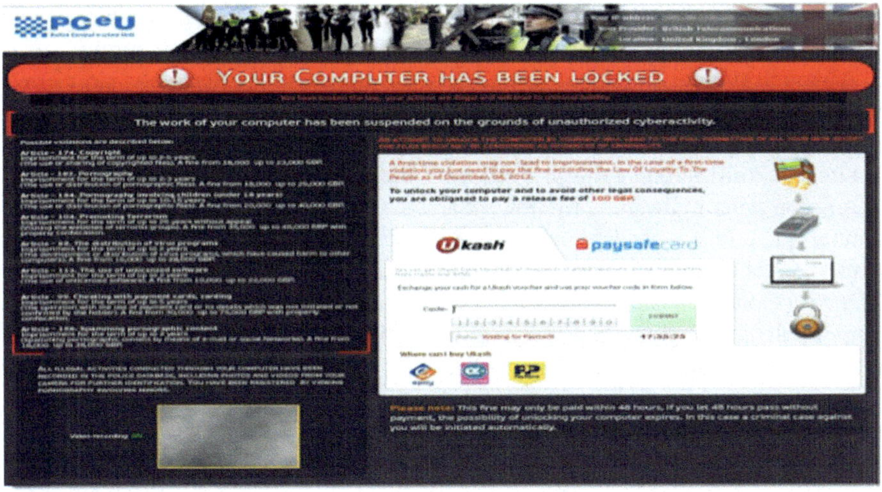

Fig. 16 Lock screen ransomware

5 Analysis Between Biological Virus and Computer Virus

The words "computer virus" was given by computer scientist Fred Cohen in 1984. The biological virus is inactive until it binds to a specific type of host cell, which causes the disease and reproduces using the cell's proteins. Similarly, a computer virus is a computer code that connects to a particular type of computer program, causing damage and reproduction (often via email) when the program is shared. Bharat Mistry, Principal Security Strategist at Trend Micro, affirms that "the underlying infiltration of both computer and biological viruses, damage and impact is very similar."

In the decades, the malware threat became a balloon. "The first big difference between malware and biological viruses is the large amount of new specialized computer malware on a daily basis," says Mistry. "The other big difference is the speed of transmission or transformation. Biological infections start in one area and stay there until the infected people can physically leave. It can take days, maybe weeks. Campaigns to the side" [27].

Malware has become sophisticated, attacking vulnerabilities in many ways. This includes newer, more dangerous types of insects (named after the human-parasitic worm), Trojans and ransomware—which, by strict definition, are not computer viruses, but are commonly known as huh. "We have some real demons out of hell." Viruses often mutate, but have the same functionality. People who use encryption, use stealth techniques—so the antivirus cannot detect it before it does—and use metamorphoses to evolve the Darwinian or randomly attack their prey, such as Stuxnet. "Biological viruses look much simpler than modern computer malware. "If SARS-CoV-2 [a virus that causes COVID-19 and/or similar diseases] becomes malware, it looks like an old-fashioned PC virus," Jelinka who has contributed many papers developing malware and solutions, as well as the use of AI in cybersecurity.

Although simple, biological viruses have developed quite effectively and there is nothing straightforward to predict how SARS-COVID-2/COVID-19 has any effect on the human body. Or how to fix it. The fall of the virus, the death of the disease, the deaths and political and cultural impacts of the global economy, anything dwarfed by any computer malware… till now. "Saras-COV-2 is really tight – it's just 30,000 symbols [12]. It is equivalent to 7 kb to 8 kb of data. I do not know of any computer virus and it is very achievable," says Anniv Ehrlich, a former professor of computer science at Columbia University and a former professor of computer science. "If you combine all the computer security break-ins, I think this is not part of all the hardships and monetary losses that have taken place."

Despite the cyber-attack tsunami of the last four decades, due to the interconnectedness of the IT world, there has been no decrease in the epidemic proportion due to a single cyberpathogen (yet). This may be a testament to the effectiveness of the security profession, or because the perpetrator is still there. The comparison on the basic structure of biological and computer virus is shown in Fig. 17.

After understanding the computer viruses and biological viruses individually, what helps us even more is, developing an understanding of how these viruses are similar. This in turn gives us valuable information and provokes our minds to think about the growing possibilities of the convergence technology and humans, which might be the way to the future.

The comparison between the biological and computer virus on various parameters is analyzed and detailed in Table 1. Similarly, the common traits between the biological and computer virus is described in Table 2.

A PC infection can be incredibly perfect at stowing away itself in the background for quite a while before it begins to grab hold and does any harm, which is the same

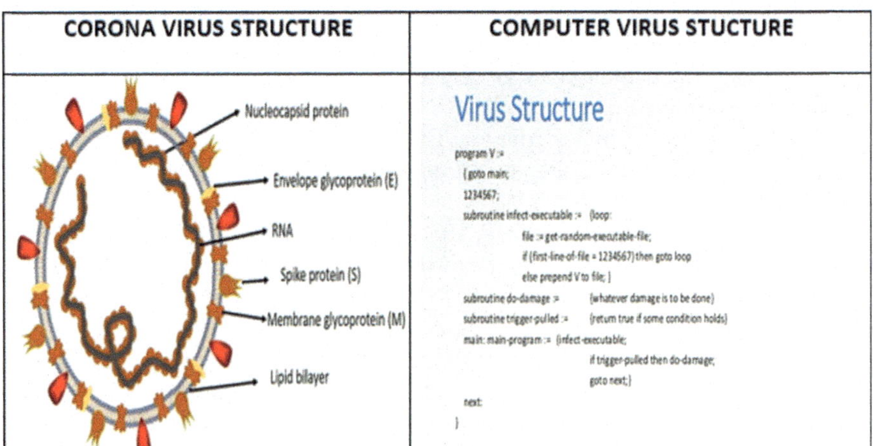

Fig. 17 Comparison on the structure of biological and computer virus

Table 1 Comparison between biological and computer virus on various parameters

Parameters	Biological virus	Computer virus
Origin	Evolution and complex form of proteins	Man-made
Work	Rely on the resources on host cells, develop itself	Are executable files and run on host when activated
Propagation	In forms of micro droplets, expelled by the host. Physical contact or in close surrounding, from person-to-person	From system to system via routing in form of executable files traveling in packets
Difficulty faced	Symptoms takes time to show which may result the spreading this incubation period. Vaccines may not prove effective. Communicable in nature, so problem in controlling it to spread	Executable files are disguised as harmless txt files. Denial of service causes shutdown. Corrupting systems and modifying changes in database causing inconsistency
Prevention	Avoiding contact from infected person. Maintaining proper hygiene and boosting up immunity. Covering up mouths and nose to restrict entry of virus in body. Quarantine of infected person	Updated antivirus in use. Getting files and services from reliable sources only. Not to fall for folders and spams available online. Quarantine of infected file
Target	Infects hosts cells	Infects computer files
Possess	Contains genetic code	Contains executable files
Size	Small but comparable size to genome	Relatively small size to host software
Protection	Vaccination and strong immunity	Antivirus software
Form	Always 3D and complex	No 2D or 3D form
Hitting Time	Virus is seasonal or comes out via evolution	Virus is active according to dataset
Composition	Up to 10^9 or 10^{11} virus particles per mL in host	No huge amount of virus in host computer

as organic viruses, for example Ebola that can lay lethargic for an exceptionally prolonged stretch of time prior showing up, anyway the two sorts can be dealt with and even relieved at an early stage before they grab hold with the assistance of an antivirus.

PC infections can come in a wide range of types (species) simply like their profile legitimate partner, such models incorporate Trojans and other viruses from mails which overwrite small virus to give some examples. Also, it is important to notice that both these viruses have specific targets too.

PC infections can come in a wide range of types (species) simply like their profile legitimate partner, such models incorporate Trojans and other viruses from mails which overwrite small virus to give some examples. Also, it is important to notice that both these viruses have specific targets too.

Table 2 Common traits between the biological system and computer networks

Biological systems	Computer networks
High complexity, high connectivity, extensive interaction between components, numerous entry points	High complexity, high connectivity, extensive interaction between components, numerous entry points
Vulnerability to intentionally or unintentionally introduced alien microorganisms that can quickly contaminate the system resulting in its performance degradation and collapse	Vulnerability to malicious codes (including computer viruses) that being introduced in the system result in unauthorized access to information and services and/or denial of service
Alien microorganisms as well as cells of a biological system are composed of the same building blocks—basic amino acids	Malicious codes as well as the operational software of a computer network are composed of the same building blocks—basic macro commands
The difference between alien microorganisms and the healthy cells of a biological system is in the gene sequencing of their building blocks	The difference between malicious codes and the operational software of a computer network is in the sequencing of their building blocks
Biological immune systems are capable of detecting, recognizing and neutralizing most alien microorganisms in a biological system	Information security systems should be capable of detecting, recognizing and neutralizing most attacks on a computer network

Deriving inspiration from the biological immune systems will also help in building the security patches that can deal with different pathogens and mutations or rather variation of malware. Understanding the biological and computer viruses similarities, dissimilarities, propagation, etc., is also important in determining and deciding human activities, isolation/quantitative detection and response strategies, etc. We can derive several parallel algorithms between biological and computer viruses and build systems that derive techniques from artificial intelligence (AI) and machine learning (ML).

For analyzing both biological and computer viruses, key is the data which needs to be analyzed by the machine learning techniques. In most of the cases, the availability and collection of data in computer viruses is easy compared to biological viruses. However, the strategies adopted for zero-day attacks, etc., may benefit the data starving scenarios of biological viruses. Hence, in the future both fields will gain support and benefits from each other with the help of the AI and ML techniques.

6 Conclusion

Both biological and computer viruses can be managed and even eliminated when taken care. PC virus can be forestalled by guaranteeing by having the most recent antivirus program present, for example AVG, Avast and a large number of free and solid programs to utilize. There are antibodies and antiviruses created for natural infections as well.

All things considered, taken the similarities among the two kinds of viruses, the inquiry that the researchers are attempting to reply is whether the separation or gap between the two can be obscured enough later on to permit organic infections to influence machines and PC ones' harm individuals? Although biological infections have been effectively integrated by researchers, PC infections that advance without support of anyone else have still not been seen in nature. They have been occasions where analysts made PC infections that develop along the Darwinian principles, yet they were never discharged to the world from a laboratory. With the utilization of electronic gadgets (clinical or something else) implanted in the human and their unavoidable need to speak with outside gadgets, a PC infection can truly influence and infect people [28]. Likewise, analysts and researchers use PCs to code manufactured infections. Thus, this chapter compares the biological and computer viruses and provides its detailed analysis in terms of their pattern, mutation, propagation, impact of infect, detection, emergence and its prevention. Further, it bring out the analogy between the biological viruses and computer viruses experienced in the past and their existence at present.

References

1. There's now COVID-19 malware that will wipe your PC and rewrite your MBR. ZDNet. https://www.zdnet.com/article/theres-now-covid-19-malware-that-will-wipe-your-pc-and-rewrite-your-mbr/
2. Baize, S., Pannetier, D., Oestereich, L., Rieger, T., Koivogui, L., Magassouba, N. F., Soropogui, B., Sow, M. S., Keïta, S., De Clerck, H., & Tiffany, A. (2014). Emergence of Zaire Ebola virus disease in Guinea. *New England Journal of Medicine, 371*(15), 1418–1425.
3. Kirk, A. D. (2019). Artificial intelligence and the fifth domain. *AFL Rev., 80*, 183.
4. Helmreich, S. (2000). Flexible infections: Computer viruses, human bodies, nation-states, evolutionary capitalism. *Science, Technology, & Human Values, 25*(4), 472–491.
5. Kleinberg, J. (2007). The wireless epidemic. *Nature, 449*(7160), 287–288.
6. Paul, G. L. (2014). Systems of evidence in the age of complexity. *Ave Maria L. Rev., 12*, 173.
7. Wessner, D. R. (2010). The origins of viruses. *Nature Education, 3*(9), 37.
8. Dubey, V. P., Kumar, R., & Kumar, D. (2020). A hybrid analytical scheme for the numerical computation of time fractional computer virus propagation model and its stability analysis. *Chaos, Solitons & Fractals, 133*, 109626.
9. Smith, M. W. (2020). *Coronavirus and COVID-19: What you should know*. WebMD.
10. Koret, J., & Bachaalany, E. (2015). *The antivirus hacker's handbook*. Wiley (Incorporated).
11. Goldenthal, K. L., Midthun, K., & Zoon, K. C. (1996). Control of viral infections and diseases. *Medical Mircrobiology*.
12. Lau, S. K., Che, X. Y., Woo, P. C., Wong, B. H., Cheng, V. C., Woo, G. K., Hung, I. F., Poon, R. W., Chan, K. H., Peiris, J. M., & Yuen, K. Y. (2005). SARS coronavirus detection methods. *Emerging Infectious Diseases, 11*(7), 1108.
13. Feldmann, H., & Geisbert, T. W. (2011). Ebola haemorrhagic fever. *The Lancet, 377*(9768), 849–862.
14. Henderson, R. (2020). Using graph databases to detect financial fraud. *Computer Fraud & Security, 2020*(7), 6–10.

15. Cohen, F. (1987). Computer viruses: Theory and experiments. *Computers & Security, 6*(1), 22–35.
16. Barak, L. (2020). Preventive medicine is the best method for computer hygiene. *Computer Fraud & Security, 2020*(1), 9–11.
17. Scaife, N., Carter, H., Traynor, P., & Butler, K. R. (2016, June). Cryptolock (and drop it): Stopping Ransomware attacks on user data. In *2016 IEEE 36th International Conference on Distributed Computing Systems (ICDCS)* (pp. 303–312). IEEE.
18. Patel, A., & Tailor, J. (2020). A malicious activity monitoring mechanism to detect and prevent Ransomware. *Computer Fraud & Security, 2020*(1), 14–19.
19. Willems, E. (2019). Thirty years of malware: A short outline. In *Cyberdanger* (pp. 1–12). Springer.
20. Cohen, F. B. (1994). *A short course on computer viruses*. Wiley.
21. Ludwig, M. A. (1993). *Computer viruses, artificial life and evolution*. Macmillan Heinemann.
22. How does anti-malware work? MalwareByteLabs. https://blog.malwarebytes.com/101/2015/12/how-does-anti-malware-work/
23. del Rey, A. M. (2015). Mathematical modeling of the propagation of malware: A review. *Security and Communication Networks, 8*(15), 2561–2579.
24. Newman, M. E., Forrest, S., & Balthrop, J. (2002). Email networks and the spread of computer viruses. *Physical Review E, 66*(3), 035101.
25. Top five dangerous computer virus with I LOVE YOU virus. INextLive. https://www.inextlive.com/top-five-dangerous-computer-virus-with-i-love-you-virus-201701310015
26. O'Gorman, G., & McDonald, G. (2012). *Ransomware: A growing menace*. Symantec Corporation.
27. D'Onofrio, D. J., & An, G. (2010). A comparative approach for the investigation of biological information processing: An examination of the structure and function of computer hard drives and DNA. *Theoretical Biology and Medical Modelling, 7*(1), 1–29.
28. Otten, E. J. (2016). Ciottone's disaster medicine. *Journal of Emergency Medicine, 50*(5), 801.

Role of AI and AI-Derived Techniques in Brain and Behavior Computing

Om Prakash Yadav, Yojana Yadav, and Shashwati Ray

1 Introduction

The electroencephalography (EEG) captures electric potentials of the brain in non-invasive manner [1–3]. Other non-invasive techniques are magnetoencephalography (MEG), positron emission tomography (PET), functional magnetic resonance imaging (fMRI) as well as optical imaging. Limited spatial resolution of EEG limits its use as compared to high-resolution techniques like fMRI and computed tomography (CT) [4]. Resolution of EEG signals is in millisecond range and is easily and real-time available, hence it continues to be a valuable tool for brain–computer interface (BCI) [5–7].

The EEG record the brain's spontaneous electrical activity and focuses on electric potential through the placed electrodes on the scalp (100 μV) or on the outer layer of the brain (1–2 mV) over a period of time [7]. The effective bandwidth of these signals is approximately 100 Hz. EEG signals are basically recorded at sampling rates in between 250 and 2000 Hz for clinical purposes. However, high-resolution modern EEG devices (for real-time applications) can record even above 20,000 Hz [1, 2]. Clinical features of EEG signals mainly depend upon the event potentials time and frequency characteristics [8]. These signals are also used for diagnosis of sleep disorders, brain tumors, anesthesia depth, stroke coma, brain dysfunction (encephalopathies), brain damage, brain death, and other focal brain disorders [9, 10].

An EEG is typically expressed in the form of rhythmic activity and transients. This rhythmic activity actually represents frequency bands. Details about the band (δ, θ, α, β, γ, μ) of the human EEG waves can be obtained from [11–13]. Clinical information of EEG signals is present within a bandwidth 0.5 Hz–100 Hz. For an EEG signal, a

O. P. Yadav · Y. Yadav (✉)
PES Institute of Technology and Management, Shivamogga, Karnataka, India

S. Ray
Bhilai Institute of Technology, Durg, Chhattisgarh, India

A. K. Tyagi et al. (eds.), *Intelligent Interactive Multimedia Systems for e-Healthcare Applications*, https://doi.org/10.1007/978-981-16-6542-4_4

resolution of 16 or more bits is preferable. However, the standard resolution required for clinical equipment (or high-resolution EEG devices) is minimum 24 bits [14].

The history of artificial intelligence (AI) joints the connections between brain science study and AI. The mesh of neurons available in human brain has been discovered by microscopes that inspired the artificial neural network (ANN). Similarly, the brains convolution property and multilayer structure are discovered by using electronic detectors, inspired by convolutional neural network (CNN) and deep learning (DL). Although AI and brain science community both are directly unconnected, the results obtained of brain science disclose important and unique issues related to principles of intelligence which lead to significant breakthrough in AI.

1.1 EEG Artifacts

An EEG is highly non-stationary weak signal with noises (artifacts) contaminating their characteristics to significant levels [15, 16]. These artifacts are categorized as physiological and non-physiological. Physiological artifacts (due to ocular, muscular, cardiac activity, perspiration, and respiration) are internal, i.e., through human body itself whereas non-physiological (includes disturbances due to electrode pop, cable movement, reference placement, electrical and electromagnetic interferences, and body movements) artifacts are external to the human body [17–19].

These artifacts degrade the quality of EEG signal and thus prevent correct diagnosis. Comprehensive knowledge about the artifacts affecting EEG is primarily required to them significantly. However, still this area is challenging for researches to completely model the noise signals and it the preliminary stage for almost all biomedical field. Existing brain signal enhancement methods can be obtained from [20–23].

1.2 Brain–Computer Interface (BCI)

A BCI is an interface system to extract and translate the EEG signals obtained from brain into messages to control machines. The EEG signals are required to be processed and then decoded into control signals so that it can be easily perceived by any mechanical, electrical or electronic device [24]. Weak strength and sensitivity to artifacts make BCI stages more complicated.

Typical features of EEG utilized in BCI include event-related potential, steady-state visual evoked potential with sensorimotor rhythm, and time–frequency features [25]. Existing medical applications of BCI are utilized for analysis of sleep pattern, epilepsy, disorders of consciousness, mental fatigue and workload, emotions, depth of anesthesia, mental state monitoring, etc. [26–28]. BCI is also found useful for persons severely disabled by clinical disorders like brainstem stroke, spinal cord injuries, muscular and chronic peripheral neuropathies, etc. [29]. Other non-clinical

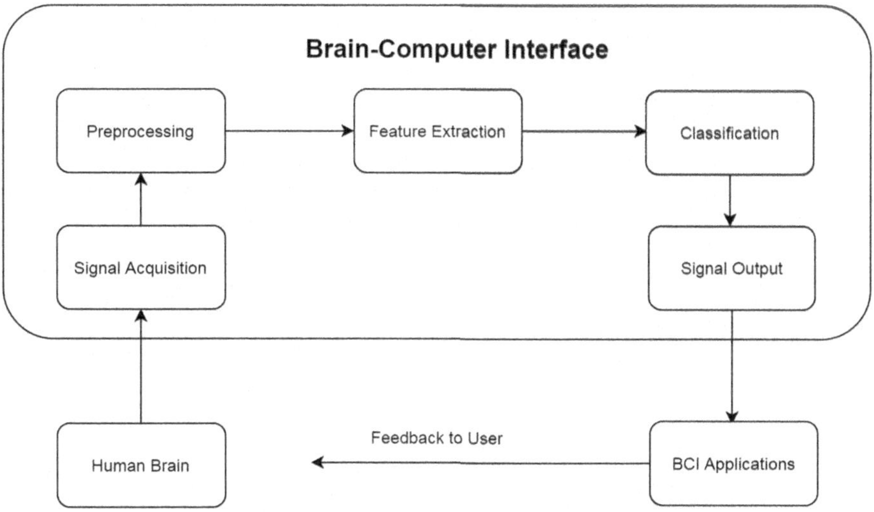

Fig. 1 Brain–computer interface

applications of BCI include machine control, environmental control, cognition of music, media, games, etc. Details of these applications can be obtained from [30].

There are currently two approaches to BCIs: invasive and non-invasive. Invasive or direct normally requires electrodes to be implanted under scalp for brain signals and extracts more informative and accurate signals with risks like brain surgery; non-invasive structures typically records using head-worn sensors. However, non-invasive method is consumer-friendly but lowers the performance [30, 31].

A brain–computer interface system consists of some important stages: data acquisition, preprocessing, feature extraction with feature translation, and device output [24, 32]. General steps involved in BCI applications are shown in Fig. 1.

The data acquisition system is accountable for collecting the EEG signals. Then task of preprocessing is to reduce noise contents in brain signals to further enhance signal-to-noise ratio, i.e., SNR of recorded signals, i.e., to reduce artifacts without compromising clinical information available in the brain signal. Then the preprocessed signal is given to the specific feature extraction algorithmic rule. Here, feature extraction algorithm extracts suitable information for the brain signals. The feature translator transforms the features to other domains so that it can be easily interpreted by the classifier. Since brain signals are highly dynamic and changes with behavior, a suitable translator is required so that classification can easily be achieved. The classifier output classifies the translated information into groups that be fed as different signals to control BCI systems [27, 33, 34].

In short, BCIs when clubbed with AI will show the feelings that are felt without narrating and hence AI facilitates BCI in a number of ways.

1.3 Challenges in the Field of BCI Implementation

The foremost challenge for BCI systems is its dependency on data acquisition and deciphering brain activity. For every activity, brain can produce different signals and also these signals are dependent upon emotional and mental states which make the interfacing more difficult. Even the recorded brain signals are weak in magnitude and are also sensitive to noises. Traditional approaches are based on frequency spectrum of EEG signals for BCI systems [35]. Also, EEG signals are highly user-specific making BCI implementation more complicated. Since BCI domain involves other domains like neuroscience, cognitive science, physics, biology, etc. [36], this further makes this field difficult. Recently, machine learning algorithms are gaining popularity for the development of BCI applications particularly in medical and robotic fields which makes them the most efficient tool for BCI systems.

1.4 EEG Databases

A number of sparsely populated EEG repositories are available online. But lack of open-source software for standard EEG limits biomedical research. Updated EEG data for public use is available from https://sccn.ucsd.edu/~arno/fam2data/publicly_available_EEG_data.html. Available EEG sparsely populated online EEG data, patient-specific online repository, multipurpose data repositories, and analytic tools facilitating large-scale data mining can be found in [37]. A variety of online databases under different conditions along with their description for specific research can also be obtained from https://github.com/meagmohit/EEG-Datasets. Pediatric subject brain signals of Children's Hospital Boston can be found in [38]. Open access online EEG records for different mental states, application-specific can also be collected from http://bnci-horizon-2020.eu/database/data-sets.

Formats, duration, sampling frequency, number of channels, etc., play very important role in assessment of algorithms. So, for comparison of algorithms, same set of data may provide robust comparison. However, algorithms should be designed in such a way that they should be applicable to any data.

2 Machine Learning

ML is the most popular subset of AI that predicts the future by automatically learning and improving from experience, i.e., ML algorithms use input data and use it for learning and training to analyze the behavior of data to make predictions about the future on an autonomous basis [39, 40].

Data is the core part of ML algorithms, and hence it has opened up a vast potential for BCI applications. The ML algorithms because of its capability to learn from data in an efficient, systematic, and fast manner have given another dimension to the way we perceive information [41]. Data generated from EEG signals is voluminous. For complete diagnosis of EEG-related diseases, continuous monitoring of EEG signals is required which in turn requires large volume of data. Hence, it can be observed that the ML models can effectively be useful for analysis of EEG signals. All ML models are accessed through accuracy and if the accuracy is within acceptable limits, the ML model is deployed else, the model is trained again and again with the training data with different parameters of the model. Optimization of the models is also required to produce accurate results [42, 43].

In ML algorithms, the input data can be broadly divided into two types: labeled data and unlabeled data. As far as labeled data is concerned, it has both inputs as well as corresponding outputs and hence a lot of efforts are required to label the data. Unlike labeled data, unlabeled data only has only inputs and hence requires more complex solutions [44]. Normally classification is done on labeled data whereas clustering is done on unlabeled data.

There are mainly three subcategories of ML algorithm, i.e., supervised, unsupervised, and reinforcement learning.

2.1 Supervised Learning

Supervised ML algorithms are designed for labeled data, and hence accurate labeling of data is required to obtain correct results. In supervised learning, the ML model is fed with input data, i.e., training data to work with. This training data provides necessary information like the problem and required solution associated with the data pattern [45]. The model then finds relationships between the input and output training data by establishing a cause and effect relationship between them [39, 42]. This trained model then can be utilized for unknown data. The advantage with this algorithm is that it will continue to improve discovering new relationships in every training [46, 47].

Popular supervised ML models include linear regression, backpropagation neural network, decision trees, support vector machine, deep learning, or a more sophisticated combination of methods. Supervised learning mainly used to develop model that can classify, predict, or identify the EEG patterns based on the extracted features [39, 45, 48]. This ML algorithm is easy to implement; however, it is limited to labeled data only and it may not produce expected results for complex tasks [38]. Deep learning models versus traditional machine learning technique approaches are indicated in Fig. 2.

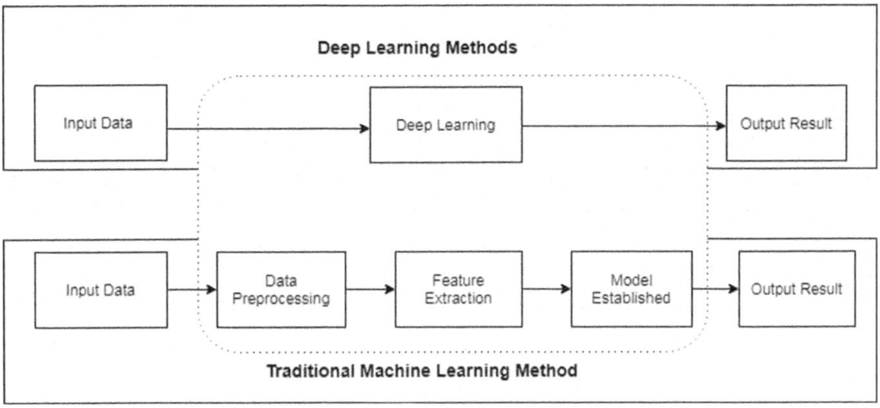

Fig. 2 Deep learning versus traditional machine learning

2.2 Unsupervised Learning

Unsupervised ML models work with unlabeled data, and hence human labor is not required for labeling of data. However, the complexity of such model increases as it has to deal with unlabeled data [40]. In this type of learning, the behavior of data pattern is perceived in an abstract manner through hidden structures which makes these models versatile [45]. An unsupervised learning algorithm learns data patterns by dynamically changing hidden structures and thus finds more applications in clustering/classification algorithms [41, 45, 49]. Unsupervised ML algorithms are usually deployed for clustering and association. Popular unsupervised algorithms existing in literature are: clustering, K-means clustering, KNN, mixture models, singular value decomposition, and self-organizing maps [45, 50]. Advantage associated with unsupervised learning is that it can even hidden pattern of brain signals and is useful for real-time applications.

2.3 Reinforcement Learning

Reinforcement learning is reward–punishment-based training of models to make a sequence of decisions based on a trial-and-error method. Desirable outputs are endorsed, and undesirable outputs are discouraged [39, 45]. This type of ML is required where we are not sure about the result of any action. These kinds of situations are surprisingly common in BCI applications, and hence this learning algorithm is found to be well suited. Two widely used reinforcement ML models are Markov decision process and Q learning. Reinforcement learning algorithms are categorized as: model-free and model-based. Current action is based on some trial-and-error experience in model-free learning whereas in model-based learning current action is dependent upon previously learned lessons. This type of learning is generally deployed for closed-loop brain-controlled interfaces [39, 51, 52].

3 Available Tools for ML and BCI

ML algorithms can be executed on a number of platforms. Depending upon the accessibility and requirement, any of the one or more ML platforms may be utilized: MATLAB, Alteryx Analytics, RapidMiner, H2O.ai, SAS TIBCO software, Databricks Unified Analytics Platform, Domino Data Science Platform, Microsoft's Azure Machine Learning Studio, OpenNN, Apache Spark MLlib, Neon, DiffBlue, TensorFlow, Protege, Eclipse Deeplearning4j, IBM Watson Studio, Google Cloud AI Platform, IBM Decision Optimization, Anaconda Enterprise, TensorFlow, BigML, DataRobot, Deep Cognition, RStudio Team, Petuum, etc. Details about licensing, price, and installation about these platforms can be obtained from respective Web sites.

The BCI toolbox facility is to provide toolboxes that provide data, methods, research with evaluation to have the pace of innovation in the BCI field. The publically available software platforms for BCI community are as follows: (1) BCI2000, (2) BCI2000Web (3) OpenViBE, (4) TOBI Common Implementation Platform (CIP), (5) WebFM (6) BCILAB, (7) BCI++, (8) xBCI, (9) BF++, (10) Biosig, and (11) Fieldtrip [53].

4 Classification Algorithms in Machine Learning

A classifier utilizes signal characteristics (parameters) as inputs to predict a class. During training a classifier, model maps inputs to outputs, and once trained, the model is capable of predicting classes to testing data. ML classifiers are binary classification (two class labels), multiclass classification (more than two class labels), multilabel classification (two or more class labels wherein each label has different labels), and imbalanced classification is multilabel classification with each label unequally distributed [54]. A mostly ML application for BCI belongs to imbalance classifications. The performance tools for imbalance classifiers are accuracy, recall, precision, and F-measure.

4.1 Performance Parameters

Once a classifier algorithm is applied to any data, it classifies the given data and then model can be tested for its accuracy with which the model is capable of classifying the data. A true positive (TP) observes a positive class whereas a true negative (TN) correctly observes a negative class. A false positive (FP) wrongly predicts the positive class whereas a false negative (FN) wrongly observes the negative class [55, 56].

Accuracy is defined as the ratio that indicates true predictions about the classifier model.

$$\text{Accuracy} = \frac{\text{TP} + \text{NP}}{\text{TP} + \text{TN} + \text{FP} + \text{FN}} \tag{1}$$

Precision represents proportion of true positives which were actually true.

$$\text{Precision} = \frac{\text{TP}}{\text{TP} + \text{FP}} \tag{2}$$

Recall evaluates ratio of actual positives identified correctly.

$$\text{Recall} = \frac{\text{TP}}{\text{TP} + \text{FN}} \tag{3}$$

All the parameters, i.e., accuracy, precision, and recall are positive-oriented parameter, and model producing higher value will be considered better. Care should be taken while improving precision as precision and recall are inversely proportional [55].

F-measure balances both the precision and recall in one number.

$$\text{Fmeasure} = \frac{2 * \text{Precison} * \text{Recall}}{\text{Precison} + \text{Recall}} \tag{4}$$

F-measure is also positive-oriented parameter and model yielding higher value would be considered better classifier.

These parameters, however, change with the size of data, i.e., more samples will produce concrete results. In order to compare ML classification algorithms, same number of samples must be taken.

4.2 Existing Machine Learning-Based BCI Classification Methods

The task of classification assigns an object to one of several classes on the basis of some rule. In BCI, generally linear classifiers simple models are used. However, the classification in presence of noises makes even simple classification more difficult.

Support vector machine, i.e., SVM prepares a set of hyperplanes that too in an infinite-dimensional space which can further be used for classification; even this can also be used for artifact reduction. Le et al. [57] developed SVM model to classify motor imagery (MI) dataset III for problem in BCI Competition II by transforming two optimal points to hyperplane and obtained promising results. The accuracy of

SVM classification algorithms mainly depends on the kernel function and penalty parameters. This dependency has been overcame by using SVM with particle swarm optimization and has been tested over MI data obtained from the BCI Competition Datasets [58]. Semi-supervised SVM with batch-mode incremental learning method is found to reduce computation training time for BCI interfacing [59]. Classification accuracy of SVM algorithms was also improved by using common spatial pattern (CSP) as well as chaotic particle swarm optimization (CPSO), i.e., twin SVM (TWSVM) for MI EEG [60]. SVM has also been used for the recognition of the will of a human being [61], removal of noises from EEG signals [62], classification of mental and cognitive task [63, 64], and P300-based cursor movement control [65]. The popularity of SVM-based classifiers is due to its simplicity and robustness with regard to dimensionality but at the cost of execution time.

The k-nearest neighbor (KNN) identifies *k*-nearest samples from training set. This classification technique assigns a point value to the dominant class among its *k*-nearest neighbors. BCI applications, the KNN, are mainly achieved using a metric distance [35]. With a significantly high neighbors and training samples, KNN can actually approximate any function even for nonlinear classification. KNN algorithms are very efficient with low-dimensional feature vectors of BCI signals [66]. KNN classification technique has been applied for Concealed Information Test (CIT) and reported an accuracy of 96.7% [67]. Spark and rule KNN-based scalable framework has been utilized for deceit identification using BCI P300 and even reported an accuracy of 92.46% [68].

Multilayer perceptron (MLP) consists of three sequential layers: input, hidden, and output, which help in transmitting data from input to output layer. MLP techniques have already been applied to binary, multiclass, synchronous, asynchronous BCI [69–72]. MLP model may suffer from overfitting due to less or excess number of neurons. Giovanni et al. in [73] compared MLP and fuzzy C-means and reported MLP to be better in terms of training data size. Sridhar et al. utilized MLP to model nonlinear relationship of EEG signal. Rate of convergence of MLP is relatively slow and often yields suboptimal solutions. MLP has also been utilized to categorize emotional states like joy, angry, sadness, and happiness on the basis of EEG signal [74]. Hamedi et al. [75] compared MLP and radial basis function (RBF) with SVM over motor-related EEG and reported accuracy much higher for SVM-RBF.

The Naive Bayes (NB) is very simpler and efficient probabilistic multiclass classifier and it classifies by assuming that the extracted features are independent which is actually not possible with EEG signals. Juliono et al. [76] have used data of University of Technology for the BCI Competition II with the spectral estimation by periodogram and the distribution of imaginary EEG using Naïve Bayes classifier and reported accuracy of 80%. They further compared LDA and the NB EEG-based classifiers to analyze movement of both right as well as left hand [77]. LDA and NB results are almost same with an accuracy of 70%. The results of classification for imaginary movement control using NB are further increased to 85% by using EMOTIV cap-based system in [78]. NB classifier has been used to classify mental status on the basis of EEG recording of subjects. The classification is performed on

IVa and IVb datasets of BCI Competition and results are found be improved up to 21% [79].

The algorithm takes decision on randomly selected trees by means of voting. The random forest (RF) classifiers prevent overfitting of the model and are considered to be more accurate for real-time classification but suffers from high computational time and complexity. Okumu et al. have used Fast Walsh Hadamard transformation with Fourier and Wavelet transform along with RF algorithm to improve classification results over Dataset III in BCI Competition 2003 [80]. RF algorithms were successfully used to classify mental status, i.e., concentration and meditation in [81]. David et al. proposed RF models as compared to LDA for classification-based sensorimotor rhythms [82].

Logistic regression (LR) utilizes logistic function to classify the possible binary outputs for inputs. It assumes predictors to be independent of each other without any missing data. LR algorithms may result in overfitting for sparsely and highly dense data (as brain signals). So, LR algorithms are not found to be suitable for brain signals; however, few applications in motor imagery classification are found in literature. Suily et al. [83] proposed cross-correlation-based LR model to classify motor imagery (MI) data IVa with respect to BCI Competition III and recorded better results. LR models were even found to perform better without any prior feature extraction or noise removal steps in [84]. Only 65% accuracy is reported for classification of targeted finger movements in [85].

5 Clustering Algorithms in BCI

Clustering is unsupervised form of learning wherein similar data are grouped on the basis of homogeneity properties. Since brain shows different characteristics for different emotions, mental activities, health conditions, life styles, etc., these characteristics can be clustered and utilized in an organized manner for any specific application in BCI.

5.1 Performance Parameters in Clustering Algorithms

There is no reasonable way to determine the validity of cluster predictions. However, following matrices may be utilized to evaluate the relative performance of cluster models.

The Davies-Bouldin (DB) index is the ratio of similarity within-cluster distances to between-cluster distances. It can be evaluated as

$$\mathrm{DB} = \frac{1}{n}\sum_{i=1}^{N} \max{}_{j \neq i}\left(\frac{\sigma_i + \sigma_j}{d(c_i, c_j)}\right) \tag{5}$$

where n represents total count of clusters and σ_i is the average distance of all points in cluster i from c_i, i.e., the cluster centroid. This is negative-oriented parameter and algorithm producing lower DB would be considered better [86].

This Dunn index (DI) is the proportion of minimum of intercluster distance to the maximum cluster size [87]. It can be evaluated as

$$\mathrm{DI} = \frac{\min_{1 \le i \le j \le N} d(i, j)}{\max_{1 \le k \le N} d'(k)} \tag{6}$$

where i, j, and k are individual clusters, whereas d is the intercluster distance and d' is the intracluster difference. Higher the value of DI, better the clustering algorithm.

The silhouette coefficient (SC) can be calculated like

$$s(i) = \frac{b(i) - a(i)}{\max\{a(i), b(i)\}} \tag{7}$$

where $a(i)$ is nothing but the average of the distance of one point from other points in its cluster $b(i)$ is the smallest average distance of i to all other points in any other cluster. Its range is from $-1 \mathrm{to} 1$. Higher positive would produce better clusters [88].

The Calinski–Harabasz index (CHI) is used when the knowledge of labels are not known in advance like EEG signals. It is defined in terms of dispersion as ratio of sum of dispersion between and within clusters.

$$\mathrm{CHI} = \frac{\mathrm{D}(b_n)}{\mathrm{D}(w_n)} \mathrm{X} \frac{N - n}{n - 1} \tag{8}$$

where (b_k) is dispersion between clusters and $\mathrm{D}(w_k)$ is dispersion within clusters and n represents the count of clusters similarly N is to represent the total size of the data [89]. This parameter is also positive-oriented, and higher value is expected for better clustering algorithms.

5.2 The Existing Clustering Method in BCI

The k-means-based clustering algorithm basically divides data (n elements) to k clusters such that each element is a member of the cluster having nearest mean. This algorithm also suffers from the convergence of the local minima. This local convergence problem has been resolved by Jaya optimization method for the selection of initial cluster and has been applied to MI task, which showed promising results [90]. Annushree Bablani et al. used k-means algorithm to classify EEG data into three clusters for concealed information test [91]. K-means algorithms were successfully applied to classify cognitive activity based on math activity for data extracted from a single EEG sensor [92]. K-means algorithm is applied to cluster EEG signal according to their frequency and temporal characteristics. The accuracy of clustering is increased by preprocessing the EEG signals before application of *k*-means clustering algorithm [93].

A Gaussian mixture model (GMM) consists of Gaussian distributions with unknown parameters. Classical GMM models in BCI suffer due to the presence of noises. However, GMM models based on the genetic algorithm and expectation–maximization method produced reliable results in [94]. The time as well as frequency analysis of EEG records event-related desynchronization (ERD) which can further be used for reaching control. Khatami et al. developed GMM based an online BCI system using ERD to turn on and off the system with an average accuracy of 99.3% and 96.3%, respectively [95]. GMM model was successfully applied for depicting stroke patients' imagery EEG distribution features [96]. An integrated layered GMM to predict alertness level depending upon EEG recordings has been presented by Gu et al. in 2011. In their article, they have developed hierarchical GMM that can automatically remove noises, quantify vigilance, and discover underlying patterns of EEG. Results claimed are found to be better than SVM and LDA under complicated probability distributions [97].

A self-organizing map (SOM) produces a low-dimensional data (maps) through competitive learning on input data. Spectral frequency characteristics of EEG signals from the 3-class identification problem of the BCI Competition [98] have been utilized to segregate EEG signals using SOM neural networks and achieved hit ratio of 60% [99]. Zeehan et al. [100] used wavelet transform along with spectral coefficients to further enhance the hit ratio to 84.17%. SOM classifier is also utilized for mental tasks classification and achieved average accuracy about 91% [101]. A SOM algorithm based on subattribute information (SOMSA), i.e., differences in individual's EEG (specifically θ, α, and β) data has been presented in [102]. The results claimed are found to be superior to traditional SOM classifiers. SOM is even successfully used in single EEG channels with the P300 component detection [103].

Linear discriminant analysis (LDA) linearly splits features into two or more classes. The LDA algorithm assumes Gaussian distribution of the data for the concerned classes which is not actually possible for BCI applications. Hence, versions of LDAs are used in BCI applications. Once such version like z-score (based mean and standard deviation)-based LDA has been used to classify Iva data of BCI Competition III and reported high accuracy than traditional LDA algorithms [104]. BCI-based hand gesture and finger movement are also found to be controlled through a time-variant-based linear discriminant analysis, i.e., TVLDA [105]. Linear discriminant analysis is also sensitive to training data because training data may be imprecise. The problem has been addressed and resolved by Onishi et al. in [106]. The regularized LDA along with principal component analysis (PCA) is suitably applicable for the classification of the P300-based BCI.

Fuzzy c-means (FCM) allows one data from two or more clusters. Hsu et al. used discrete wavelet transform (DWT) to extract data using amplitude modulation technique and then used these features to discriminate left finger lifting and resting from EECG signals using FCM method. Results obtained are found to be superior to k-means and LDA classification methods [107]. Empirical wavelet transform (EWT) is found to be capable of decomposing EEG signal. This feature of EWT has been successfully used for mental task classification model using FCM in [108].

6 Deep Learning

Deep learning (DL) has multiple hidden neural layers networks that can learn even through unlabeled data. Although ML learning BCI systems have made tremendous developments, actually BCI faces significant challenges as mainly brain signals are weak in magnitude and are highly affected by different types of artifacts during recording and transmission. Addition of artifacts reduces SNR which further deteriotes signal strength. So, preprocessing of brain signal is primary requirements. Moreover, EEG data collection methods are still expensive due unavailability of cheaper recorders and time-consuming. Even online data have small number of participants and are specific to particular conditions. DL has two advantages for BCI implementations, i.e., firstly, it works directly on raw brain data and secondly it captures both features and dependencies through hidden structures. DL models are categorized into four classes based on the aim: discriminative, representative, generative, and hybrid DL models. Discriminative DL models work by learning discriminative features adaptively. Representative model learns from pure features of the input data. Generative models learn from the joint probability distribution of the input data along with the target label. Hybrid DL models are combinations two or more DL models.

6.1 Popular DL Models in Machine Learning

Recurrent neural network (RNN) is a recurrent network whose present output depends upon the past output and inputs. For, BCI application, it utilizes the temporal structure and frequencies of brain signals during training and produces the output. RNN has been implemented to distinguish the visual objects using brain waves by Palazzo et al. [109]. The RNN algorithms suffer from vanishing gradient problem which limits its application for long EEG signals. The long short-term memory (LSTM) algorithms can determine long-term dependencies and are replacement for RNN for BCI models. Kumar et al. used classified real-time motor imagery tasks with high accuracy in [110].

Convolution neural networks (CNNs) are inspired from biological process and a regularized versions of fully connected networks. This deep learning is now gaining popularity for processing of time varying series data. Since these architectures learn from raw data, they are prone to overfitting data. Zhang et al. analyzed left- and right-hand MI tasks through CNN. Authors have used different function, i.e., rectified linear unit (ReLU), exponential linear unit (ELU) also scaled exponential linear unit (SELU) and reported SELU function to produce better results [111]. CNNs for P300-based BCIs can also be obtained from [112, 113].

A restricted Boltzmann machine (RBM) is random networks of neuron shaving capability to extract internal characteristics, i.e., probability distribution of brain signals independently in generative sense. This feature of RBN has been successfully implement over 9 subjects to extract the features of motor rhythm and obtained overall median-accuracy of 88.7% with a standard error of 6.6% as compared to Naive classifier wherein median accuracy and standard error reported is 83.5% and 6.6%, respectively [114]. RBM is also found to produce comparable decoding performance even with missing motor imagery ECG data. The algorithm is also capable of smooth operation for the online BCI system [115]. RBMs are also successfully utilized to identify networks and their temporal activations in [116].

A deep belief network actually combines directed and undirected networks in such a way that upper layer is undirected RBM and the bottom layer directed RBM. These directed and undirected networks help in pretraining and fine-tuning. DBN was found to be superior to SVM, LDA, and extreme learning machine (ELM) in classifying EEG data according to channel fusion levels [117]. Sobhani reported 97% accuracy in classifying P300 data by using four-layer DBN in which last layer is logistic regression layer [118]. Lu et al. [119] first extracted the time and spatial features of input data and then used softmax-based DBN classifier for P300 data. Wavelet packets were used to extract time–frequency characteristics and the features extracted were used for MI EEG signals identification and classification in [120]. Other applications of DBN for brain signals analysis can be obtained from [121]. DBN may also be applied for multimodal data and large datasets.

An autoencoder learns by copying input to output by transforming the connection weights that minimizes the error between input and outputs. It has an encoder–decoder and a hidden layer. Encoder transforms the input data to a code that is further mapped to output through decoder. Li et al. [122] developed an autoencoder to extract information from scarce EEG signals. Autoencoder also finds applications for seizure prediction using EEG datasets. Autoencoders were also utilized for effective data compression of EEG signals in [123].

6.2 Long Short-Term Memory

The long short-term memory (LSTM) is a RNN which has capability to remember longlasting dependencies in data. LSTM networks are designed to overcome respective drawbacks of RNN. Raghda et al. [124] classified MI EEG signals using LSTM and autoencoders based on a sequence-to-sequence architecture. Mental work load classification into four classes was done using LSTM with 89.31% average accuracy for BCI [125]. Left/right-hand movement classification from EEG signals using LSTM has also been found in [126]. A most common hybrid method includes RNN and CNN. Shah et al. [127] have utilized CNN-based LSTM network for detection seizure detection. A variant of LSTM, i.e., bidirectional (BiLSTM) which can extract dependencies in an adaptive manner is found useful to recognize different imagery actions from MI-EEG signals [128].

7 Conclusion

EEG signals are still very easily available tool for BCI applications as compared to other brain signals. However, preprocessing of these signals is essential because of poor SNR, inter- and intravariability. A number of online databases of brain signals are available for BCI applications; however, care should be taken while downloading signals as performance of algorithms depend upon sample format, sample size, sampling rate, and sample specifications. ML algorithms learn from the past experiences and are able to predict future and hence find applications in BCI domain. Dependency of ML algorithms on true data, time, resources, and error susceptibility hinders its use on BCI applications. However, a number of classification and clustering algorithms are available in literature with pros and cons utilizing benefits of existing ML algorithms. DL methods are gaining popularity because of their classification accuracy over large dataset. Currently Internet of things, BCI, and AI are clubbed and are utilized for the betterment of society.

References

1. Bashashati, A., Fatourechi, M., Ward, R. K., & Birch, G. E. (2007). A survey of signal processing algorithms in brain–computer interfaces based on electrical brain signals. *Journal of Neural Engineering, 4*(2), R32.
2. Huang, W., Goldsberry, L., Wymbs, N. F., Grafton, S. T., Bassett, D. S., & Ribeiro, A. (2016). Graph frequency analysis of brain signals. *IEEE journal of selected topics in signal processing, 10*(7), 1189–1203.
3. Sanei, S. (2013). *Adaptive processing of brain signals*. Wiley.
4. Wolpaw, J. R., & Boulay, C. B. (2009). "Brain signals for brain–computer interfaces". In *Brain–computer interfaces* (pp. 29–46). Springer.
5. Wolpaw, J. R. (2013). "Brain–computer interfaces: Signals, methods, and goals". In *First international IEEE EMBS conference on neural engineering, 2003. Conference proceedings* (pp. 584–585).
6. Maiorana, E., La Rocca, D., Campisi, P. (2015). "On the permanence of EEG signals for biometric recognition". *IEEE Transactions on Information Forensics and Security*, 163–175.
7. Pei, X., Hill, J., & Schalk, G. (2012). Silent communication: Toward using brain signals. *IEEE Pulse, 3*(1), 43–46.
8. Niedermeyer, E., & da Silva, F. L. (2005). *Electroencephalography: Basic principles, clinical applications, and related fields*. Lippincott Williams & Wilkins.
9. Chernecky C. C., Berger, B. J. (2012). *Laboratory tests and diagnostic procedures-e-book*. Elsevier Health Sciences.
10. Rubio, J. D. J., Vázquez, D. M., & Mújica-Vargas, D. (2013). "Acquisition system and approximation of brain signals." *IET Science, Measurement and Technology, 7*(4), 232–239.
11. Deuschl, G., & Eisen, A. (1999). "Recommendations for the practice of clinical neurophysiology: Guidelines of the international federation of clinical neurophysiology." *52*.
12. Da Silva, F. L. (2009). "EEG: Origin and measurement." *EEg-fMRI*, 19–38.
13. Murugappan, M., Rizon, M., Nagarajan, R., Yaacob, S., Hazry, D., Zunaidi, I. (2008). "Time-frequency analysis of EEG signals for human emotion detection". In *4th Kuala Lumpur international conference on biomedical engineering 2008* (pp. 262–265).
14. Uktveris, T., & Jusas, V. (2018). Development of a modular board for EEG signal acquisition. *Sensors, 18*(7), 21–40.

15. Chang, C.-Y., Hsu, S.-H., Pion-Tonachini, L., & Jung, T.-P. (2018). "Evaluation of artifact subspace reconstruction for automatic EEG artifact removal". In *2018 40th Annual international conference of the IEEE engineering in medicine and biology society (EMBC)* (pp. 1242–1245).
16. Jung, T.-P., Makeig, S., Humphries, C., Lee, T.-W., Mckeown, M. J., Iragui, V., & Sejnowski, T. J. (2000). Removing electroencephalographic artifacts by blind source separation. *Psychophysiology, 37*(2), 163–178.
17. Islam, M. K., Rastegarnia, A., & Yang, Z. (2016). Methods for artifact detection and removal from scalp EEG: A review. *Neurophysiologie Clinique/Clinical Neurophysiology, 46*(4–5), 287–305.
18. Minguillon, J., Lopez-Gordo, M. A., & Pelayo, F. (2017). Trends in EEG-BCI for daily-life: Requirements for artifact removal. *Biomedical Signal Processing and Control, 31*, 407–418.
19. Urigüen, J. A., & Garcia-Zapirain, B. (2015). EEG artifact removal—State-of-the-art and guidelines. *Journal of neural engineering, 12*(3), 031001.
20. Al-Ani, T., Trad, D., & Somerset, V. S. (2010). "Signal processing and classification approaches for brain–computer interface". *Intelligent and Biosensors*, 25–66.
21. Brunner, C., Allison, B. Z., Krusienski, D. J., Kaiser, V., Muller-Putz, G. R., Pfurtscheller, G., & Neuper, C. (2010). Improved signal processing approaches in an offline simulation of a hybrid brain–computer interface. *Journal of neuroscience methods, 188*(1), 165–173.
22. Lotte, F. (2014). "A tutorial on EEG signal-processing techniques for mental-state recognition in brain–computer interfaces". *Guide to Brain–Computer Music Interfacing*, 133–161.
23. Sanei, S., & Chambers, J. A. (2013). *EEG signal processing*. Wiley.
24. Buttfield, A., Ferrez, P. W., & Millan, J. R. (2006). Towards a robust BCI: Error potentials and online learning. *IEEE Transactions on Neural Systems and Rehabilitation Engineering, 14*(2), 164–168.
25. Wolpaw, J. R., Birbaumer, N., Heetderks, W. J., McFarland, D. J., Peckham, P. H., Schalk, G., Donchin, E., Quatrano, L. A., Robinson, C. J., & Vaughan, T. M. (2000). Brain–computer interface technology: A review of the first international meeting. *IEEE Transactions on Rehabilitation Engineering, 8*(2), 164–173.
26. Santhanam, G., Ryu, S. I., Byron, M. Y., Afshar, A., & Shenoy, K. V. (2006). A high-performance brain–computer interface. *Nature, 442*(7099), 195–198.
27. Allison, B. Z., Wolpaw, E. W., & Wolpaw, J. R. (2007). Brain–computer interface systems: Progress and prospects. *Expert Review of Medical Devices, 4*(4), 463–474.
28. Fazel-Rezai, R., Allison, B. Z., Guger, C., Sellers, E. W., Kleih, S. C., & Kübler, A. (2012). P300 brain–computer interface: Current challenges and emerging trends. *Frontiers in Neuroengineering, 5*, 14.
29. Wolpaw, J. R., Loeb, G. E., Allison, B. Z., Donchin, E., do Nascimento, O. F., Heetderks, W. J., Nijboer, F., Shain, W. G., & Turner, J. N., (2006). BCI meeting 2005-workshop on signals and recording methods. *IEEE Transactions on Neural Systems and Rehabilitation Engineering, 14*(2), 138–141.
30. Mak, J. N., & Wolpaw, J. R. (2009). Clinical applications of brain–computer interfaces: Current state and future prospects. *IEEE Reviews in Biomedical Engineering, 2*, 187–199.
31. Waldert, S. (2016). "Invasive versus non-invasive neuronal signals for brain–machine interfaces: Will one prevail?" *Frontiers in Neuroscience, 10.*
32. Shih, J. J., Krusienski, D. J., & Wolpaw, J. R. (2012). March. Brain–computer interfaces in medicine. *Mayo clinic proceedings, 87*(3), 268–279. Elsevier.
33. Pfurtscheller, G., Neuper, C., & Birbaumer, N. (2005). *Human brain–computer interface.* CRC Press.
34. Vallabhaneni, A., Wang, T., & He, B. (2005). Brain–Computer interface. In Neural engineering (pp. 85–121). Springer.
35. Blankertz, B., Curio, G., & Müller, K. R., (2002). Classifying single trial EEG: Towards brain–computer interfacing. In *Advances in neural information processing systems* (pp. 157–164).
36. Murphy, M. D., Guggenmos, D. J., Bundy, D. T., & Nudo, R. J. (2016). Current challenges facing the translation of brain–computer interfaces from preclinical trials to use in human patients. *Frontiers in Cellular Neuroscience, 9*, 497.

37. Cavanagh, J. F., Napolitano, A., Wu, C., & Mueen, A. (2017). The patient repository for EEG data+ computational tools (PRED+ CT). *Frontiers in Neuroinformatics, 11*, 67.
38. Goldberger, A. L., Amaral, L. A., Glass, L., Hausdorff, J. M., Ivanov, P. C., Mark, R. G., Mietus, J. E., Moody, G. B., Peng, C. K., & Stanley, H. E., (2000). PhysioBank, PhysioToolkit, and PhysioNet: Components of a new research resource for complex physiologic signals. *Circulation, 101*(23), e215–e220.
39. Alpaydin, E. (2020). *Introduction to machine learning*. MIT press.
40. Marsland, S. (2015). *Machine learning: An algorithmic perspective*. CRC press.
41. Gutierrez, D. D. (2015). *Machine learning and data science: An introduction to statistical learning methods with R*. Technics Publications.
42. Flach, P. A. (2001). On the state of the art in machine learning: A personal review. *Artificial Intelligence, 131*(1–2), 199–222.
43. Torrey, L., & Shavlik, J. (2010). "Transfer learning". In *Handbook of research on machine learning applications and trends: Algorithms, methods, and techniques* (pp. 242–264). IGI Global.
44. Zhu, X., & Goldberg, A. B. (2009). Introduction to semi-supervised learning. *Synthesis Lectures on Artificial Intelligence and Machine Learning, 3*(1), 1–130.
45. Ayodele, T. O. (2010). Types of Machine Learning Algorithms, *New Advances in Machine Learning*, 19–48.
46. Kotsiantis, S. B., Zaharakis, I., & Pintelas, P. (2007). Supervised machine learning: A review of classification techniques. *Emerging Artificial Intelligence Applications in Computer Engineering, 160*(1), 3–24.
47. Osisanwo, F. Y., Akinsola, J. E. T., Awodele, O., Hinmikaiye, J. O., Olakanmi, O., & Akinjobi, J. (2017). Supervised machine learning algorithms: Classification and comparison. *International Journal of Computer Trends and Technology (IJCTT), 48*(3), 128–138.
48. López-Larraz, E., Sarasola-Sanz, A., Irastorza-Landa, N., Birbaumer, N., & Ramos-Murguialday, A. (2018). Brain–machine interfaces for rehabilitation in stroke: A review. *NeuroRehabilitation, 43*(1), 77–97.
49. Zhang, D. (2006). *Advances in machine learning applications in software engineering*. Igi Global.
50. Ghahramani, Z. (2003). "Unsupervised learning". In *Summer school on machine learning* (pp. 72–112).
51. Harrington, P. (2012). *Machine learning in action*. Manning Publications Co.
52. Jordan, M. I., & Mitchell, T. M. (2015). Machine learning: Trends, perspectives, and prospects. *Science, 349*(6245), 255–260.
53. Brunner, C., Andreoni, G., Bianchi, L., Blankertz, B., Breitwieser, C., Kanoh, S. I., Kothe, C. A., Lécuyer, A., Makeig, S., Mellinger, J., & Perego, P. (2012). BCI software platforms. In *Towards practical brain–computer interfaces* (pp. 303–331). Springer.
54. Brownlee, J. (April 2020). https://machinelearningmastery.com
55. Javaid, A., Niyaz, Q., Sun, W. & Alam, M. (2016). A deep learning approach for network intrusion detection system. In Proceedings of the 9th EAI international conference on bio-inspired information and communications technologies (formerly BIONETICS) (pp. 21–26).
56. Vafeiadis, T., Diamantaras, K. I., Sarigiannidis, G., & Chatzisavvas, K. C. (2015). A comparison of machine learning techniques for customer churn prediction. *Simulation Modelling Practice and Theory, 55*, 1–9.
57. Le, T., Tran, D., Hoang, T., Ma, W. & Sharma, D. (2011). Generalised support vector machine for brain–computer interface. In *International conference on neural information processing* (pp. 692–700). Springer.
58. Ma, Y., Ding, X., She, Q., Luo, Z., Potter, T., & Zhang, Y. (2016). Classification of motor imagery EEG signals with support vector machines and particle swarm optimization. *Computational and Mathematical Methods in Medicine, 2016*, 1–8.
59. Qin, J., Li, Y., & Sun, W. (2007). "A semisupervised support vector machines algorithm for BCI systems". *Computational Intelligence and Neuroscience, 2007*.

60. Duan, L., Hongxin, Z., Khan, M. S., & Fang, M. (2017). Recognition of motor imagery tasks for BCI using CSP and chaotic PSO twin SVM. *The Journal of China Universities of Posts and Telecommunications, 24*(3), 83–90.
61. Costantini, G., Todisco, M., Casali, D., Carota, M., Saggio, G., Bianchi, L., Abbafati, M., & Quitadamo, L. (2009). "SVM classification of EEG signals for brain–computer interface". In *Proceedings of the 2009 conference on Neural Nets WIRN09: Proceedings of the 19th Italian workshop on neural nets, vietri sul mare, Salerno, Italy, May 28–30 2009* (pp. 229–233).
62. Halder, S., Bensch, M., Mellinger, J. (2007). Online artifact removal for brain–computer interfaces using support vector machines and blind source separation. Computational Intelligence and Neuroscience, 2007.
63. El Bahy, M. M., Hosny, M., Mohamed, W. A., & Ibrahim, S. (2016). "EEG signal classification using neural network and support vector machine in brain–computer interface. In *International conference on advanced intelligent systems and informatics* (pp. 246–256).
64. Li, X., Chen, X., Yan, Y., Wei, W., & Wang, Z. J. (2014). Classification of EEG signals using a multiple kernel learning support vector machine. *Sensors, 14*(7), 12784–12802.
65. Ma, Z., Gao, X., & Gao, S. (2007). "Enhanced P300-based cursor movement control". In *International conference on foundations of augmented cognition* (pp. 120–126).
66. Borisoff, J. F., Mason, S. G., Bashashati, A., & Birch, G. E. (2004). Brain–computer interface design for asynchronous control applications: Improvements to the LF-ASD asynchronous brain switch. *IEEE Transactions on Biomedical Engineering, 51*(6), 985–992.
67. Bablani, A., Edla, D. R., & Dodia, S. (2018). Classification of EEG data using k-nearest neighbor approach for concealed information test. *Procedia Computer Science, 143*, 242–249.
68. Thakur, S., Dharavath, R., & Edla, D. R. (2020). Spark and Rule-KNN based scalable machine learning framework for EEG deceit identification. *Biomedical Signal Processing and Control, 58*, 101886.
69. Palaniappan, R. "Brain–computer interface design using band powers extracted during mental tasks".
70. Anderson, C. W. & Sijercic, Z. (1996). Classification of EEG signals from four subjects during five mental tasks. In *Solving engineering problems with neural networks: Proceedings of the conference on engineering applications in neural networks (EANN'96)* (pp. 407–414).
71. Haselsteiner, E., & Pfurtscheller, G. (2000). Using time-dependent neural networks for EEG classification. *IEEE Transactions on Rehabilitation Engineering, 8*(4), 457–463.
72. Chiappa, S., & Bengio, S. (2003). *HMM and IOHMM modeling of EEG rhythms for asynchronous BCI systems.*
73. Saggio, G., Cavallo, P., Ferretti, A., Garzoli, F., Quitadamo, L. R., Marciani, M. G., Giannini, F., & Bianchi, L. (2009). Comparison of two different classifiers for mental tasks-based brain–computer interface: MLP neural networks versus fuzzy logic. In *2009 IEEE international symposium on a world of wireless, mobile and multimedia networks and workshops* (pp. 1–5).
74. Lin, Y. P., Wang, C. H., Wu, T. L., Jeng, S. K., & Chen, J. H. (2007). Multilayer perceptron for EEG signal classification during listening to emotional music. In *TENCON 2007–2007 IEEE region 10 conference* (pp. 1–3).
75. Hamedi, M., Salleh, S. H., Noor, A. M., & Mohammad-Rezazadeh, I. (2014). Neural network-based three-class motor imagery classification using time-domain features for BCI applications. In *2014 IEEE region 10 symposium* (pp. 204–207).
76. Machado, J., Balbinot, A., & Schuck, A. (2013). A study of the Naive bayes classifier for analyzing imaginary movement EEG signals using the periodogram as spectral estimator. In *2013 ISSNIP biosignals and biorobotics conference: Biosignals and robotics for better and safer living (BRC)* (pp. 1–4).
77. Machado, J., & Balbinot, A. (2014). Executed movement using EEG signals through a Naive bayes classifier. *Micromachines, 5*(4), 1082–1105.
78. Stock, V. N., & Balbinot, A. (2016). Movement imagery classification in EMOTIV cap based system by Naïve bayes. In 2016 38th annual international conference of the IEEE engineering in medicine and biology society (EMBC) (pp. 4435–4438).

79. Wang, H., & Zhang, Y. (2016). Detection of motor imagery EEG signals employing Naïve bayes based learning process.
80. Okumuş, H. & Aydemır, Ö. (2017). Random forest classification for brain–computer interface applications. In *2017 25th signal processing and communications applications conference (SIU)* (pp. 1–4).
81. Edla, D. R., Mangalorekar, K., Dhavalikar, G., & Dodia, S. (2018). Classification of EEG data for human mental state analysis using random forest classifier. *Procedia Computer Science, 132*, 1523–1532.
82. Steyrl, D., Scherer, R., Förstner, O., & Müller-Putz, G. R. (2014). Motor imagery brain–computer interfaces: Random forests versus regularized LDA-non-linear beats linear. In Proceedings of the 6th international brain–computer interface conference (pp. 241–244).
83. Li, Y., Wu, J. & Yang, J. (2011). Developing a logistic regression model with cross-correlation for motor imagery signal recognition. In *The 2011 IEEE/ICME international conference on complex medical engineering* (pp. 502–507).
84. Tomioka, R., Aihara, K., & Müller, K. R. (2007). Logistic regression for single trial EEG classification. *Advances in Neural Information Processing Systems, 19*, 1377.
85. Javed, A., Tiwana, M. I., Tiwana, M. I., Rashid, N., Iqbal, J., & Khan, U. S. (2017). Recognition of finger movements using EEG signals for control of upper limb prosthesis using logistic regression. *Biomedical Research, 28*(17), 7361–7369.
86. Davies, D. L., & Bouldin, D. W. (1979). A cluster separation measure. *IEEE Transactions on Pattern Analysis and Machine Intelligence, 2*, 224–227.
87. Ansari, Z., Azeem, M. F., Ahmed, W., & Babu, A. V. (2015). Quantitative evaluation of performance and validity indices for clustering the web navigational sessions. *World of Computer Science and Information Technology Journal (WCSIT), 1*(5), 217–226.
88. De Amorim, R. C., & Hennig, C. (2015). Recovering the number of clusters in data sets with noise features using feature rescaling factors. *Information sciences, 324*, 126–145.
89. Caliński, T., & Harabasz, J. (1974). A dendrite method for cluster analysis. *Communications in Statistics-theory and Methods, 3*(1), 1–27.
90. Sinha, R. K., & Ghosh, S. (2016). Classification of two class motor imagery task using Jaya based k-means clustering. In 2016 international conference on global trends in signal processing, information computing and communication (ICGTSPICC) (pp. 175–179).
91. Bablani, A., Edla, D. R., Kuppili, V., & Ramesh, D. (2020). A multi stage EEG data classification using k-means and feed forward neural network. *Clinical Epidemiology and Global Health, 8*(3), 718–724.
92. Azhari, A., & Hernandez, L. (2016). Brainwaves feature classification by applying k-means clustering using single-sensor EEG. *International Journal of Advances in Intelligent Informatics, 2*(3), 167–173.
93. Asanza, V., Ochoa, K., Sacarelo, C., Salazar, C., Loayza, F., Vaca, C., & Peláez, E. (2016). Clustering of EEG occipital signals using k-means. In *2016 IEEE ecuador technical chapters meeting (ETCM)* (pp. 1–5).
94. Wang, B., Wong, C. M., Wan, F., Mak, P. U., Mak, P. I., & Vai, M. I. (2010). Gaussian mixture model based on genetic algorithm for brain–computer interface. In *2010 3rd international congress on image and signal processing* (Vol. 9, pp. 4079–4083).
95. Khatami Firoozabadi, S. F., & Erfanian, A. (2010). "An online BCI system for reaching control using Gaussian mixture model classifier with adaptive learning". *Medical Engineering and Physics*, 730–739.
96. Zhang, H., Liu, Y., Liang, J., Cao, J., & Zhang, L. (2013). "Gaussian mixture modeling in stroke patients' rehabilitation EEG data analysis". In 2013 35th annual international conference of the IEEE engineering in medicine and biology society (EMBC) (pp. 2208–2211).
97. Gu, J. N., Liu, H. J., Lu, H. T., & Lu, B. L. (2011). An integrated hierarchical Gaussian mixture model to estimate vigilance level based on EEG recordings. In *International conference on neural information processing* (pp. 380–387).

98. Blankertz, B., Muller, K. R., Krusienski, D. J., Schalk, G., Wolpaw, J. R., Schlogl, A., Pfurtscheller, G., Millan, J. R., Schroder, M., & Birbaumer, N. (2006). The BCI competition III: Validating alternative approaches to actual BCI problems. *IEEE Transactions on Neural Systems and Rehabilitation Engineering, 14*(2), 153–159.
99. Bueno, L., & Bastos, T. F. (2015). A self-organizing maps classifier structure for brain–computer interfaces. *Research on Biomedical Engineering, 31*, 232–240.
100. Baig, M. Z., Ayaz, Y., Gillani, S. O., Jamil, M., & Naveed, M. (2015). Motor imagery based EEG signal classification using self organizing maps. *Science International, 27*(2), 1165–1170.
101. Liu, H., Wang, J. & Zheng, C. (2005). Using self-organizing map for mental tasks classification in brain–computer interface. In International symposium on neural networks (pp. 327–332).
102. Ito, S. I., Sato, K., & Fujisawa, S. (2012). Learning algorithm for self-organizing map classification of electroencephalogram patterns with individual differences. In *The 2012 international joint conference on neural networks (IJCNN)* (pp. 1-6).
103. Vařeka, L., & Mautner, P. (2014). Self-organizing maps for event-related potential data analysis. In International conference on health informatics (HEALTHINF-2014) (pp. 387–392).
104. Zhang, R., Xu, P., Guo, L., Zhang, Y., Li, P., & Yao, D. (2013). Z-score linear discriminant analysis for EEG based brain–computer interfaces. *PLoS ONE, 8*(9), e74433.
105. Gruenwald, J., Znobishchev, A., Kapeller, C., Kamada, K., Scharinger, J., & Guger, C. (2019). Time-variant linear discriminant analysis improves hand gesture and finger movement decoding for invasive brain–computer interfaces. *Frontiers in Neuroscience, 13*, 901.
106. Onishi, A., & Natsume, K. (2013). Ensemble regularized linear discriminant analysis classifier for P300-based brain–computer interface. In 2013 35th annual international conference of the IEEE engineering in medicine and biology society (EMBC) (pp. 4231–4234).
107. Hsu, W. Y., Li, Y. C., Hsu, C. Y., Liu, C. T., & Chiu, H. W. (2012). Application of multiscale amplitude modulation features and fuzzy c-means to brain–computer interface. *Clinical EEG and Neuroscience, 43*(1), 32–38.
108. Gupta, A., & Kumar, D. (2017). Fuzzy clustering-based feature extraction method for mental task classification. *Brain Informatics, 4*(2), 135–145.
109. Palazzo, S., Spampinato, C., Kavasidis, I., Giordano, D., & Shah, M. (2017). Generative adversarial networks conditioned by brain signals. In Proceedings of the IEEE international conference on computer vision (pp. 3410–3418).
110. Kumar, S., Sharma, A., & Tsunoda, T. (2019). Brain wave classification using long short-term memory network based OPTICAL predictor. *Scientific Reports, 9*(1), 1–13.
111. Zhang, J., Yan, C., & Gong, X. (2017). Deep convolutional neural network for decoding motor imagery based brain–computer interface. In 2017 IEEE international conference on signal processing, communications and computing (ICSPCC) (pp. 1–5).
112. Liu, M., Wu, W., Gu, Z., Yu, Z., Qi, F., & Li, Y. (2018). Deep learning based on batch normalization for P300 signal detection. *Neurocomputing, 275*, 288–297.
113. Manor, R., & Geva, A. B. (2015). Convolutional neural network for multi-category rapid serial visual presentation BCI. *Frontiers in Computational Neuroscience, 9*, 146.
114. Kobler, R. J., & Scherer, R. (2016). Restricted Boltzmann machines in sensory motor rhythm brain–computer interfacing: A study on inter-subject transfer and co-adaptation. In 2016 IEEE international conference on systems, man, and cybernetics (SMC) (pp. 469–474).
115. Chu, Y., Zhao, X., Zou, Y., Xu, W., Han, J., & Zhao, Y. (2018). A decoding scheme for incomplete motor imagery EEG with deep belief network. *Frontiers in Neuroscience, 12*, 680.
116. Hjelm, R. D., Calhoun, V. D., Salakhutdinov, R., Allen, E. A., Adali, T., & Plis, S. M. (2014). Restricted Boltzmann machines for neuroimaging: An application in identifying intrinsic networks. *NeuroImage, 96*, 245–260.
117. Al-kaysi, A. M., Al-Ani, A., & Boonstra, T. W. (2015). A multichannel deep belief network for the classification of EEG data. In *International conference on neural information processing* (pp. 38–45).

118. Sobhani, A. (2014) "P300 classification using deep belief nets". In *European symposium on artificial neural networks (ESANN).*
119. Lu, Z., Gao, N., Liu, Y., & Li, Q., (2018). The detection of p300 potential based on deep belief network. In *2018 11th international congress on image and signal processing, biomedical engineering and informatics (CISP-BMEI)* (pp. 1–5).
120. Li, M. A., Zhang, M., & Sun, Y. J. (2016). A novel motor imagery EEG recognition method based on deep learning. In *Proceedings of the 2016 international forum on management, education and information technology application.* (pp. 728–733).
121. Movahedi, F., Coyle, J. L., & Sejdić, E. (2017). Deep belief networks for electroencephalography: A review of recent contributions and future outlooks. *IEEE Journal of Biomedical and Health Informatics, 22*(3), 642–652.
122. Li, F., Zhang, G., Wang, W., Xu, R., Schnell, T., Wen, J., McKenzie, F., & Li, J. (2016). Deep models for engagement assessment with scarce label information. *IEEE Transactions on Human-Machine Systems, 47*(4), 598–605.
123. Hosseini, M. P., Pompili, D., Elisevich, K., & Soltanian-Zadeh, H. (2017). Optimized deep learning for EEG big data and seizure prediction BCI via internet of things. *IEEE Transactions on Big Data, 3*(4), 392–404.
124. Elessawy, R. H., Eldawlatly, S., & Abbas, H. M. (2020). A long short-term memory autoencoder approach for EEG motor imagery classification. In *2020 international conference on computation, automation and knowledge management (ICCAKM)* (pp. 79–84).
125. Asgher, U., Khalil, K., Khan, M. J., Ahmad, R., Butt, S. I., Ayaz, Y., Naseer, N., & Nazir, S. (2020). Enhanced accuracy for multi-class mental-workload detection using LSTM for BCI. *Frontiers in Neuroscience, 14*, 584.
126. Zhang, G., Davoodnia, V., Sepas-Moghaddam, A., Zhang, Y., & Etemad, A. (2019). Classification of hand movements from EEG using a deep attention-based LSTM network. *IEEE Sensors Journal, 20*(6), 3113–3122.
127. Shah, V., Golmohammadi, M., Ziyabari, S., Von Weltin, E., Obeid, I., & Picone, J. (2017). Optimizing channel selection for seizure detection. In *2017 IEEE signal processing in medicine and biology symposium (SPMB)* (pp. 1–5).
128. Lin, J. S., & She, B. H. (2020). A BCI system with motor imagery based on bidirectional long-short term memory. In IOP conference series: Materials science and engineering (Vol. 719, p. 012026).

Applications of Intelligent System in Healthcare

Innovative Services Using Cloud Computing in Smart Health Care

V. Malathi and V. Kavitha

1 Introduction

Well-being is a condition for the prosperity of the body, humanity, and public activity, enabling everyone to be socially and financially remunerated. For improving security, worthy, and proficiency of patient consideration and lessening medical services conveyance costs, both electronic clinical records (ECRs) and electronic prosperity records (EPRs) are essential to the impressive idea of medical care digitalization. To give a reported record of care that upholds both current and upcoming consideration got by the patient from the equivalent or different clinicians or care suppliers is the primary role of the EPR. The EPR provides procedures for patient and clinicians matching. For ECRs to arrive their maximum capacity to reforming the medical care conveyance with high caliber and moderate spending, the interoperability of EPRs is a crucial empowering innovation.

Today, progress in innovation is exceptionally clinical sciences that have transformed medical services associations into client-arranged conditions. These associations are increasing quality. It will not be done without sufficient time to access data. As shown by the International Organization for Standardization (ISO) importance, electronic prosperity record (EPR) is limit, confident interchange, and induction to understanding information in mechanized plan a few affirmed customers. These data integrate the patient previous, current, and forthcoming data. The primary focus of the EPR is to assist in supporting coordinated, competent, and quality well-being.

In another clarification, EPR joins all information related to the inhabitants' prosperity from prior birth (information about pre- and post-pregnancy fetuses) to after death (data got from postmortem and so). This information sets aside incessantly and automatically over the long run. On the possibility that essential, no communication with the region or time, all or a portion of this information will be open

V. Malathi (✉) · V. Kavitha
Department of Computer Science and Applications, Hindusthan College of Arts and Science, Coimbatore, India

A. K. Tyagi et al. (eds.), *Intelligent Interactive Multimedia Systems for e-Healthcare Applications*, https://doi.org/10.1007/978-981-16-6542-4_5

to endorsed individuals. In general, the planned EPR financial backers are individual from the board audience. Every medical care benefactor is an accomplices and customers. The EPR has a significant adjustment in conveying clinical consideration, reducing mistakes, and developing wellness care. Simple entry of all patient history data enhances care, concentrates on data, and decreases clinical analytical mistakes. Synchronous access to dedicated EPR is clinical centers is an impressive advantage. Also, it is crucial for keeping and safeguard data from crumbling, degradation, and decimation in at any rate.

The creation of EPR advantage is the experience of certain obstacles, which may be classified as specialized, hierarchical individual, monetary, and morally legitimate boundaries. In terms of obstructions in HER execution, the use of innovation, for example, cloud computing is powerful in its practical use. Cloud computing is the calculus that was ended with a gathering of distant servers who structure an organization. It promotes information capacity and online access data, and online admittance to administrations and PCs; cloud computing is essentially obtaining figurative assets over the Internet. Today, numerous medical care suppliers and coverage agencies utilize few types of EPR, most of which will store unified datasets. In general, the patient may rely on various medical suppliers. Besides, a patient may use separate medical coverage agencies; the distribution of data between medical suppliers across authoritative boundaries encourages correspondence between these domains.

A designer will have the opportunity to create more secure, less expensive, and higher quality through cloud computing capabilities and strengths, such as financial adaptability. It is easier to redesign these projects than existing systems. Every program that explodes in demand for one of the PCs in the association can refresh itself. It is a simple and rapid innovation. The sharing of information in the cloud is accessible to all gadgets associated with the server anywhere and any structure. The reason for this inquiry was to investigate effectively directed examinations in cloud computing.

2 Cloud Computing

Cloud computing has recently emerged as alternative state which communicates and encourages Web-based information technology (IT) administrations. It offers types of support that are on-demand, adaptable, and multioccupying at pay review site. A few definitions have been provided for cloud computing model, yet nobody is the standard definition that fully portrays it. Nonetheless, the National Institute of Standards and Technology (NIST) characterizes it as "Cloud computing is a model for engaging all around masterminded, on-request network admittance to an assembled gathering of configurable enrolling resources like organizations, servers, stockpiling, applications, and administrations which can be immediately provisioned and conveyed with insignificant administration exertion or expert center correspondence." The NIST cloud structure additionally portrays five key credits, three assistance models, and four deployment models (Fig. 1).

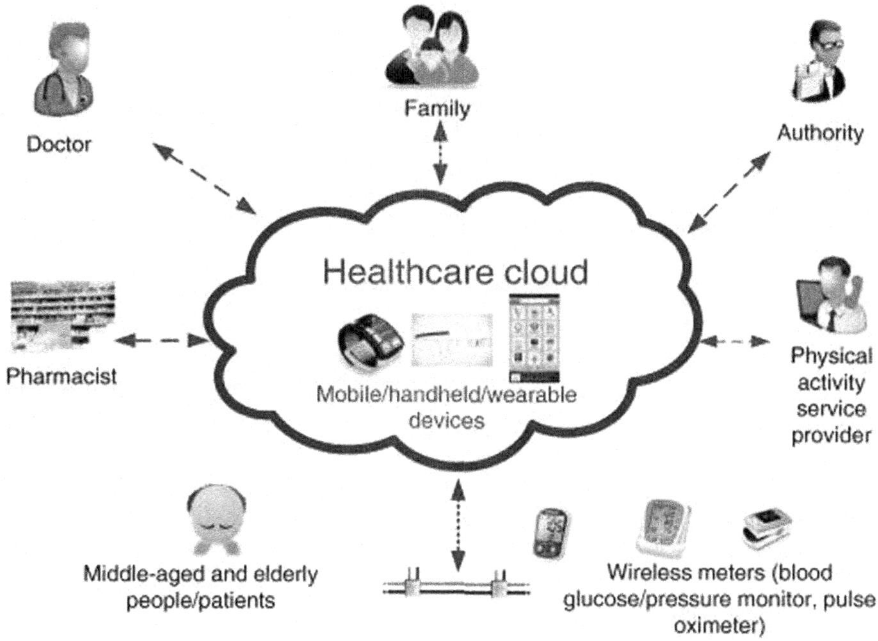

Fig. 1 Architecture of healthcare cloud

2.1 *Features of Cloud Computing*

- **On request self-management**—A buyer can obtain allegorical force only and generally without the requirements of any human mediation of the specialized organization.
- **Comprehensive network access**—Computing capabilities are open over the Internet in standard segments.
- **Pooling assets**—Customers believe that the resource available is limitless and can be purchased at any cost and anytime. Physical and virtual goods are powerfully designated and reallocated to the buyer, given their demands.
- **Fast elasticity**—Resources can be readily and flexibly distributed.
- **Measured services**—As a result, cloud frameworks control and advance assets utilization by assessing proper limitations. (e.g., capacity, force preparation, data transmission, and dynamic customer accounts).

2.2 *Cloud Service Models*

Cloud computing can be separated into three processing models. There are.

- Software as a service (SaaS),

- Infrastructure as a service (IaaS),
- Platform as a service (PaaS).

All cloud models have their arrangement of central focuses that could serve the necessities of dissimilar associations.

2.2.1 Infrastructure as a Service (IaaS)

IaaS outfits a relationship with the typical structure for keeping up its activities. These may involve system administration, assets determination, for example, servers or capacity and staff control. In those cases, the association usually controls the work environment, applications, and frameworks. For example, a clinical facility may utilize the cloud for illustrative imaging fiasco recuperation. The cloud specialist organization has little collaboration with the day-by-day occasions at the medical clinic. Admitted to this information is restricted to a depending on the situation premise despite calamity.

2.2.2 Platform as a Service (PaaS)

PaaS is a support model that enables clients to process requests sent, but not the hidden frame. It is most normal in creating programming applications where architects address enhancement instruments, databases, and middleware as core programming. Medical services providers who use IT improvement personnel can use this model to build an electronic clinical record in the vicinity.

2.2.3 Software as a Service (SaaS)

SaaS is transforming into a model that enables medical service providers to rapidly embrace new advancements without capital expenditures or disproportionate availability efforts. SaaS provides the customer with very distant access to the application, typically via the Internet browser. Offices do not stress capacity or application as only explicit limits frames are empowered for the customer. The association would settle for compensation for the application's use and compensation for every survey or model in gigabytes. The SaaS can be immediately sent and used without capital expenses, realizing the most extreme availability and innovation advantage.

2.3 Cloud Deployment Model

The most remote cloud communities have an immense number of servers and stacking gadgets to permit rapid stacking. It is occasionally possible to show a geographical region to reconcile customer data. Thus, cloud computing templates are organized according to their region. Cloud layout templates demonstrate how cloud services are made available to clients. The four deployment models identified with cloud computing are depending on the following:

2.3.1 Public Cloud Deployment

A public cloud is the best convenient organizational model, as economies of scale are increased. The public cloud is accessible to all individuals and is completely supervised by the cloud cooperative. Clients typically purchase an application utilized from a public cloud supplier. Public cloud instances are Amazon.com or salesforce.com. The customer transfers his data in this total environment. The servers, stockpiling, and systems administrations are divided between all supporters' and applications are transmitted on the Web. Public cloud schemes are more perilous because they are available to anyone, and the discernment is that security and protection penetrate with public clouds.

Calamity recuperation for medical care associations could be appropriate for a public cloud model. There are restricted passageways to the information, stockpiling is more expense adequately oversaw, and access has been just due to the crisis. (see Fig. 2) Policy frameworks are not dependent on this information; thus, service-level agreements (SLAs) can be insignificant.

2.3.2 Private Cloud Deployment

Private clouds are mainly that: a private cloud model that a solitary association works. The innovation resides within the server farm of an association, and they can convey the assets depending on the situation to the different divisions. Private clouds are relied upon to be the most probable model embraced by medical services suppliers until cloud suppliers have exhibited how to beat the numerous difficulties related to other cloud models. In private clouds, the ability to monitor and control delicate patient information stay within the organization (see Fig. 3). Private clouds are more costly because economies of scale are rather lost; however, confidence in deployment is higher. This trade-off must be weighed as part of the cloud strategy.

2.3.3 Hybrid Cloud Deployment

A hybrid cloud joins at least two clouds, yet they stay extraordinary elements. A hybrid cloud distribution will share innovation; however, data, applications, and so on will remain separate. Using inhabitance and namespaces gives the divisions clients running on the equivalent "box". Healthcare suppliers can transmit a hybrid cloud for fiasco retrieval of demo images or clinical framework (see Fig. 4). The use of hybrid clouds is less danger with associations because members are more aware of who is

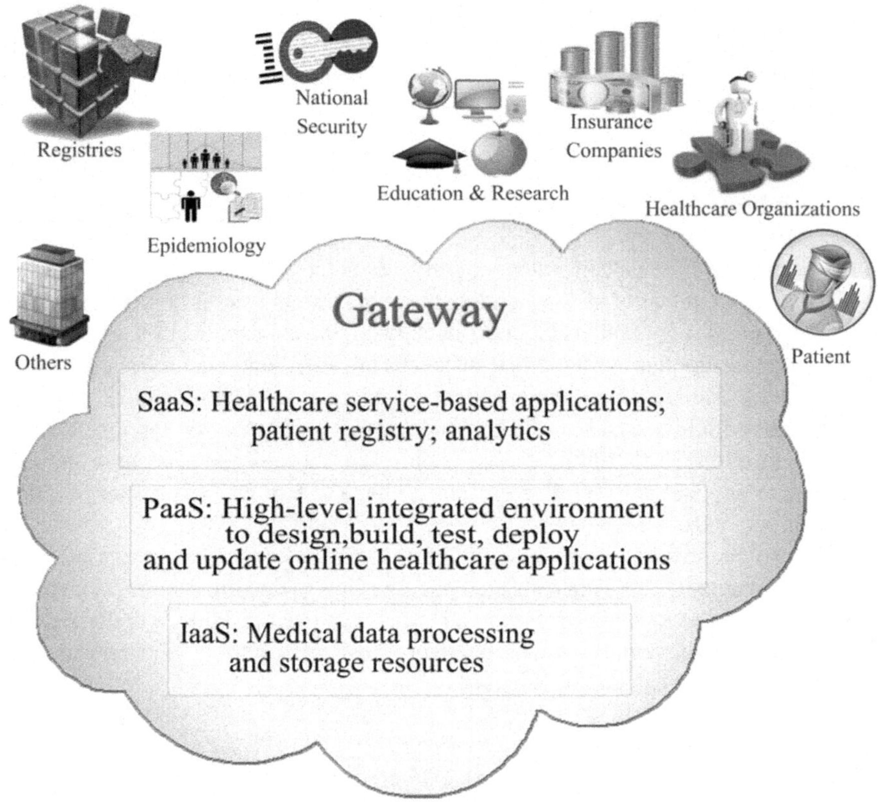

Fig. 2 Cloud architecture for health care

using the facilities. Expanded degrees of authority over the information are more apparent in a hybrid model, as requests keep a level of partition between amenities while using economies of scale in the framework.

2.3.4 Community Cloud Deployment

A community cloud is a smaller public (see Fig. 5). It will be aimed at a few establishments that assist particular local clients. For example, a Linux community cloud would allow designers to share tools to improve Linux. The association would not have to spend the capital that would somehow, or another, be needed to acquire a customary software permit. They would just compensate for the utilization of the product as the designers utilized it (Fig. 6).

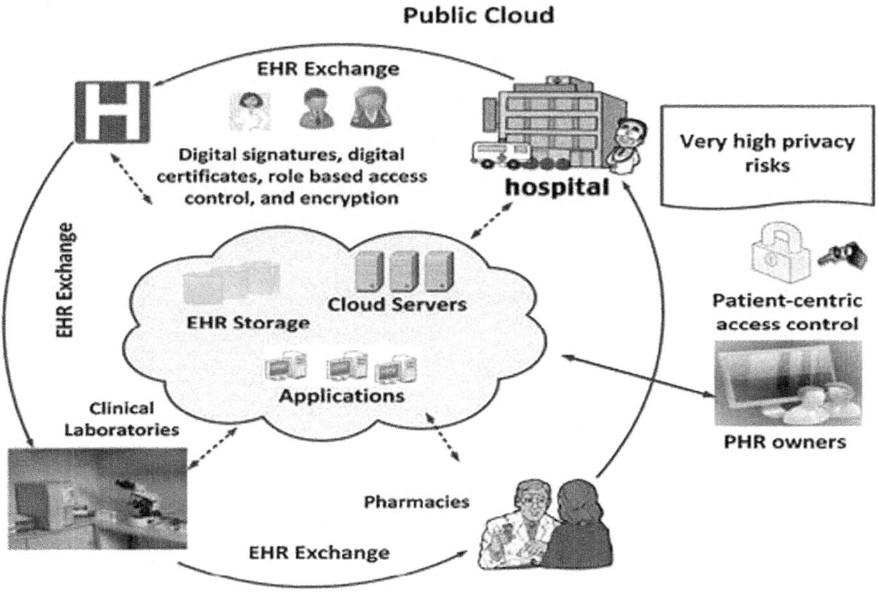

Fig. 3 Public cloud environments

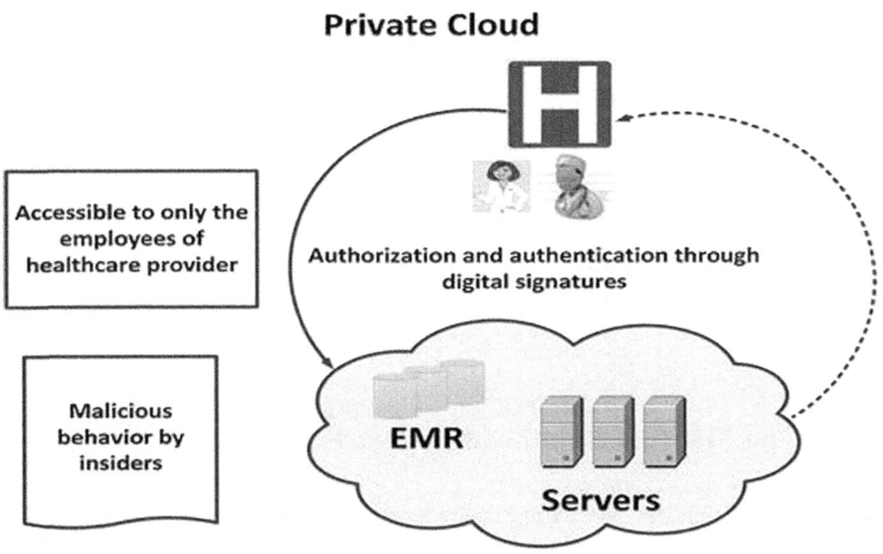

Fig. 4 Private cloud environments

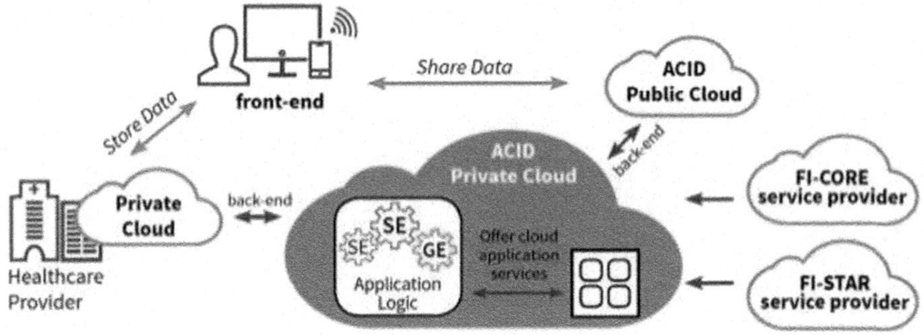

Fig. 5 Hybrid cloud environments

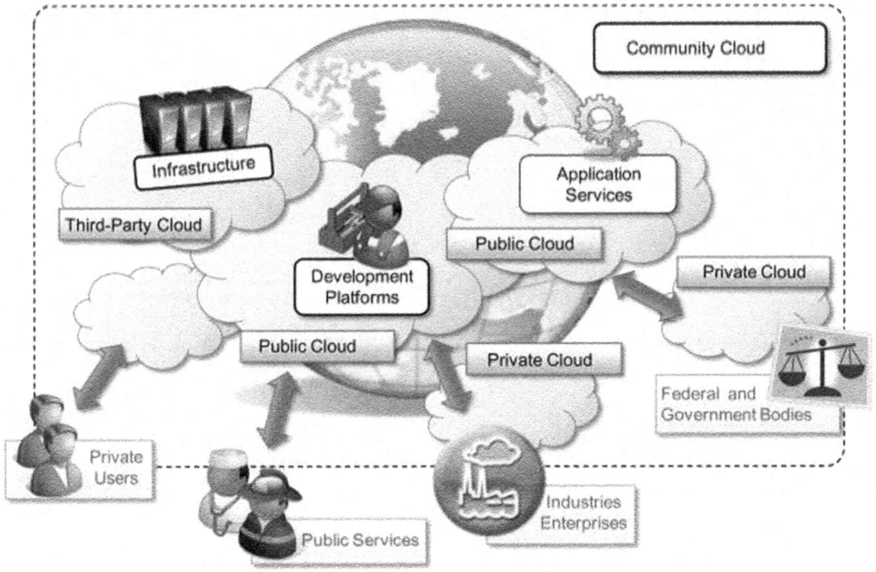

Fig. 6 Community cloud environments

3 Present Status of Healthcare Industries

The healthcare industry has ordinarily underused advancement as a technique for improving patient inclusion. In facts, even today, associations rely on hard copy clinical records and transcribe notes to educate and decide. Mechanized information is sold in offices and applications, making it harder to access a patient's longitudinal record troublesome, if this is certainly possible. This absence of admittance costs the medical care industry a significant amount of money every year to copy and leftover. The exchange of patient information across clinicians, offices, and even patients is unusual and complex. The clinic's dependence on vendors to joint their different advances leads to costly and questionable information tests that neglect to transmit expected results.

Different nations have unexpectedly moved this problem, from the focal public clearinghouse (UK) to territorial well-being habitats (Canada) to more granular fitness information exchanges; all are acknowledged with different level achievement. Those nations that have skirted hardcopy records and begun with indicative imaging appear to have had more accomplishment in a restricted way yet still cannot seem to progress with the more significant segments of the patient record.

As electronic prosperity records, picture archiving and communication system (PACS), and progressive clinical structures develop and become more visible, and current storage assets are expanded. Running an advanced pathology framework could put petabyte-level claims on the current basis right away. Today, patients rely on funder for their medical services; they are more aware of their illnesses and are progressively demanding admission to the most recent advances. Simultaneously, they search for the best consideration at the best price and will explore their alternatives. After that, applications for admission to individual patient registers are increased, and associations must follow.

Many emerging countries are building information centers about medical services that can help make information more versatile. Canada has developed analytical imaging warehouses that provide benefits to patient and reserve funds. Nations around the planet continue promoting new abilities that will improve patient consideration, moreover where cloud computing can help boost our business. In the fifth planning stages, 25% are being updated. Just 5% have recently accepted cloud computing, but they collect an expected 20% of reserve funds for updating applications. The next step is to change all the applications more clinically involved in the cloud.

In contrast to different firms, the clinical benefits industry has underutilized advancement to improve operational profitability. Most medical care settings rely on hardcopy clinical records. Digitized data is not ordinarily compact, which stifles data sharing between medical service artists. The utilization of development to cultivate collaboration and arrange care among patients and specialists and the clinical neighborhood confined. Medical care modification has ordered that it is energy for healthcare information technology (HIT) to be restructured around the planet. Cloud computing is at the focal point of this change. Cloud computing gives a framework that allows emergency clinics, clinical practices, insurance agencies, and research facilities to benefit from improved asset registration at lower initial capital expenditures (Fig. 7).

Also, cloud environments will reduce barriers to advancing and modernizing HIT frameworks and solicitations. Cloud computing recognizes the critical innovation needs of the medical care industry.

- Allows admission to check-in and substantial storage spaces that are not given under conventional IT conditions.
- Supports key indicators for electronic prosperity records (EPR), radiology pictures, and genomic offloading relief, a problematic undertaking from medical clinic IT departments.

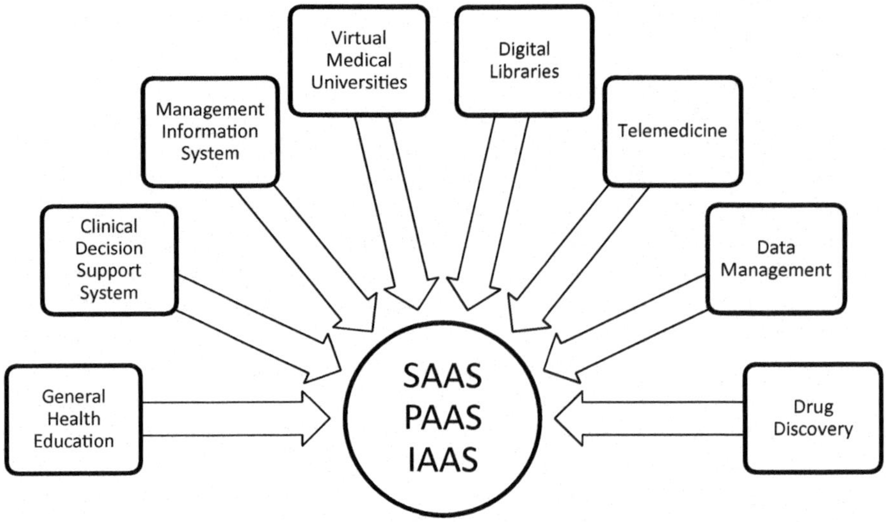

Fig. 7 Cloud-driven healthcare services

- Encourages the sharing of EPRs between doctors and clinics approved by geologies, making the admission of indispensable information considerably more convenient and reducing the need for copy testing.
- Enhances the capacity to decompose and track data so that information on medicines, expenditures, and execution and viability studies can be reviewed and tracked.

4 Cloud Computing in Medical Services

Cloud computing in the clinical consideration area opens novel entrances for clinical specialists. They have the adaptive ability to control the versatility of information, rapid access to clinical records, and an enormous limit on hospital files' storage. The medical care industry has used new advanced to smooth cycles, bring new considerations to patient, applications and at least improve the administration of medical services. Despite IT plans, clinical consideration affiliations face challenges, for instance, the excellent establishment of the board budgets, dynamic necessities for computational resources, the flexibility of HR, inescapable access, multiresidency, and extended interest for collaboration. These legitimizations of critical challenges introduce cloud computing in clinical benefits affiliations.

As reaction healthcare establishments depend on the usage of information and communication technologies (ICTs) to defeat challenges and fulfill patients' requests practically, they receive new advances to improve, expand, and rethink how medical services have been conveyed for quite a long time. The grouping of cloud computing and medical care services can probably enhance various medical care capabilities such as telemedicine, post-hospital care plans, and virtual medication compliance. Besides, it improves access to medical care by telehealth.

According to the new review report, cloud computing represented 7.6% of the global information and communications technology (ICT) innovation market valued at $3 trillion in 2017. While the worldwide information innovation market is the figure to develop at a compound annual growth rate (CAGR) of 10.1% somewhere in the range of 2018 and 2022, **cloud computing** incomes, which passed $233B in 2017, are developing at over 25%. In principle, the whole IT market could move to the cloud, so the disturbance yet to be released onto the worldwide programming and IT administration area will probably be considerable.

Lately, the allocation of resources to cloud computing innovation has increased importance for medical associations and networks. In any case, there is still idleness to defeat because of information security and protection anxieties, framework accessibility, administrative consistence stresses, and an absence of the staff abilities needed to oversee and keep up the innovation. Accepting and approving a cloud-based model can be valuable for medical care, as cloud arrangements offer adaptability, versatility alternatives, and remote admission to administrations and data. They likewise ensure significant designs are as yet running if there should be an event of a solitary point disappointment, and they make the frame recovery much simpler and quicker (Fig. 8).

The cloud administrations that are likely to change existing medical services frameworks work and connect are EPR. An EPR is an advanced document containing residents/patient's very own information (name, image, address, DOB, so forth) and well-being history (existing sicknesses, earlier surgical treatment, allergies, blood type, injections, so on). One of the drivers for the use of cloud computing in health care is to increase cost appropriateness. When using the cloud, the profitability of medical

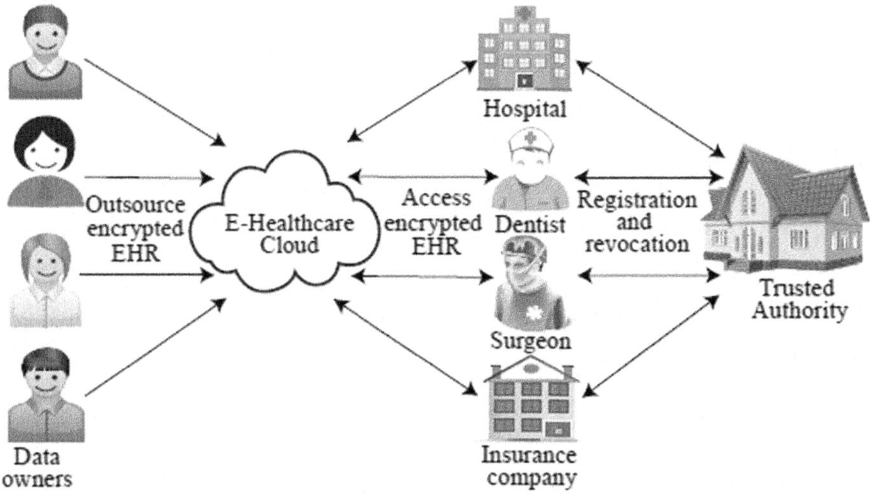

Fig. 8 Architecture of the e-healthcare cloud system

service providers has a higher rate of return. Cloud arrangements would support a shift in attendants' hours of work from reduced organization operations to direct patient consideration. It would be essential if distinctive medical service companies embrace various clouds that are viable with each other to address interoperability trials among executives.

For instance, a patient comes to the hospital's casualty department and shows her/his ID. Just with that, the attendants would have the option to get to the EPR of the patient whenever the patient agrees on access, and afterward diverted to the correct treatments, skirting tedious enrollment cycles, and clinical tests that are not required because all the most recent data is now appearing in the EPR. It is a given that the significant worry of medical care experts is to give acceptable quality consideration to their patients, making their involvement in the medical care system is as "charming" as could be expected, with an explicit concentration to patient-security. Medical assistants should be placed in the co-creation of driving seats, planning of "fit-for-reason" arrangements, deployable arrangements, and displacement bleeding edge back to coordinate patient consideration.

5 Benefits of Cloud Computing in Healthcare Industry

Health care in the age of computerization has become an area where a vast amount of information is produced consistently. The patient's clinical and monetary subtleties, just as any exploration, are only a portion of the created information, and keeping a speedy and safe database is of most significance. The epidemic of COVID-19, clinics, and doctors are stunned by patients. Medical service experts are constrained by the measurement of information that should be created or shared, and the rate at which it should occur. Fortunately for them, cloud provides a speedy, protected, and convenient setting. Cloud computing accompanies an extraordinary combination of benefits that can contribute significantly to the healthcare sector.

- **Management of servers**

The benefit of cloud framework for medical services is that information oversight is not the healthcare supplier's work. With IT experts able to oversee and handle the framework, healthcare providers can focus on other essential healthcare features.

- **Cost benefits**

In cloud computing, it is simpler to lead the service area you pay and make practical choices. By making a customized arrangement that meets our needs, we can discuss a much more economical deal than setting up your structures.

- **Intended to manage a tremendous amount of data**

As previous stated, health and its related fields create a ton of information. For instance, clinical pictures like scans are tremendously in-depth and produce high-resolution images using various information. Much of this information should be kept for the patient's lifetime too, to be protected. Actual capacity is inconvenient, and cloud computing offers a more accessible option.

- **Quick velocities**

With increasing numbers of patient, speed is of extreme significance. The availability of quicker cloud servers simplifies the transfer, sharing, and retrieving of information quickly. It also allows for rapid change. Interchange of information and message between medical services labors, clinics, investigation hubs, and funding authorities such as grants to clinical groups creates a higher medical care atmosphere. Time is the incarnation in medical services and the cloud; we would now be significantly more time-competent.

- **Security and protection**

Cloud computing has made remarkable progress concerning security anxieties. The use of private and hybrid cloud framework has guaranteed that the clinical and monetary complexities remain secure. For instance, if a clinic has a patient who needs rising subsidizes utilizing a group financing stage, there can be a safe exchange of information between the raised and the clinic using cloud frameworks. Besides, remote servers keep it safer from anything on the spot, perilous and further reduce problems when retrieving information.

The opportunities that Cloud computing gives to the Healthcare systems:

- **Adaptability**

The demands of the medical care organization may change over time. It is easy to adapt cloud to your needs. The cloud permits you to increase meet your current needs, prevent unnecessary consumption, and take future development.

- **Ability to update**

The ability to refresh innovation is in constant evolution. As the frameworks are revised, the information should be changed or updated. When this happens, it will be much easier and faster to refresh information with the cloud. Having a cloud-based framework will help you refresh your information, applications, and framework as fast as possible.

- **Permitting easier collaborations**

In later life, resource sharing is essential to opening better doors for patients, e.g., teaming up with other medical care suppliers can offer better assistance while working together with swarm financing and other elective subsidizing alternatives empowers patients to manage their costs. Group efforts like these make a superior medical services framework for everybody.

Using cloud data in telemedicine practices

During this epidemic, specialists and patients themselves are at risk of becoming infected in medical clinics. In this crucial period, telemedicine practices can help medical care employees provide safe remote medical services. These advanced clinical frameworks need to move the patient information to and fro at extraordinary fast, something that cloud can be utilized effectively, while likewise keeping up the doctor–patient protection. By including cloud computing as part of a telemedicine setting, we could now have a protected framework, both substantially and digitally.

6 Cloud Computing Services to Medical Services Industry

With an immense number of cloud computing benefits in medical services, the market is likely to exceed $40 billion by 2026. Zymr gives full-stack cloud programming improvement for the medical care sector. Our medical care administrations incorporate Patient Apps, Medical Apps, EPR Incorporation, Well-being Analytics, and Healthcare IoT.

- ***Patient-centric apps*** have become an excellent focal point for Healthcare Delivery Organizations (HDO). Our emphasis is on these apps to safely coordinate with the EPR framework and environment of care suppliers. Patients can undoubtedly get to their clinical records and well-being reports, track interactive well-being, plan arrangements and specialists.
- ***Clinical apps*** can help doctors and healthcare groups give non-stop attention. Doctors and nurses can reach patients, files, and reports. Our center is the HIPAA consistency and safety concerns to open up these applications more coordination with medical care's biological IT system.
- ***EPR integration*** is linked to apps' coordination with the HDO EPR/ECR framework to deliver specific medical service suppliers' benefits. Our emphasis is on organizing healthcare administration, understanding integration and adherence to EPR framework, integrating clinical resources and FHIR recharging, combining ECR and Epic heritage, MEDITECH, CoCENTRIX, and Training Synthesis.
- ***Health analytics*** provides significant experiences in informing medical services to improve the information about medical services. Our attention is on the enormous investigation of information, revealing the isolated aid by HDO, the safety of EPR, consistency, clinical errors, and benefit reports of saving money.
- ***Healthcare IoT*** involves IoT-based apps for patients and HDOs to encourage the transport of medical services. Our emphasis is on the patient IoT-based observing framework, medication following, and fall location apps, hospital IoT-based hardware tracing, ecological apps, and lab upkeep, just as on medical IoT-based consideration robotization apparatuses.

7 Importance of Cloud Adoption in Health Care

Cloud computing in health care reinforces the company's competence while reducing expenditures. Cloud computing simplifies and secures clinical records, simplifies robot background activities , and even promotes telehealth apps' creation and maintenance. Global medical cloud is needed for a $35 billion market by 2022, developing 11.6% annually. Though assumption, 83% of the healthcare zone is now utilizing the cloud for their central tasks. Better information control for patients and less support and cost investment funds on the association side add to increased cloud selection in health care.

The various elements that support cloud adoption in health care are:

(1) **Simplified Data Access**

Collecting patient data has been a tedious task. With all the information transferred to the cloud, wellness experts now think it is easier to follow a patient's wellness file and stick to informed choices.

(2) **Data Storage and Management**

Loading and retaining a vast amount of information require more care for IT personnel, programming, equipment, resulting in additional use. Currently, the cloud does everything for you, reducing your additional spending.

(3) **Backup and Recovery data**

Information loss is the most astonishing part of any organization today. Here, the cloud gives some leeway to ideal reinforcements and recovery choices, limiting the chances of essential information misfortune.

(4) **Smart Data Potential**

Cloud promotes the use of brilliant information arrangements such as big data and machine learning that enhance the ability to recognize, separate, anticipate, and respond quickly to information data needs.

(5) **Data Interoperability**

Portable gadgets, IoT-enabled gadgets, and online wellness tracking apps, combined in the cloud, have shown the benefits of information interoperability in health care.

(6) **Better Information, Better Treatment**

Before the beginning of innovation and, all the more significantly, the Web, the medical services industry was about pantries and work areas with many documents. As the twenty-first-century approaches, these documents are currently available on PCs and are effectively adapt too many regions with the cloud's help. Manually written reports can cause doctors to shift in making the following strides. It could be agonizing to shuffle between a few documents spread across a table for examining numerous records. With cloud-based applications, the review of information becomes safe and error-free and doctors can make informed decisions for patients contingent on that information.

(7) **Extensive Research is Good Research!**

Cloud computing administrations force specialists and welfare specialists to make available world -class solutions. Big data is shared and obtained from different places.

It is rapidly handled into compact, easy-to-refer data through user-friendly cloud applications that help reviewers make a good decision and give all around guided treatments.

(8) **Telehealth Services**

Efficient freedom for both patients and clinical experts adds to the rise of online health advice and remote coherent medical services. The cloud is at the core of e-health administration.

8 COVID-19 Impact on Cloud Computing in Healthcare Industry

The COVID-19 outbreak has reshaped the standard procedures of healthcare associations amid overcrowding and lack of resources. Market players that were exclusively reliant on facilitated IT foundation and insufficient cloud structure are hooking to keep tasks smooth, particularly as the requirement for virtual counseling m-healthcare & telemedicine is expanded. On the other hand, the new frontline organizations who took the cloud development way before the COVID-19 crisis highlighted their priorities even under current conditions. Giving a response to the constraints facilitated foundation, the cloud has given a platform to agree with the safety guidelines in medical services, made it more straightforward to conform to operational work measure change, and ensure a steady patient-supplier composed exertion aided handle another well-being climate reality. Subsequently, cloud computing ended up immense use of the medical services industry under circumstances such as present.

Cloud computing is also considered an essential part of the sharing of information. During the COVID-19 epidemic, the requirement to share patient information across the healthcare system is higher than at any other time. Furthermore, healthcare settings and its connected parts do a lot of data. For example, clinical images and patient wellness data are huge data load. These data for the patient's entire life must be stored, kept safe, and communicated to the highest unbreakable quality.

The exchange of information and communication between medical clinics, medical procedure centers, crisis clinics, and other health care a supplier has been simplified with the cloud computing selection. During the pandemic, there is considerable time and cloud computing can save time. Cloud computing is maybe the best tools to investigate the COVID-19 crisis. Cloud speedily empowered us to work, conserve, shop, and play indirectly, sitting in the safe confines of our homes. Since the international pandemic, the advancement of cloud computing has become the proper foundation of some of the fundamental advances and healthcare enhancement.

1. **Data investigation and prescient models**:

Information has arisen as an incredible weapon in the battle against the epidemic. Hearty bits of knowledge driven from vast volumes of information are utilized across the lifespan of epidemic administration from analyzing to treat to fix and, above all, for examination and medication disclosure. Based on insights, 2300 Exabyte's of medical service information will be delivered in 2020 (as indicate by pre-COVID gauges). The present test is the separated and partitioned nature of these collections of information. Cloud-based information lakes contribute to unifying and facilitating access to examination information. As of late, AWS transformed its COVID-19 information lake to state-of-the-art data warehouse and organized epidemic datasets for analysts and medical service providers. The cloud company also worked closely with the WHO to use cloud progress to build various jurisdictions. WHOs Conservatoire app, its occasional dashboard, Open WHO information transmission boards, its initial framework of warning worked with the help of AWS cloud advancements and various devices.

2. **Telehealth through cloud**:

Remote medical services or virtual medical care is the most significant change the medical care sector has adopted. Gradually, suppliers are beholding new healthcare conveyance simulations and healthcare administration, including telemedicine and telehealth facilities. The telehealth services market was emerging at an impressive 65% in 2020. Remote consulting frameworks based on cloud computing powered by artificial intelligence can relieve doctors and clinics by providing clinical data to patients, evaluating indications and threat factors. Cloud-facilitated telemedicine and remote monitoring become increasingly regular for treating COVID-19 patients who are isolated at home. Telecounseling helps reduce the danger of irresistible openness, a significant burden on clinicians, and greater consideration of the patient.

3. **Cloud-fueled bots**:

Inquiries and solicitations have swamped medical clinics and contact centers across the world since the outbreak. General welfare associations medical care specialists must react quickly to deliver exact data, new emergency patients, and accelerate activity. Numerous medical care organizations are taking a gander at healthcare robots and emergency robots to broaden those energies and commitment with residents.

The majority of these devices can be immediately sent to sites or applications and transmit a common self-administration and discussion experience to people. It accomplishes something beyond giving the correct data. Bots can responds to urgent patient needs, check indications, reserve arrangements, and deliver coordinated clinical databases and conventions. Few clinics use chat robots to address the psychological wellness issues due to COVID-19.

9 Deal with the Cloud Environment

The board of cloud conditions is like overseeing conventional IT conditions. Again, the cloud should do it across the limit between the cloud administration client and the cloud specialist organization. The customary administrative boundaries for IT conditions like expense, support, administration of the executives, security, effectiveness, staffing is generally legitimate for the administration of cloud conditions. A couple of driving edge parts of IT may represent a specific test in a cloud setting.

These incorporate the administration of.

- Electronic well-being records (counting sharing),
- Automation of associated Web gadgets with constant information,
- Field gadgets (counting doctor/medical caretaker's tablet for catching or showing information),
- Intelligent psychological partners (general practitioner assistant) and so forth, etc.

1. **Electronic Prosperity Records**

EPR is currently used in a limited way in different world pieces, and there is an overall development toward embracing them. The accompanying qualities of EPRs present explicit administration worries in a half and half cloud environment:

- Recovering and communicating well-being information for patients to/from outer sources with security, protection, and provenance issues.
- Dealing with the protection and security of patient well-being information by and large.
- Guaranteeing the accessibility of patient well-being information.
- Guaranteeing ideal synchronization of patient well-being information.

These apprehensions recorded above require the cloud environment to be steady of the particular capacity recorded. Frameworks should be accessible, associated, got and fittingly observed, and logged for the appropriate execution of administrative, consistent, and interior security and confidentiality controls. Explicit controls are ordinarily needed by the essential administrative system, like HIPAA in the USA.

2. **Web of Things**

Patients outfitted with associated gadgets for computerized checking requires particular cloud administration the executives support. These medical services gadgets support a broad scope of capabilities, counting:

- Fall discovery for elderly patients.
- Well-being checking for patients with persistent issues likes diabetes and coronary illness.
- Location of raising side effects for patients with mental problems.

Gadgets of these sorts are ordinarily associated with the Web and are fit for telling/alarming an assigned medical care administration focus with information and other relevant episode data. It will require the cloud environment to address framework accessibility, availability, protection, and security. The security challenge of any gadgets associated with the Web is of specific concern. Information should take care of to get the endpoints concerned and guarantee the patient data's secrecy. Utilization of more specific transmission conventions, for example, MQTT, might be fitting alongside encryption of the information traffic.

3. **Field Devices**

These gadgets (generally PDAs, tablets, laptops, and so on) are utilized by medical care staff to recover and record patient information on the spot. These gadgets require an offbeat information transfer system to forestall information misfortune and keep the worldwide EPR store refreshed. Here are a couple of board contemplations that should be tended to for these gadgets,

- Ensure gadgets and organization assets against interference and suspended administrations brought about by assaults on the emergency clinic or gadget maker's Web workers, when the progression of outside correspondence solicitations will deter and not permit reactions to genuine assistance demands.
- Regularly update clinical gadgets and organization programming. It is pivotal to set up a confided in upkeep environment, setting up access with support and backing administrations.
- Provide security insurance for Android gadgets and applications that utilize powerless passwords, making a straightforward access way for programmers to take broadband signals and misuse VPN associations. There is no equipment information encryption on Android gadgets, so there is more severe, recognizable information that data might put away on the gadget.
- Set up secure correspondences through an assortment of systems administration components. Information should get communication ways among gadgets and frameworks. In both HTTP-based and occasion-based models, the utilization of SSL/TLS to set up ensured interchange is inescapable. Give solid cryptographic algorithms to build up a protected correspondences channel; this permits most of the rationale running on gadgets, accesses, and cloud-facilitated frameworks to expect a safe interchanges channel and zero in on giving the capacity of the gadget or application.

4. **Shrewd Automated Assistance**

Doctors, medical attendants, and other medical services suppliers can utilize quite a few psychological arrangements that help dissect an immense measure of unknown information from worldwide sources, connect against particular information hailed on the patient, and give the specialist dynamic co-op. It would be conceivable on account of cloud associated frameworks. It is additionally expected that such a framework would, by and large, require Web access (i.e., cloud conveyed) and, in this manner, require materialness of all cloud executives standards.

5. Frameworks Maintenance

Support of data frameworks applies to cloud administrations as it never really house frameworks. The distinction that a few parts of the cloud administration environment are the cloud specialist provider's obligation. It is fundamental for the cloud administration client to have affirmation about the cloud merchant's ability for:

- Fixing of programming and frameworks to manage known issues conveniently, fundamental security weaknesses.

- Support and tuning, for example, information-based ordering and reserve resets.
- Framework refreshes, especially of seller created refreshes.
- Framework updates, including moving to more current variants of software with added highlights and usefulness.

The cloud service customer must have assurance about the cloud vendor's capacity for:

- Patching of software and systems to deal with known issues promptly, particularly critical security vulnerabilities.
- Maintenance and tuning, such as database indexing and cache resets.
- System updates, particularly vendor-generated updates.
- System upgrades, including moving to newer versions of software with added features and functionality.
- Synchronizing maintenance activities with the cloud service customer's IT management plan, typically through a system of notifications.
- Ensuring availability and performance service-level objectives (SLOs) are met even during maintenance cycles.

HCOs must ensure that the SLA is met for each cloud service while keeping in mind the criticality of specific service-level objectives and the consequences of failure to meet those objectives. For many cloud services, the onus is on the cloud service customer to detect if the SLOs are not satisfied and to demand action on the part of the cloud service provider to rectify the situation.

10 Conclusion

There are massive opportunities and inspirations to pick cloud innovation in clinical benefits. The opportunity has arrived to clasp hands with clinicians and Pc specialists to keep on executing the wide advancement, which suits little practices to tremendous clinics. The COVID-19 epidemic can use the good conditions that cloud-based systems offer. It tends to be reasoned that such systems can profoundly diminish the number of resources needed by in-house groups to administer data. The availability of cloud grants medicinal services organizations to emphasis on contributing better administrations, which is their central part instead of contributing time and assets on IT. The early adopters of cloud-based facilities are obtaining the rewards of it for a long time. During the pandemic, the requests ascended during the COVID-19 flare-up have shown that cloud-based medical care administrations are achievable and essential. Cloud computing should also be embraced in the contemporary state's medical services industry like never before. Subsequently, we can securely presume that cloud-based administrations have upheld the well-being area by making data more open, interoperable, secure electronic prosperity record (EPR) stockpiling, and community-oriented patient consideration increasingly.

References

1. Agarkhed, J., Ramegowda, A., & Patil, S. (2019). Smart healthcare systems using cloud computing environments. *Proceedings of ICCDN 2018*. https://doi.org/10.1007/978-981-13-3450-4_59.
2. Cloud Standard Customer Council. (2017). Impact of cloud computing on healthcare version 2.0. Retrived March 26 2017, from https://www.omg.org/cloud/deliverables/CSCC-Impact-of-Cloud-Computing-on-Healthcare.pdf.
3. Chatman C. (2010, June). How cloud computing is changing the face of health care information technology. *Health Care Compliance, 12*(3), 37–70.
4. Cloud Computing. Clear Benefits: The emerging role of cloud computing in healthcare information systems. Available online: http://www.techrepublic.com/whitepapers/cloud-computing-clear-benefits-theemerging-role-of-cloud-computing-in-healthcare-informationsystems/2384337. (accessed on 28 June 2012).
5. Chen, P., Freg, C., Hou, T., Teng, W.-G. (2010, December). Implementing RAID-3 on cloud storage for EMR system. In *Proceedings of the 2010 International Computer Symposium (ICS)*, Taiwan, pp. 850–853.
6. Davidson, E., Heslinga, D. (2006). Bridging the IT adoption gap for small physician practices: An action research study on electronic health records. *Information Systems Management, 24*, 15–28.
7. Goldschmidt, P.G. (2005). HIT and MIS: implications of health information technology and medical information systems. *Communications of the ACM, 48*, 69–74.
8. Guo, L., Chen, F., Chen, L., Tang, X. (2010). The building of cloud computing environment for e-health. *Proceedings of the 2010 International Conference on E-Health Networking, Digital Ecosystems and Technologies (EDT), The IEEE International Conference on E-Health Networking*, July 1–3, 2010; Lyon, France. New York, NY: IEEE; 2010.
9. Horowitz, B. (2011). Cloud computing brings challenges for health care data storage, privacy. Retrieved from http://www.eweek.com/c/a/Health-Care-IT/Cloud-Computing-Brings-Challenges-for-Health-Care-Data-Storage-Privacy-8516081. (accessed on 23 July 2013).
10. Haughton, J. (2011). Year of the underdog: Cloud-based EHRs. *Health Management Technology, 32*(1), 9.
11. Javaid, M., Haleem, A., Vaishya, R., Bahl, S., Suman, R., & Vaish, A. (2020). Industry 4.0 technologies and their applications in fighting COVID-19 pandemic. *Diabetes & Metabolic Syndrome: Clinical Research & Reviews, 14*, 419–422.
12. Kaplan, M., Kneifel, C., Orlikowski, V., Dorff, J., Newton, M., Howard, A., Shinn, D., Bishawi, M., Chidyagwai, S., Balogh, P., et al. (2020). Cloud computing for COVID-19: lessons learned from massively parallel models of ventilator splitting. *Computing in Science & Engineering, 22*, 37–47.
13. Li, M., Yu, S., Ren, K., & Lou, W. (2010, September). Securing personal health records in cloud computing: patient-centric and fine-grained data access control in multi-owner settings. In *Proceedings of the 6th International ICST Conference on Security and Privacy in Communication Networks (SecureComm 2010)*, Singapore, pp. 89–106.
14. Lo, O., Fan, L., Buchanan, W., Thümmler, C., Khedim, A., Lawson, A., Uthmani, O., & Bell, D. (2011, May). Patient simulator: Towards testing and validation of e-Health infrastructures. In *Proceedings of the Pervasive Health*, Dublin, Ireland.
15. Mell, P., Grance, T. (2011). The NIST definition of cloud computing.
16. Rosenthal, A., Mork, P., Li, M. H., Stanford, J., Koester, D., & Reynolds, P. (2010, April). Cloud computing: a new business paradigm for biomedical information sharing. *Journal of biomedical informatics, 43*(2), 342–53.
17. Saranummi, N. (2011). In the spotlight: Health information systems: Mainstreaming mHealth. *IEEE reviews in biomedical engineering, 4*, 17–19.
18. Schweitzer, E. J. (2011, July). Reconciliation of the cloud computing model with US federal electronic health record regulations. *Journal of the American Medical Informatics Association.*

19. Mukherjee, S., Dolui, K., & Datta, S. K. (2014). Patient health management system using e-health monitoring architecture, *IEEE International Advance Computing Conference (IACC)*, Gurgaon, pp. 400–405.
20. Wang, X., & Tan, Y. (2010). Application of cloud computing in the health information system. *Proceedings of the 2010 International Conference on Computer Application and System Modeling (ICCASM), International Conference on Computer Application and System Modeling*, Taiyuan, China. New York, NY: IEEE; 2010.
21. Terry, K. (2013). Why telemedicine should be integrated with EHRs, ACOs. *Information Week*. http://www.informationweek.com/interoperability/why-telemedicine-should-be-integrated-with-ehrsacos/d/did/1109882?.
22. Zhang, T., Liu, L. (2010, July). Security models and requirements for healthcare application clouds. In *Proceedings of the IEEE 3rd International Conference on Cloud Computing*, Miami, FL, USA, pp. 268–275.
23. Google Privacy Center Google. (2010). Oct 3, [2011-08-06]. Webcite privacy policy http://www.google.com/google-d-s/intl/en/privacy.html.
24. Amazon Web Services. (2008). Oct 01, [2011-08-05]. Webcite AWS privacy notice. http://aws.amazon.com/privacy/.

Toward Healthcare Data Availability and Security Using Fog-to-Cloud Networks

K. A. Sadiq, A. F. Thompson, and O. A. Ayeni

1 Introduction

The global population increase in patients seeking medical services has created enormous challenges for healthcare providers. Medical facilities such as hospital beds, workforce, patient observation, patient monitoring, and drug management have become complex tasks and require much cheaper solutions [1]. Healthcare providers widely adopt the IoT to provide solutions to the challenges mentioned earlier. The IoT collects, processes, stores, and monitors patients' data using sensors embedded in electronic devices and communicates such data through the network, using communication protocols like the Internet, Bluetooth, and Zigbee to a remote cloud server for timely decision making [1–3]. IoT has also demonstrated other benefits in online medical consulting from a remote location, patients contact tracing in epidemic and pandemic situations, and real-time monitoring and treatments of patients' heart rates and sugar level. All these benefits of IoT in healthcare IoHT has projected its global market from \$72.5 billion in 2020 to \$188.2 billion in 2025, which will produce 79.4 zettabytes (ZB) of data [4–6]. The introduction of IoT in healthcare had shifted medical data processing, analysis, and storage to the cloud networks, owned private or public service providers, and available on measured payments. However, the security and reliability of the medical data generated by IoHT devices in third-party hands have become a global concern for academia, healthcare providers, and the patient. It is worth knowing that medical data are confidential to both IoHT providers and patients

K. A. Sadiq (✉)
Department of Computer Science, Kwara State Polytechnic, Ilorin, Nigeria

A. F. Thompson · O. A. Ayeni
Cyber Security Science Department, Federal University of Technology, Akure, Nigeria
e-mail: afthompson@futa.edu.ng

O. A. Ayeni
e-mail: oaayeni@futa.edu.ng

A. K. Tyagi et al. (eds.), *Intelligent Interactive Multimedia Systems for e-Healthcare Applications*, https://doi.org/10.1007/978-981-16-6542-4_6

but valuable to cyber-criminal for perpetrating fraud, such as using patient social security number SSN and medical history for insurance claims. Also, medical service availability is crucial in IoHT as patients on real-time monitoring, online medical consultation, and patient contact tracing cannot tolerate network degradation.

The DDoS stands out among cyber-attacks. An attacker sends unsolicited messages using compromised legitimate users' devices to the cloud server with the intention of either degrade and make the IoHT cloud server unavailable for legitimate activities or steal by impersonating legitimate patients to steal information [7, 8]. Mostly, DDoS also takes advantage of network and users' device hardware and software vulnerabilities to install malicious software called malware that makes them captive and act like "Zombies" to perform illicit acts [7–9]. The DDoS has various variants such as the ping of death attack, hypertext transfer protocol HTTP flood attack, synchronize SYN flood attack, user datagram protocol UDP attack, Internet control message protocol ICMP attack, slowloris attack, and smurf attack. The SYN attack is considered the most famous DDoS, with an attack projection of 15 million by 2023 from 7.9 million attacks in 2018 [10]. Putting the DDoS in perspective in the IoHT cloud server, the chapter contribution proposes fog computing introduced by CISCO network in 2012 to perform packet filtering for the IoHT cloud server. The fog node situated between the IoHT devices and the IoHT cloud servers performs few computational processes like analysis and data storage. Also, it reduces network latency, and mobility supports challenges associated with the cloud network. The fog node computes the network delay, the server response time and compares it with the cloud server's threshold value during data transmission. If the network delay and the server response time are higher than the initial threshold value, the packet is considered suspicious. Captcha is sent to the packet source to avoid Bonet; otherwise, the packet is normal. The remainder of the research is as follows; 1.2 discusses IoHT systems, cloud characteristics, service, deployment, challenges, and DDoS attacks. 1.3 looked at related literature. 1.4 discussed the fog and cloud computing differences and challenges. 1.5 and 1.6 discuss the proposed framework and the conclusion, while 1.7 mentioned the references.

2 Background

This section provides insights on IoHT concepts, cloud network, and DDoS in IoHT.

2.1 IoHT Systems

The introduction of IoHT provides both healthcare providers and patients the opportunities to access medical services from remote locations and monitor patients and chronic diseases from different geographical areas. Medical decisions in real time and drug management are also carried remotely, thereby strengthening medical services' efficiency and productivity at a cheaper rate. The IoT collects, processes, stores, and monitors patients' data using sensors embedded in electronic devices and communicates such data through the network, using communication protocols like the Internet, Bluetooth, and Zigbee to a remote cloud server for timely decision making [1–3]. The IoHT architecture consists of application, network, and perception layers. The application layer, as regards IoHT, is responsible for delivering medical services to the patients. In contrast, the perception layer uses sensors to collect data about its physical environment and passes such data through the transceivers for processing using protocols. The network layer establishes a connection between the application and perception layer and ensures smooth and secured data communication using Wi-Fi, Bluetooth, Ethernet, Cellular, Satellite, and XBee (Fig. 1).

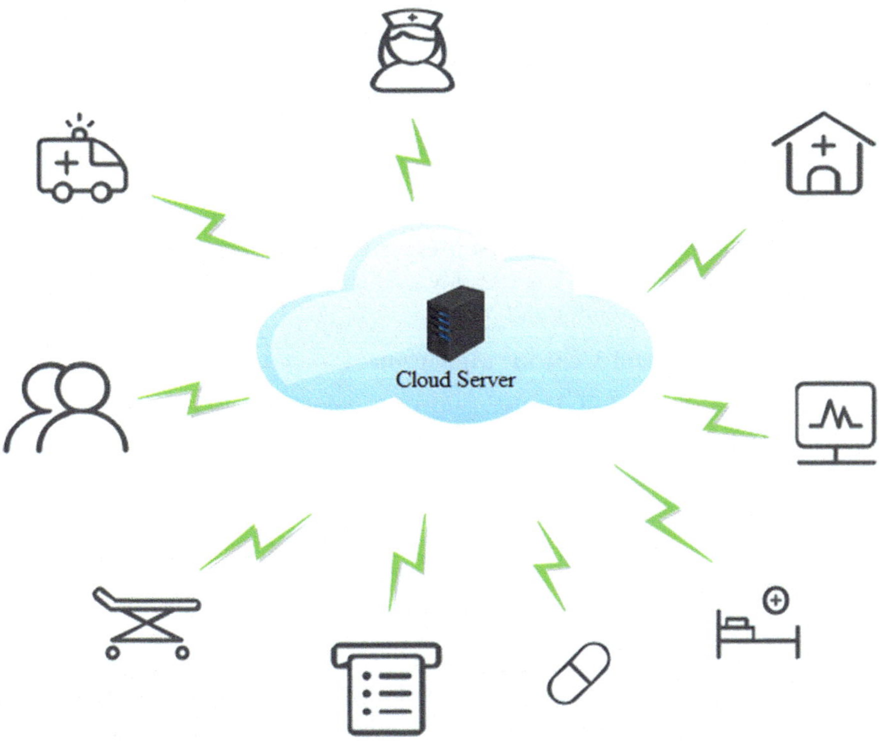

Fig. 1 IoT devices and personnel connect to the cloud server

2.2 *Benefits of IoHT*

Real-Time Monitoring

The real-time monitoring of patients using IoHT devices saves patients' lives in emergencies like heart attack, diabetics, cancer, and asthma attack. They collect patients' data like glucose level, blood pressure level, oxygen, patient weight, and communicate to the IoHT providers for diagnosis and decision making. The patients' data collected by these devices are primarily stored, processed, and accessed on the cloud networks.

Patients Contact Tracing

The IoHT enables us to perform contact tracing of patients in emergencies. Each patient's data resides on the cloud or the network, and IP address triangulation can allow us to know patients' physical locations. The IoHT can prove to be a great technology to collect, analyze, and monitor patients' data in hazardous and infectious situations.

Online Medical Assistance

The IoHT has reduced doctors' and patients' communication barriers by providing alternatives like online communication irrespective of geographical distance. Also, medical services through IoHT are readily available anytime at a cheaper, speedy, and reduced emergency room wait time.

Better Patient Drug and Medicine Management

The IoHT enables healthcare practitioners to remotely detect if the patient has taken medicine using physicians' medical applications. The therapist will call and remind a patient of that or, even more, if not. It is possible to automate this entire operation.

2.3 *Cloud Network*

Constraints like limited power, computational ability, and storage characterize the IoHT with all the advantages mentioned above [8]. Researchers widely adopt the migration of IoHT significant data computation and storage to the cloud network to minimize the computational and storage burden on IoHT devices, thereby strengthen their overall performance [2, 10]. Cloud computing is the technology of storing and accessing computing powers like storage, network, memory over a network, typically, the Internet from a remote server/location on a pay-as-you-use service [8]. Cloud computing provides IoHT technology with benefits like:

1. Cloud computing reduces costs, both capital and operating cost;
2. Cloud computing provides measured service for resource usage;
3. Cloud computing resources are scalable;

4. Environmentally friendly sensors/devices deployments;
5. Provides big data aggregation.

2.3.1 Characteristics of Cloud Computing

Cloud computing is distinct from the traditional client/server network because of its specific features, like; broad network access, rapid elasticity, resource pooling, on-demand self-service, and pay-as-you-use service [8] (Fig. 2).

1. **Broad Network Access**

The broad network access allows access to various cloud services across multiple locations simultaneously using various devices.

2. **Rapid Elasticity**

With cloud computing, users can adjust to their workload variations by automatically supplying and de-provisioning services without user awareness.

3. **Resource Pooling**

Multiple cloud users can use the same physical infrastructure and maintain high security and better hardware utilization through a multi-tenant model.

4. **On-Demand Self-Service**

Cloud users can perform all the actions needed to set up a cloud service on their own instead of going through an IT department. The cloud user request is handled automatically without human involvement.

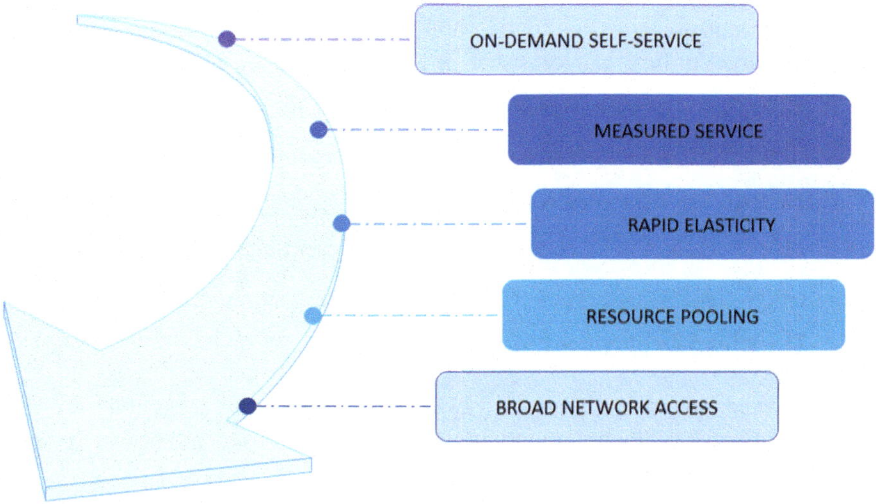

Fig. 2 Cloud network features

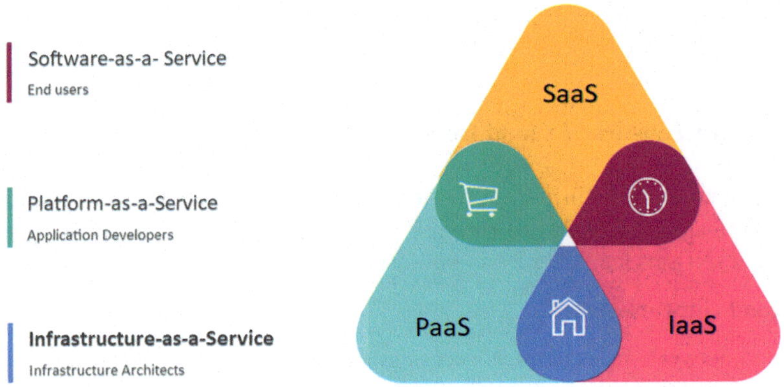

Fig. 3 Cloud service model

5. **Pay-As-You-Use**

Unlike traditional client/server networks, cloud networks use cloud application software that measures and charges each cloud user based on the service's usage.

2.3.2 The Cloud Service Models

The service model defines the types of services available to cloud users. Three distinct service models are available to cloud users, namely software-as-a-service (SaaS), platform-as-a-service (PaaS), and infrastructure-as-a-service (IaaS) [8] (Fig. 3).

1. **Software-as-a-service**

SaaS allows cloud users to use software applications over the Internet via subscription or free of charge for limited access such as Salesforce, Yahoo Mail, and Gmail.

2. **Platform-as-a-service (PaaS)**

Allows cloud users or vendors to create and host their applications.

3. **Infrastructure-as-a-service (IaaS)**

IaaS involves outsourcing IT equipment used for supporting cloud operations.

2.3.3 The Cloud Deployment Models

The cloud deployment models define how cloud services are accessible to cloud users. The primary deployment models available to cloud users are private, public, community, and hybrid clouds (Fig. 4).

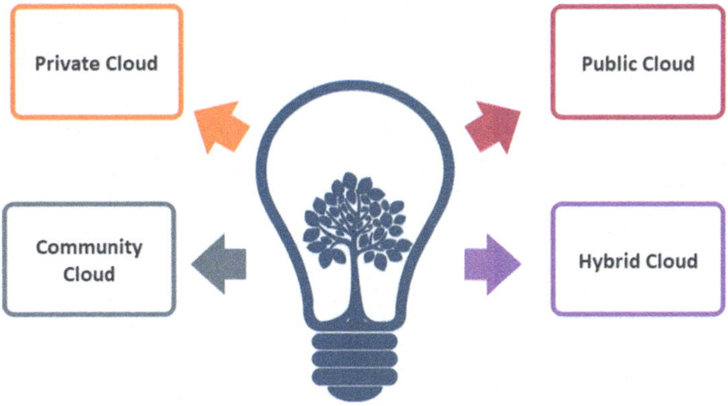

Fig. 4 Cloud deployment model

1. **Private Cloud**

A private cloud is a cloud provisioned for a single organization, a business enterprise with numerous users to meet their computational needs. This cloud infrastructure may reside on-site or off-site.

2. **Public Cloud**

A public cloud is a cloud provisioned for public usage. The infrastructure resides on the premises of cloud service providers.

3. **Community Cloud**

The community cloud is a private cloud for organizations, academia, and a government that shares a common interest in IT requirements.

4. **Hybrid Cloud**

The hybrid cloud combines two or more different cloud deployments. Each cloud deployment remains a distinct entity but bound together by the proprietary technology.

2.4 *The Cloud Challenges*

1. **Security**

Cloud resources are only accessible through a network, typically the Internet, making cloud user data vulnerable to cyber-criminals. DDoS creates the most severe threats to cloud service availability, integrity, and confidentiality among all cyber threats [11]. The DDoS attacks prevent legitimate users from accessing the server resources by over-flooding the server with illegal requests, thereby making cloud resources unavailable or degrade its services. A DDoS also takes advantage of legitimate users' hardware and software vulnerabilities to install malicious software called malware that makes the victims captive and act like "Zombies" to perform illicit acts [9].

2. **High Latency**

The cloud network latency is the rate of delay between users' requests and the server's response time. Cloud user services are often challenged with high latency because data processing requests might occur in a cloud server with a far geographic distance from where the data is needed [7]. The longer the distance cloud users' requests travel, the higher the cloud latency, which significantly affects cloud effectiveness and efficiency.

3. **Service Level Agreement**

The adoption of cloud networks brings about many legal challenges, such as data privacy and data jurisdictions [8]. Cloud processing, data analysis, and data storage are only achievable through the Internet and physical storage distributed across multiple geographic locations. Each location has different laws governing data security, privacy, and usage. The SLA has been a massive challenge for cloud service providers and cloud users.

4. **Real-Time Response**

The increase of IoT devices characterized by limited resources necessitated outsourcing their computational requirements to the cloud network and required real-time response. However, the latency issue associated with the cloud network does not provide a guarantee for time-sensitive applications.

5. **High Bandwidth Demand**

Ample data transportation in and out of the cloud servers comes with both technical and financial sacrifices. The bandwidth of the cloud network is the total amount of data the network connection can manage successfully at a given time. As the IoT devices kept growing, as stated in [5–7], this creates a massive bottleneck for the cloud platform.

6. **Interoperability**

The interoperability among cloud vendors has created a significant setback for cloud users. Cloud users cannot migrate from one service provider to another, even if the cloud users' operational and business demands require such change, such as migrating existing application stacks and servers from Amazon cloud to Microsoft Azure.

2.5 DDoS in IoHT

The DDoS attacks prevent legitimate cloud service users from accessing Cloud resources by over-flooding the server with illegal requests, making Cloud resources unavailable. A DDoS uses IoHT device software or hardware vulnerabilities to install its malicious software called malware, making the victims captive and act like "Zombies" to perform illicit acts on the attacker's instructions [12]. The cloud attackers are motivated by various incentives, such as revenge, ideological belief, financial or economic gains, cyber-warfare, and intellectual contest among cyber-attackers [11]. DDoS attackers mainly target either the application or communication (network/transport) layer. The communication layer attacks use Transmission Control Protocol (TCP), User Datagram Packets (UDP), Internet Control Message Protocol (ICMP), and Domain Name Service (DNS) to initiate the DDoS attacks. The DDoS attacks categories include flooding attacks, protocol exploitation, reflection-based attacks, and amplification-based attacks [10, 12]. The application-level flooding attacks target the hypertext transfer protocol HTTP and session initiation protocol SIP [12]. Detecting DDoS attacks is difficult because attackers mostly impersonate legitimate nodes to send packets and make it difficult to detect or trace back [10]. DDoS attacks can render cloud services unavailable or degrade their performance due to spike packet requests. Various methods like intrusion detection and anomaly detection using numerous machine learning algorithms have been proposed in the past [12].

The DoS has various variants such as the ping of death attack, hypertext transfer protocol HTTP flood attack, synchronize SYN flood attack, user datagram protocol UDP attack, Internet control message protocol ICMP, slowloris attack, and smurf attack.

1. **SYN Flood Attack**

The attacker sends volumetric connection requests to the server and intentionally fails to acknowledge the connection. The server continues to wait for the sender to finalize the half-open connection. The attacker continues to recruit multiple devices to create the half-open packet requests until the server's resources become degraded or unavailable.

2. **Ping of Death Attack**

In this DDoS attack variant, the attacker sends a larger packet than the machine's buffer size forcing it to such down or crash. For example, a modern operating system buffer can only handle packet size 65,536 bytes. Any packet size greater will make it crash or shut down.

3. **Smurf Attack**

The attacker uses the IP and ICMP of a legitimate device to simultaneously send ECHO ping to the server, thereby exhausting its resources.

4. **Slowloris Attack**

The slowloris DDoS attack is capable of using a single computer system to take down a web-server. The attacker sends a half-connected HTTP request and continues sending the requests until the web-server is exhausted.

3 Literature Review

The chapter contribution review selected publications between 2015 and December 2020 on Google Scholar, IEEE, Springer, and Elsevier using keywords like IoT in healthcare, DDoS mitigation using fog computing, and IoTH benefits and security challenges. [13] states that the fog network comprises three layers; terminal, fog, and cloud layers. The work proposes a fog node as a filtering layer for the incoming traffic and resides between the IoT device and cloud servers using two phases. The first phase checks all incoming packets' IP addresses for spoofing. If the IP address is spoofed, the system updates its IP address blacklist; otherwise, the fog server process it, and a captcha test is sent to the user to avoid bot attack. If the captcha test is successful, the fog server sent it to phase two, where the protocols and test tools are analyzed. If the analysis is successful, the fog sends the user's request to the cloud; else, the fog rejects the packet. [14] proposes fog computing-based security (FOCUS), which has threefold protection approaches. The first fold introduces virtual private networks to secure all IoT communication channels using data encryption that prevents attacks like man-in-the-middle and sniff. The second fold, the traffic analysis unit, uses a machine learning technique to classify packets as trusted or suspicious based on the incoming packets' anomaly behavior. The third fold, challenge-response unit, and firewall are responsible for conducting authentication procedures on all suspicious packets in the second fold by sending a challenge question to the suspicious machine to check botnet attack. If the machine response is adequate, the server grants access to the packet. Otherwise, the packet is labeled untrusted and blacklist, and blocked by the firewall. The FOCUS experimentation was carried out in a proof-of-work prototype. Ref. [15] uses the recurrent neural network as a machine learning method to detect network intrusion in the fog layer in real-time. The authors introduced an advanced backpropagation method for error correction and new performance metrics. The work tested new performance metrics Mathew correlation and Cohen's kappa coefficient during the simulation using the NSL-KDD dataset. Ref. [16] the work proposes a software-defined network SDN solution to monitor and update flow rules or routing rules for the entire fog network against DDoS. The SDN detaches the network device's hardware and software components, making device accessing and control realistic from a remote location. The researchers introduced two algorithms to enhance the DDoS detection performance of the traditional SDN. The first algorithm uses a sequential hypothesis to decide if a connection is normal or malicious. The rate-limiting algorithm observes the nodes' connection rates since a compromised node will want to connect to multiple nodes for attack propagation. Ref. [17] uses an anomaly-based approach to defend the system from DDoS attacks. The system adopted two different machine learning approaches: Naive Bayesian classifier, hidden Markov model, and virtual honey. The Bayesian classifier calculates the packet's probabilities as normal or malicious using the packet's source and destination bytes. The packet is further sent to the Markov model to determine the packet's state. If the probability is higher than the threshold value, the server sends the packet to the VHP device responsible for managing all log activities. The network administrator uses the log activities of the VHP device to monitor the entire network. To evaluate the proposed model, parameters, like True and False Negatives, True and False Positives, were tested. [18] demonstrated a mitigating scheme that uses both fog and cloud computing architecture to build a secured system. It deploys a defensive module in the SDN controller located in the fog server. The defender analyzes, predicts, and filters incoming packets against DDoS attacks using the network traffic information. The defender adopted SVM, Naive Bayes, and KNN, all ensembles, to help make decisions. The defender passes packets found to be legitimate to the cloud; otherwise, it drops the packet. The results obtained show that the CPU utilization and memory utilization are incredibly high during and after the attack compare to before the attack. The KNN performs best with 86% accuracy, while Naive Bayes performs at least 82.01% with the WEKA tool used for the simulation. Ref. [19] evaluates the performance of different machine learning algorithms, namely J48, random forest (RF), support vector machine (SVM), and K-nearest neighbor (KNN), to detect and secure the network against DDoS attacks. The evaluation process involves training and testing all the machine learning algorithms and adopt the best model to the network design's mitigating and prevention script. The Hping3 program using python helped to produce the normal and DDoS packets. The dataset's feature selection process was carried out with tshark, while Mininet and RYU controllers were used to create the SDN topology and controller, respectively. The experiment shows J48 as the best performing machine learning algorithm for the network design. [20] In this design, every SDN controllers maintain a list of IP addresses known as blacklist and possible victim. It also monitors the rate of incoming packets to compute the threshold value of each host. The blacklist IP address contains every host that exceeds the incoming packet threshold. In contrast, the possible victim list includes IP addresses of all the servers within the network since servers are mostly DDoS attack victims. The proposed model also uses two approaches in its operations, namely the comparator and the counter. The comparator component is responsible for comparing the packet count per IP address. If this packet count is greater than the previously calculated maximum threshold value (Packet count > Max Threshold), the system sends a message alert. The controller will then install the rule to drop all the incoming packets for that destination for some time, perceiving it as "malicious." The attacker's IP addresses and the possible victim are shared with the other SDN controllers through the Ethereum blockchain. If the packet count value does not exceed the maximum threshold value (Packet count < Max Threshold), it means no attack has occurred, and it will keep on comparing the packet. During an attack, when the other SDN controller receives the list of IP addresses, it checks whether any host in the network is sending packets to the host located in the "possible victim" list. If any host is sending the packets to the server located in the possible victim list, the SDN controller installs the rule to drop that host's packets. The counter is responsible for counting the packets by using the IP addresses of the senders. The timer will start periodically after every 15 secs. It counts the number of packets from all sender IPs. We use the counter's values to determine the "Average Threshold" value by sampling incoming packets. The simulation and analysis have proved that this scheme is quite efficient in reducing SDN controller overhead and detecting slow and fast DDoS attacks. Ref. [21] proposes an SDN framework and machine learning method to detect DDoS attacks. The researchers use three frameworks for the design: the traffic collection module helps collect traffic information. It sends the information traffic to the identification module, using support vector machine (SVM) to classify the packet as normal or malicious. The RYU controller is adopted in the design of the flow table design. The experiment is validated using the sci-kit-learn and KDD99 datasets to train and test the model design. Also tested are performance matric like True Positive (TP), False Positive (FP), False Negative (FN), and True Negative. Ref. [22] divide their model into four, i.e., the IoT/device model responsible for sensing, processing, communication, and each device has a threshold. The gateway model serves as a gateway for communication purposes. The smart contract model authorities the devices and ensures that they operate within the threshold. Lastly, the server/miner model takes care of the verification parts of the smart contract. The research work eradicates single-point-of-failure problems in most centralized architectural models, using blockchain based on a decentralized approach. The work also addressed the request for device message authentication. The simulation using the Ethereum GO client (geth) and the Linux client (ubuntu) as OS. The model is not appropriate where a large connection of IoT devices is required. It also involves high computation and processing capabilities, which is an additional task for the server.

4 Fog Computing Paradigm

Fog computing offers interchangeable services. It decentralizes cloud computing operations by introducing minimal computational process, analysis, and storage at the edge closer to the cloud service rather than forward to the cloud server for the process [10]. Fog computing aim at minimizing the distance data needs to travel for processing, thereby improving the network's overall performance. Fog computing was introduced in 2012 by the CISCO network and had gained wide adoption by organizations. Based on research findings and millions of data generated by IoT devices, the global fog computing market is projected at $188.2 billion in 2025, which will produce 79.4 zettabytes (ZB) of data [4–6]. Fog computing defers from cloud computing due to its decentralized operation.

The fog network comprises three hierarchical layers: terminal, fog, and cloud layers.

1. **The Terminal Layer**

The fog architecture's primary layer is the terminal layer, consisting of all thin and thick sensor-enabled devices. The devices in this layer are responsible for sensing and capturing data and can work in a heterogeneous network environment.

2. **The Fog Layer**:

The fog node is the center layer between the terminal and cloud layers that accommodate fog servers, routers, base stations, network gateways, and switches. The fog layer has six architectures; physical and virtualization, monitoring, pre-processing, temporary storage, security, and transport layer, as shown in Figs. 5 and 6.

a. **Physical and Virtualization Layer**: This layer is responsible for sensing and capturing data before sending it to the next layer for processing via a gateway.
b. **Monitoring Layer**: This node is responsible for monitoring all the nodes connected to the fog network.

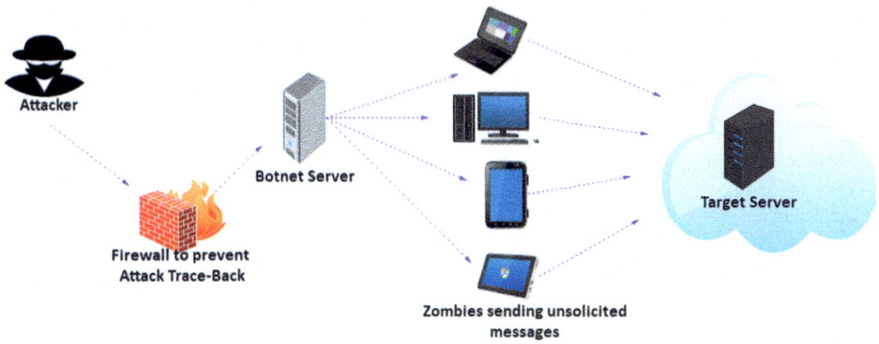

Fig. 5 DDoS attack scenario

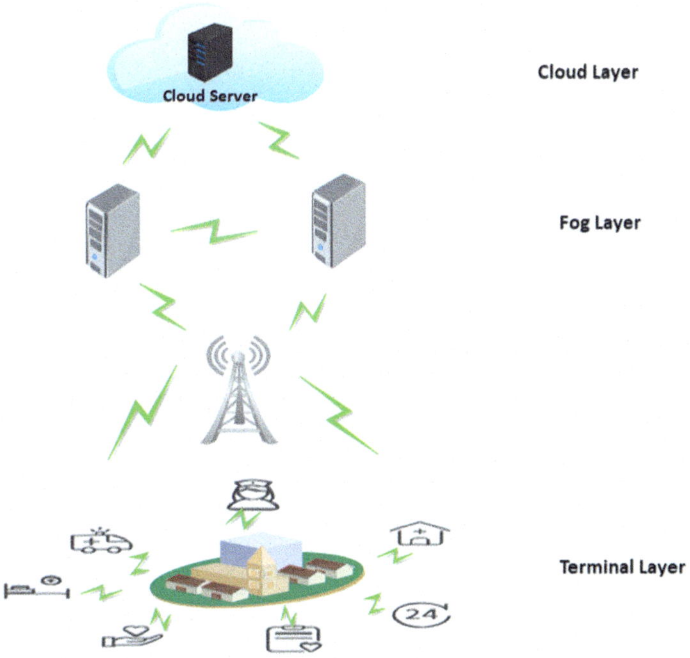

Fig. 6 Fog computer hierarchical architecture

c. **Pre-Processing Layer**: This layer performs feature extraction of meaningful information from multiple data sources within the fog network.
d. **Temporary Storage Layer**: The layer stores data temporarily before being sent to the cloud server for processing.
e. **Security Layer**: This layer ensures data integrity, accessibility, and confidentiality by providing security operations such as encryption and decryption, packet filtering.
f. **Transport Layer**: The layer establishes a secure connection between the fog server and the cloud server for data processing and storage.

3. **The Cloud Layer**:

This layer is the core of the entire network, where all devices that perform high computational processes and storage are situated and managed.

4.1 The Cloud and Fog Computing Differences

The fog node is not a substitute for the cloud network; instead, it provides complimentary service to the cloud network [10]. The deployment of a fog network is decentralized, while the cloud network provides a centralized deployment using the Internet. The figure below shows the difference and similarities between cloud and fog networks (Fig. 7).

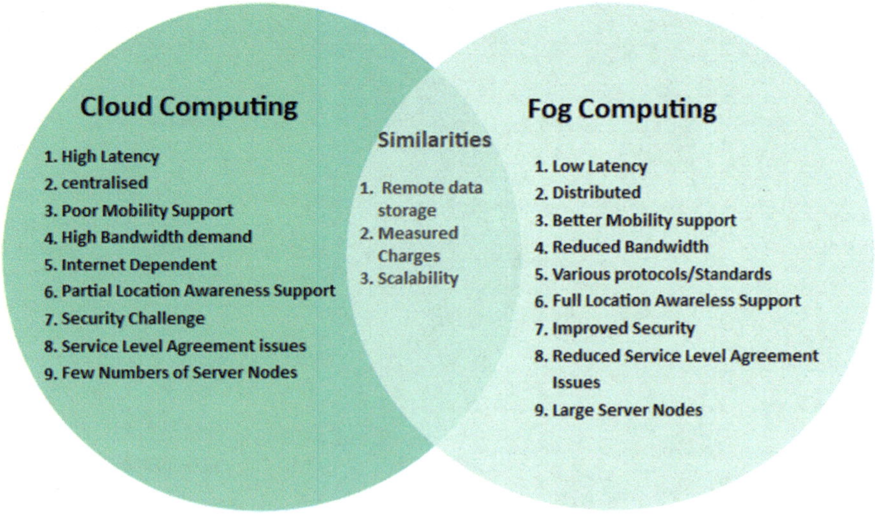

Fig. 7 Cloud and fog similarities and differences

4.2 Fog Computing Benefits in IoHT

Due to IoHT operations' sensitivity, network issues like response time delay, network connection failures, and high bandwidth affecting the IoHT service delivery are intolerable in the IoHT network. Also, the data generated by the IoHT monitoring sensors are enormous, and transferring such data to the cloud network will generate numerous challenges like bandwidth, latency, and security issues. Transferring parts of IoHT computational requirements to the fog layer closer to where the data originates will improve the IoHT service delivery efficiency and productivity. The fog network provides data aggregation to address bandwidth issues. Also, the closeness of IoHT to the fog layer reducing the distance data needs to travel for analysis and storage, thereby reducing the network latency and delay. The locator/ID separation (LISP) protocol to the fog network provides mobility support. The location awareness of fog helps in IoHT patient contact tracing and mobile monitoring. The fog also offers better security for IoHT providers and users as IoHT providers define their security requirements. The single point of failure faced by the traditional cloud networks is solved in fog networks as various protocols and standards are used to establish connections between the IoHT devices and the edge network. Among other areas of fog computing are shown in Fig. 8 below.

Fog computing areas of applications ranging from security, sensor networks, time-sensitive application [23]. Among the vital roles played by fog computing are:

1. **Vehicular Ad-Hoc Networks**

Fog computing has demonstrated a promising technique to solve time-sensitivity issues in a vehicular ad-hoc network by providing computational requirements at the network's edge, therefore satisfying the latency-sensitive tasks. The real-time

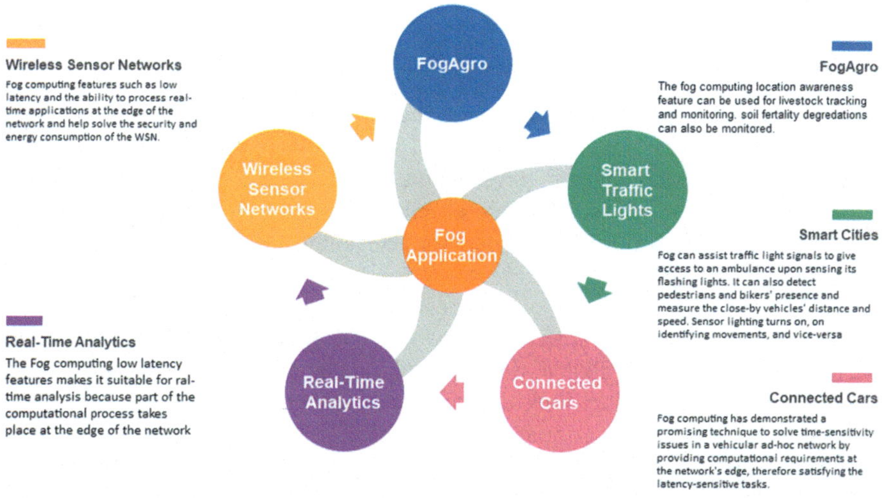

Fig. 8 Areas of applications of fog computing

interaction of fog computing can also support autonomous vehicles, which provide features such as automatic steering and self-parking.

2. **Smart Traffic Light**

Fog can assist traffic light signals to give access to an ambulance upon sensing its flashing lights. It can also detect pedestrians and bikers' presence and measure the close-by vehicles' distance and speed. Sensor lighting turns on, on identifying movements, and vice-versa.

3. **Wireless Sensors and Actuators**

The critical challenges of WSN are energy consumption and security. Fog computing features such as low latency and the ability to process real-time applications at the edge of the network and help solve the security and energy consumption of the WSN.

4. **Health Data Management**

Health data management is an excellent concern for cloud users, as health data contains crucial information that can jeopardize patients privacy when compromised. Fog computing makes it possible to realize a patient's goal of locally taking possession of part of the health data rather than pushing the entire data to the cloud.

5 Leveraging IoHT Cloud Services with Fog Network

Integrating the fog layer between the IoHT device and the cloud network has improved the efficiency and solves the challenges of the traditional IoHT cloud networks mentioned above. This integration introduced new network architecture layers to the IoHT, including medical sensors and actuators, smart e-health gateways, and a cloud platform.

1. **Medical Sensors and Actuators**

These are primarily wireless IoHT devices characterized by limited power resources and can sense medical data from the patient irrespective of location or respond to the fog networks' commands. Figure 9 below shows a sweat sensor that can detect and analyze sodium, potassium, glucose, and lactate elements found in sweat and communicate the data to IoHT providers for decision making.

2. **Smart e-health Gateways**

The Fog network supports numerous protocols, platforms, and data formats because the fog network is a distributed system, unlike a centralized cloud network [24]. This layer is an intermediary node or bridge to connect to the cloud network. Little computational activities like storage, process, and data analysis are carried out at this layer instead of pushing to the cloud, therefore improving patients' data security, latency, real-time interaction, and support data mobility (Fig. 10).

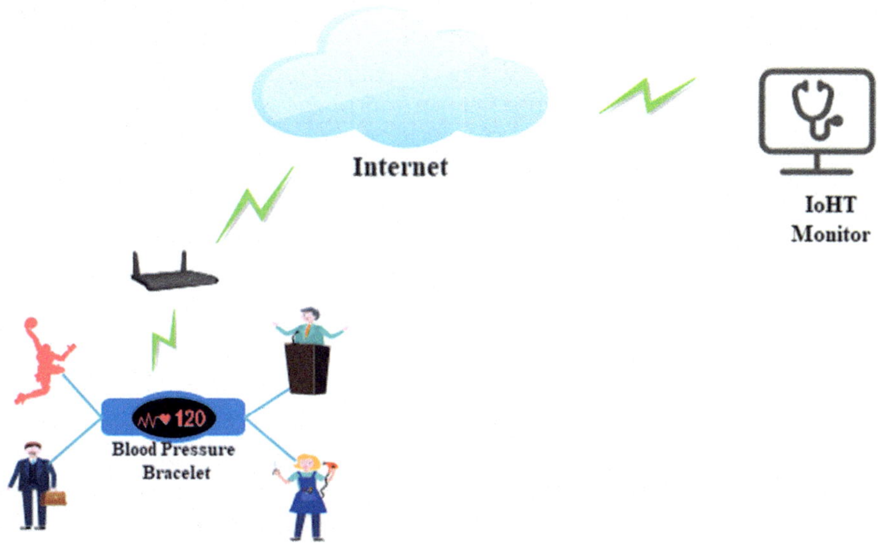

Fig. 9 Blood pressure remote monitoring

Fig. 10 Smart fog gateway

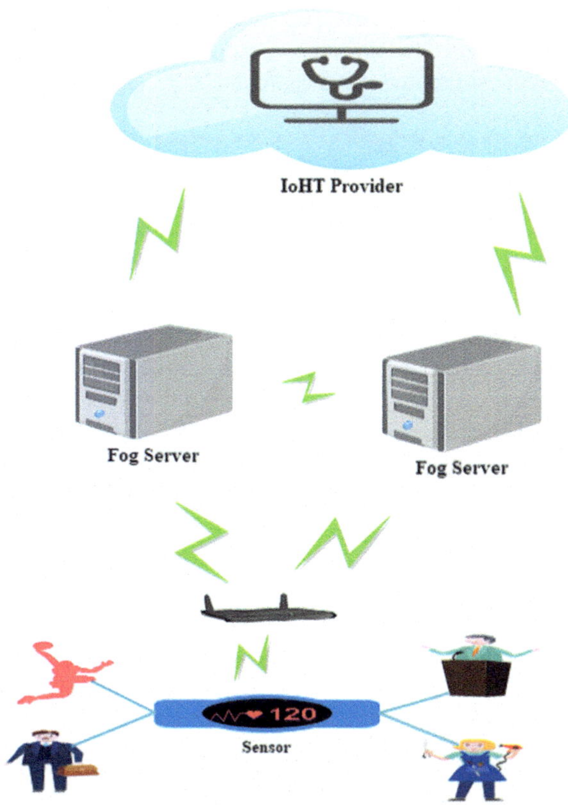

3. **Cloud Platform**

Cloud computing is storing and accessing computing powers like storage, network, memory over a network, typically, the Internet from a remote server/location on a pay-as-you-use service. The cloud can scale upward and downward resources based on users' requirements [6]. Cloud computing is distinct from the traditional client/server network because of its specific features, like; broad network access, rapid elasticity, resource pooling, on-demand self-service, and pay-as-you-use service.

6 Proposed Framework

Putting the IoHT DDoS attack challenge in perspective, researchers propose different approaches such as using a machine learning approach to differentiate normal and malicious packets, packet filtering methods, and software-defined networks SDN. However, the attack pattern of DDoS is not static, which poses a difficult challenge for the packet filtering approach, and the lack of a recent dataset to validate the machine learning approach makes is also a concern. This research proposes a packet filtering technique that computes the network delay and the server's response time and compares the medical data threshold values. If the value is higher than the server's threshold, the system sends a captcha to the incoming packets' source address and the request granted if the captcha is correct. Otherwise, the packet dropped.

6.1 Problem Formulation

Let C be medical cloud server ($k = 1, 2, 3\dots\dots.C$), F be the fog server ($g = 1, 2, 3\dots.F$), and S be the number of switches ($w = 1, 2, 3\dots\dots\dots S$) connected to the medical cloud and fog servers. Each server has a maximum number of switches connected to it as the server utilization μ is limited. The total network delay di represents the cloud server's delay to the fog Cfi and Cfi the delay from the fog to the IoHT devices i such that ($n = 1, 2, 3\dots\dots\dots i$). The server response time, which decreases beyond a threshold T during DDoS attacks, is represented as RT. The threshold T is set for every cloud and fog server, as shown in Fig. 9

The Network Delay

The total IoHT devices connected to the network is represented with i

$$i = \sum_{n=1}^{i}(J + b + c) \tag{1}$$

J, b, and c represent the IoHT device, the sensors/actuators, and the communication channel, respectively.

The network delay between the cloud SDN server and the fog server

$$C_{Fg} = \sum_{k=1}^{F} (x_{ik} - l_{ek}) \quad (2)$$

where $(x_{ik} - l_{ek})$ are the inter-arrival rate of first and second packets.

The network delay between the fog and IoHT device i (Fig. 11)

$$F_{gi} = \sum_{g=1}^{F} (y_{ig} - l_{eg}) \quad (3)$$

The total network delays

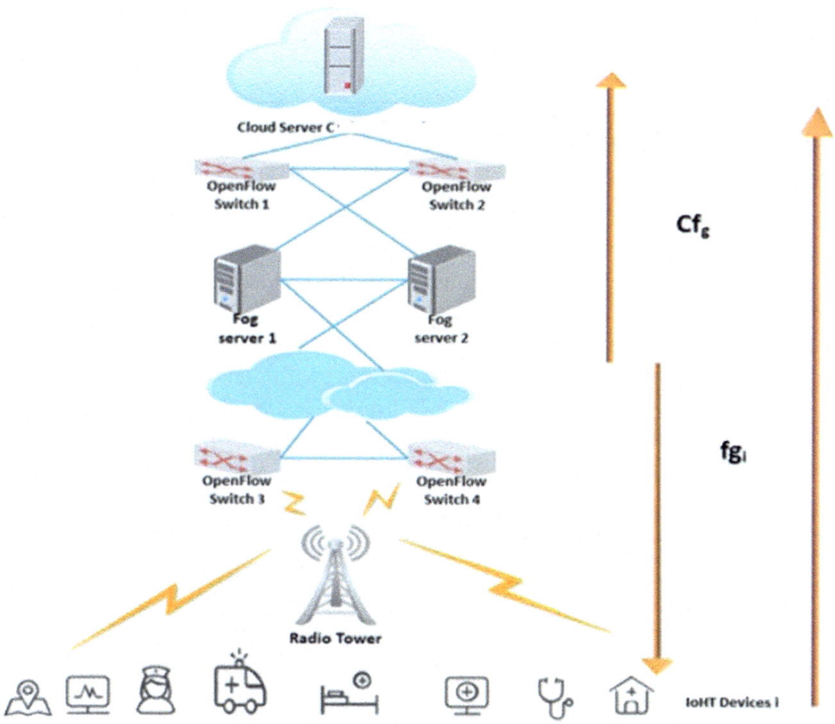

Fig. 11 Fog-to-cloud communication architecture

$$di = \sum_{k=1}^{F} (x_{ik} - l_{ek}) + \sum_{g=1}^{F} \left(y_{ig} - l_{eg}\right) \tag{4}$$

The Server Response Time

This is the total time it takes a server ($k = 1, 2, 3.........c$) to receive and respond to a packet request ($n = 1, 2, 3........i$). where packet arrival rate is β_i and server utilization μ_i

$$RT_i(\beta) = P_s/s\mu_i - \beta_i + 1/\mu_i \tag{5}$$

P_s is the server usage probability, s is the number of connection switches ($w = 1, 2, 3.... S$), and β_i is the arrival rate of all switches connected to the network server

$$\beta_i = \sum_{w=1}^{S} \beta_w \tag{6}$$

7 Result Discussion

When a packet arrives at the fog server, it compares the incoming packet's packet size with the fog server's threshold value. Suppose the compared value is lower than the fog server threshold. In that case, the fog server processes the packets, such as packet B and C in Fig. 12. When the network is under attack, the attacker sends unsolicited packet A to multiple legitimate users through a botnet server, as shown in Fig. 12. All the multiply legitimate devices from within and outside the network send unsolicited packets A to the server. The fog mitigation model proposed in this situation computes the fog and cloud server utilization and network delay. If the computed values are higher than the threshold, the fog server sends captcha Z to the user to resolve. Since the legitimate user is not aware of the packet request, such a captcha becomes unprocessed by the user, which forces the network to drop such a packet in a situation where the network is the peak of packet requests (all packets are legitimate). The request is greater than the network threshold. If users solve all the captcha requests, the cloud migrates to another cloud server between the cloud server ($k = 1, 2, 3........C$) with a higher threshold, as shown in Figure 12, to accommodate the legitimate request.

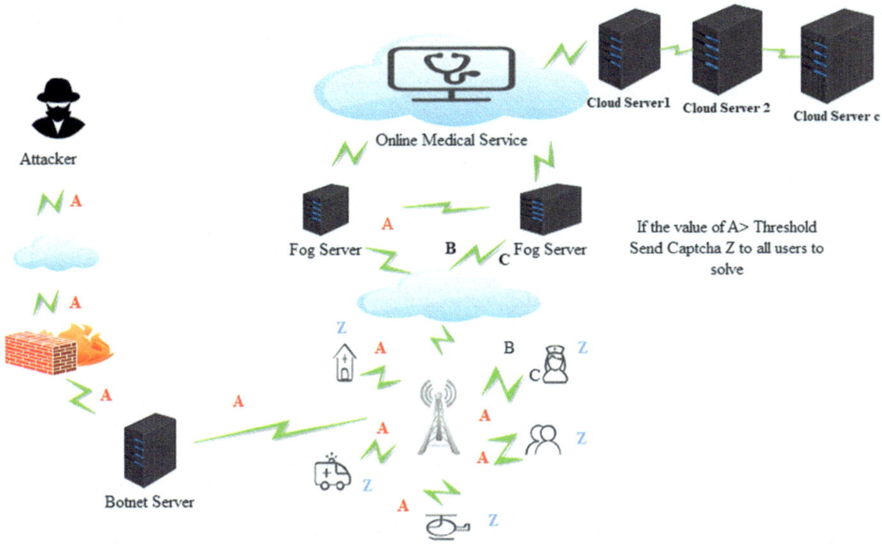

Fig. 12 DDoS mitigation architecture

8 Conclusion

The migration of parts of the IoHT service delivery from cloud to fog computing provides a vast opportunity for both IoHT service providers and patients in improving their efficiency and productivity as cloud computing faces numerous challenges like security, mobility support, and latency. Introducing fog computing to the architecture brings minimal computational requirements closer to IoHT users, reducing the cloud network latency issue and strengthening its security. Among other benefits of fog computing are mobility supports and real-time application interactions. Unfortunately, the fog is open to DDoS security challenges that pose a significant threat to IoHT data availability and integrity.

In this research, the authors describe IoT, IoHT, and its connection with the cloud network and the challenges faced by IoHT-to-cloud networks. Also, the research introduces fog nodes as an architectural framework to mitigate DDoS attacks in traditional IoHT-to-cloud server architecture. The fog node compares the incoming packets' impact with the server's utilization rate and the average network delay with its threshold. If the utilization and delay are higher than the threshold, the fog server sends a captcha to the packet's source address to resolve. If the captcha is successful, the fog forwards the packet to the cloud server and migrates the request to the cloud server with more enormous resources; otherwise, if the captcha fails, the packets are dropped. The fog node packet filtering is a promising technique with fewer computational requirements, and experimental validation of the approach can be carried out in future work.

References

1. Internet of Healthcare Things (IoHT) Trends. https://www.eseye.com/internet-of-healthcare-things-ioht-trends
2. Maksimović, M. (2017). The roles of nanotechnology and the internet of nano things in healthcare transformation. *TecnoLógicas, 20*(40), 139–153.
3. Zhou, L., Guo, H., & Deng, G. (2019). A fog computing-based approach to DDoS mitigation in IIoT systems. *Computers and Security, 85*, 51–62.
4. Benefits of Internet of Things (IoT) in our Lives and Businesses. https://www.tech21century.com/internet-of-things-iot-benefits
5. Help Net Security. https://www.helpnetsecurity.com/2019/06/21/connected-iot-devices-forecast
6. Sethi, P., & Sarangi, S. (2017). Internet of things: Architectures, protocols, and applications. *Journal of Electrical and Computer Engineering*, 1–25.
7. Reasons You Need an IoT Device Management Platform. https://behrtech.com/blog/5-reasons-you-need-an-iot-device-management-platform
8. Chandrasekaran, K. (n.d.). *Essentials of cloud computing*. 14–17.
9. Ahmed, M., & Kim, H. (2017). DDoS attack mitigation in internet of things using software defined networking. *2017 IEEE third international conference on big data computing service and applications (BigDataService).*
10. DoS (Denial of Service) Attack Tutorial: Ping of Death, DDOS. https://whyihacker.blogspot.com/2017/04/dos-denial-of-service-attack-tutorial.html
11. Osanaiye, O. (2015). Short paper: IP spoofing detection for preventing DDoS attack in cloud computing. *2015 18th international conference on intelligence in next generation networks.*
12. Zhang, P., Zhou, M., & Fortino, G. (2018). Security and trust issues in fog computing: A survey. *Future Generation Computer Systems, 88*, 16–27.
13. Paharia, B., & Bhushan, K. (2018). Fog computing as a defensive approach against distributed denial of service (DDoS): A proposed architecture. *2018 9th international conference on computing, communication and networking technologies (ICCCNT)* (p. 7).
14. Maharaja, R., Iyer, P., & Ye, Z. (2019). A hybrid fog-cloud approach for securing the internet of things. *Cluster Computing, 23*(2), 451–459.
15. Almiani, M., AbuGhazleh, A., Al-Rahayfeh, A., Atiewi, S., & Razaque, A. (2020). Deep recurrent neural network for IoT intrusion detection system. *Simulation Modelling Practice and Theory, 101*, 102031.
16. Singh, S., Kumari, K., Gupta, S., Dua, A., & Kumar, N., (2020). Detecting different attack instances of DDoS vulnerabilities on edge network of fog computing using gaussian Naive bayesian classifier. *2020 IEEE international conference on communications workshops (ICC Workshops).*
17. Priyadarshini, R., Kumar Barik, R., & Dubey, H. (2020). Fog-SDN: A light mitigation scheme for DDoS attack in fog computing framework. *International Journal of Communication Systems, 33*(9), 1–13.
18. Rahman, O., Quraishi, M., & Lung, C. (2019). DDoS attacks detection and mitigation in SDN using machine learning. *2019 IEEE world congress on services (SERVICES)*, (pp. 184–189).
19. Ahmed, Z., Afaqui, N., & Humayun, O. (2019). Detection and prevention of DDoS attacks on software defined networks controllers for smart grid. *International Journal of Computer Applications, 181*(45), 16–21.
20. Yang, L., & Zhao, H. (2018). DDoS attack identification and defense using SDN based on machine learning method. *2018 15th international symposium on pervasive systems, algorithms and networks (I-SPAN)* (pp. 174–178).
21. Javaid, U., Siang, A., Aman, M., & Sikdar, B. (2018). Mitigating loT device-based DDoS attacks using blockchain. *Proceedings of the 1st workshop on cryptocurrencies and blockchains for distributed systems* (pp.71–76).

22. Rodrigues, J., De Rezende Segundo, D., Junqueira, H., Sabino, M., Prince, R., Al-Muhtadi, J., & De Albuquerque, V. (2018). Enabling technologies for the internet of health things. *IEEE Access, 6*, 13129–13141.
23. Negash, B., Gia, T., Anzanpour, A., Azimi, I., Jiang, M., Westerlund, T., Rahmani, A., Liljeberg, P., & Tenhunen, H. (2017). Leveraging fog computing for healthcare IoT. *Fog computing in the internet of things* (pp. 145–169).
24. Hussain, M., & Beg, M. (2019). Fog computing for internet of things (IoT)-aided smart grid architectures. *Big Data and Cognitive Computing, 3*(1), 8.
25. Atlam, H., Walters, R., & Wills, G. (2018). Fog computing and the internet of things: A review. *Big Data and Cognitive Computing, 2*(2), 10.
26. Tomovic, S., Yoshigoe, K., Maljevic, I., & Radusinovic, I. (2016). Software-defined fog network architecture for IoT. *Wireless Personal Communications, 92*(1), 181–196.
27. Yassein, M., Hmeidi, I., Al-Harbi, M., Mrayan, L., Mardini, W., & Khamayseh, Y. (2019). IoT-based healthcare systems. *Proceedings of the second international conference on data science, E-learning and information systems—DATA '19.*
28. Sadiq, K., Thompson, A., & Ayeni, A. (2020). Mitigating DDoS attacks in cloud network using fog and SDN: A conceptual security framework. *International Journal of Applied Information Systems, 12*(32), 11–16.
29. Fakeeh, K. (2016). An overview of DDOS attacks detection and prevention in the cloud. *International Journal of Applied Information Systems, 11*(7), 25–34.
30. Hannache, O., & Batouche, M. (2020). Neural network-based approach for detection and mitigation of DDoS attacks in SDN environments. *International Journal of Information Security and Privacy, 14*(3), 50–71.
31. Ramesh, D., Edla, D., & Sharma, R. (2020). HHDSSC: Harnessing healthcare data security in cloud using ciphertext policy attribute-based encryption. *International Journal of Information and Computer Security, 13*(3/4), 322.
32. Liu, J., Yuan, C., Lai, Y., & Qin, H. (2020). Protection of sensitive data in industrial internet based on three-layer local/fog/cloud storage. *Security and Communication Networks, 2020*, 1–16.
33. Parameswari, R., & Vani, K. (2018). Mobile cloud-privacy and data security in healthcare environment using cloudsim simulator. *International Journal of Engineering and Technology, 7*(3.27), 220.
34. Ramasamy, B., & Hameed, A. (2019). Classification of healthcare data using hybridised fuzzy and convolutional neural network. *Healthcare Technology Letters, 6*(3), 59–63.
35. Guan, Y., Shao, J., Wei, G., & Xie, M. (2018). Data security and privacy in fog computing. *IEEE Network, 32*(5), 106–111.
36. Somani, V., & Trivedi, D. (2019). Utilizing cloud computing for stronger healthcare data security. *Journal of Advanced Research in Dynamical and Control Systems, 11*(11), 60–69.
37. Sarrab, M., & Alshohoumi, F. (2021). Assisted-fog-based framework for IoT-based healthcare data preservation. *International Journal of Cloud Applications and Computing, 11*(2), 1–16.
38. Biswas, S. (2018). Fog and cloud computing based smart healthcare: A framework. *International Journal of Computer Applications, 181*(6), 22–27.
39. Thota, C., Sundarasekar, R., Manogaran, G., Varatharajan, R., & Priyan, M. (2018). Centralized fog computing security platform for IoT and cloud in healthcare system. *Exploring the convergence of big data and the internet of things* (pp. 141–154).
40. Maragathavalli, P., Atchaya, S., Kaliyaperumal, N., & Saranya, S. (2021). Cloud data security model using modified decoy technique in fog computing for e-healthcare. *IOP Conference Series: Materials Science and Engineering, 1065*(1), 012044.
41. Singhal, A., & Singhal, N. (2021). Cloud computing versus fog computing: A comparative study. *International Journal of Advanced Networking and Applications, 12*(04), 4627–4632.

Gestation Risk Prediction Based on Feature Extraction and Neural Networks

E. Rajkumar, V. Geetha, and G. Sindhujha Sekar

1 Introduction

The inventive designing techniques have assumed a significant part in medication territory to assist specialists with accomplishing the ideal results viably. The clinical area cannot function productively, endure and enhance its reality without designing innovation mediation; if it was followed back, clinical examinations are supposed to change the human body's internal actions over the long term. A territory of medication that needs prompt care from specialized methods is looked at by women during their gestation because of distortion of organic conditions. Around 795 ladies biting the dust from gestation 4 and* childbirth avoidable wellsprings, 98 percent of which are* in developing* countries. The percentage level of maternal* mortality ratio has been reduced to about 845% in the year between 1990 and 2015. Around 20 million ladies, overall endure chronic sickness consistently because of gestation. In 1990, approximately 377,000 ladies passed on because of gestation complexity, which dropped to 293,000 every 2013. Among the 288,000* women who died* during the conveyance process, most of whom were rescued and the lion's share of them in low-office environments. Individuals that have encountered complications when conceiving their offspring or adopting a technique.

Previously, due to proper medication care, all the lives of pregnant women and babies will be over. Most maternal* deaths are escapable as* components to avoid or handle inconvenience. Fetal pulse the total FHR ranges between 120 and 155 BPM during the uterine cycle. It is visible sonographically for about a month and a half

E. Rajkumar (✉)
Department of Computer Science, Pondicherry Engineering College, Puducherry 605014, India

V. Geetha
Departement of Information Technology, Pondicherry Engineering College, Puducherry 605014, India

G. S. Sekar
Department of Obstetrics and Gynecology, Svmch & Rc, Ariyur, Puducherry, India

A. K. Tyagi et al. (eds.), *Intelligent Interactive Multimedia Systems for e-Healthcare Applications*, https://doi.org/10.1007/978-981-16-6542-4_7

and achieves shifts during the turn of events,. Normally, the FHR has been reduced to about 130 bpm at the end of the day, and then it is maximum in the morning of about 170 bpm at 70 days. Usually, at that point, the FHR beats anywhere in the range of 100 and 120 every moment (bpm). In the following 14–21 days, FHR shifts bit by bit and becomes: 5–6 weeks ~110 bpm (mean) ~170 bpm more than 9–10 weeks Usual FHR drops: ~151 bpm to 98 days ~142 bpm to 140 days ~131 bpm for each term. A beat-to-beat* variation of about 5 to 14 thumps can be allowed at any time [1], whereas the heart rate in a good embryo is usually regular.

The phase of incubation or gestation of a lady is a stage that may convey intricacies for both the mother and the hatchling. The fetal wellbeing might be influenced by the versatile maternal changes during this period, just as by the mother's clinical history and maternal/familial ascribes. Along these lines, the perception of fetal wellbeing and antenatal consideration during this stage is significant for maternal and fetal wellbeing [2]. Clinicians (particularly gynecologists) wish to educate the guardians about their unborn newborn children's prosperity, and they do, given effectively examined cases and past encounters. Consequently, characterizing the conceivable familial (overwhelmingly maternal) clinical information which is inclined to impact fetal wellbeing would help antenatal maternal consideration.

Notwithstanding, persistent situated medical services probably won't be done entirely because of specific challenges, such as an inadequate number of clinics close to the patient's whereabouts (towns remote in the provincial territories) or stuffed clinics in urban communities. In Turkey, m-Health programs that give admittance to wellbeing administrations and wellbeing data through versatile administrations are set up on a public level [3], where portable cell memberships cover 96.02%, and Internet clients cover 53.74% of the number of inhabitants in Turkey [4]. These foundations and portable administrations show the solid and essential job m-Health plays in lacking conditions.

The part of computerized reasoning in medical care for pregnant ladies. To survey AI's job in ladies' wellbeing, find holes, and examine AI's eventual fate in motherly wellbeing. An intentional survey of English papers using EMBASE, PubMed, and SCOPUS. The words of the quest included gestation and AI. Examination papers and book sections were incorporated, while the collection of papers, articles and notes were omitted from the survey. Included articles on gestation and AI methods and referred to pharmacological intercessions. We distinguished 376 detailed investigations from our inquiries. For the survey, a final arrangement of 31 papers was implemented. Included articles discussed several gestation issues and multidisciplinary applications of AI. Scarcely any tests associated with gestation, AI, and pharmacology, and we carefully survey those inquiries. Outside approval of prototypes and strategies depicted in the examinations is restricted, obstructing the investigations' generalizability [5].

Artificial intelligence (AI) is defined as the intelligence of machines, as opposed to the intelligence of humans or other living species [1, 6]. AI can also be defined as the study of "intelligent agents" that is, any agent or device that can perceive and understand its surroundings and accordingly take appropriate action to maximize its chances of achieving its objectives [2]. AI also refers to situations wherein machines can simulate human minds in learning and analysis, and thus can work in problem solving. This kind of intelligence is also referred to as machine learning (ML) [3]. Typically, AI involves a system that consists of both software and hardware. From a software perspective, AI is particularly concerned with algorithms. An artificial neural network (ANN) is a conceptual framework for executing AI algorithms [4]. It is a mimic of the human brain—an interconnected network of neurons, in which there are weighted communication channels between neurons [5]. One neuron can react to multiple stimuli from neighboring neurons and the whole network can change its state according to different inputs from the environment [7]. As a result, the neural network (NN) can generate outputs as its responses to environmental stimuli—just as the human brain reacts to different environmental changes. NNs are typically layered structures of various configurations. Researchers have devised NNs that can do supervised learning, where the task is to infer a function that maps an input to an output based on example pairs of inputs and outputs; unsupervised learning, where the task is to learn from test data that has not been labeled, classified, or categorized, in order to identify common features in the data and, rather than responding to system feedback, to react based on the existence or inexistence of identified common features in new data; and reinforced learning, where the task is to act within the given surroundings in order to maximize rewards and minimize penalties, both according to some form of accumulative nature [8]. With the advancement of computation power, NNs have become "deeper," meaning that more layers of neurons are involved in the network to mimic a human brain and carry out learning. In addition, more functions can be incorporated into the NN, such as merging feature extraction and classification functions into a single deep network—hence, the technical term "deep learning."

2 Review of Literature

The most widely used hazard prototypical for PTB in the local obstetric region relies on a mixture of obstetric history, small baby fibronectin testing, and cervical components. A woman with a past marked at 26 weeks by previous preterm transport. However, in an analysis by the National Institute of Child Health and Human Development of the Maternal-Fetal System, with a typical cervical cycle and negative fetal fibronectin status, there is an 8 percent chance of PTB in her subsequent gestation [6]. If either test was positive, PTB predictive capacity increased from 28 percent to 30%, and if both tests were positive, it grew to 66%. The most common application of fetal fibronectin testing is for: (1) suggestive patients with a cervical width of less than 3 cm and a [1] risk assessment for PTB (i.e., women experiencing compression within the 24–36 week range) and the use of cervical length or fetal fibronectin status in screening for preterm transport hazards in acceptable inhabitants [2] is not confirmed by existing evidence. The risk of PTB from gestation is often not expected in these tests; they only become more alert when PTB is calculated as the predicted date of birth methods. (Dr. C. R. Walker, neonatologist and Medical Director of Critical Care at the Children's Hospital of Eastern Ontario, and

Dr S. W. Wen, pediatric disease transmission specialist at the Children's Hospital of Ottawa, Ottawa). Before 22 weeks (23 weeks being the most timely age during which longevity usually is conceivable), the methodology should be ready to assess PTB hazards. It will be material for the whole inhabitants, not only a subcategory of suggestive patients. Fiore substantiates this knowledge: "Most medications intended to forestall preterm birth are not all-around compelling and are relevant to just a little level of ladies in danger for preterm birth. A more level headed way to deal with the mediation will require a superior comprehension of the systems prompting preterm birth" [3]. The prospect of defining women at risk of preterm birth in an even more precise way by using obstetric and socio-demographic data would make it possible to take prior deterrent measures [4]. The logarithmic impact capacity file is used to streamline both power and accuracy during the mining of slanted information [5] and the programmed collector working mark (ROC) estimate bends. Over the previous decade, with a multilayer perceptron based on feed forward back proliferation, the designers explored numerous avenues for various ANN designs. They achieved excellent neural organization learning calculations using an exaggerated digression stage to function with a weight-end choice. An ANN multilayer perceptron with one veiled level is exceptionally well known for clinical information mining procedure. Clinical knowledge is accepted as non-linear, with numerous obscure partnerships, and the enclosed layer allows higher-request measurements to be identified [7]. Moreover, there has been little proof to propose that utilizing more than one shrouded layer gives a preferable outcome over utilizing one concealed layer [8]. Nine organizational boundaries have been used to guide the accumulation of learning rate; flexible scale factors of learning rate (addition of learning rate and decrease in learning rate); steady weight-rotation, which determines how strongly burdens are punished; versatile factors of weight-rotation (constant increase in weight rot and consistent reduction in gauge rot). The boundary estimates characterize how the neural organization's loads and predispositions are adjusted from age to age as an aspect of the entire square error calculated in fully prepared cases [9]. At least 25 years of age should be needed to provide a suitable learning period. The commodity developments from one boundary to the next immediately, putting forward the best boundary esteem before hitting the stale point. The architectural advances until nine close focal topics are created, and the consequences are then discarded from the pre-eminent execution organization. As a result, all organizational structures (characterized by the number of enclosed layers and the number of enclosed hubs in the confined layers) are verified by the ANN programming: the non-attendance is to route from a solitary level without held seats to a two-level with two enclosed hubs, to a two-level with 2N+1 enclosed corners, where N is the number of info factors [10]. Based on the Kolmogorov superposition theorem, updated to the ANN setting, this furthest cut-off was chosen, suggesting that the most oversized numeral of enclosed hubs required would be no more than multiple periods the amount of information source hubs in addition to one [11].

3 Problem Statement

Decreased fetal oxygen levels can lead to fetal hazards, such as fetal hypoxia. Due to UC, the oxygen level is lowered, which can further impact FHR, directly related to the oxygen level. Early hypoxic fetus prediction will assist clinicians with a machine learning technique to save the patient's life. Fetal movement is due to fetal hypoxia as well. In worse cases, it causes permanent impairment or even death. Fetal hypoxia can affect long-term neurological problems, brain development, and increased CNS risk. Fetal hypoxia diagnosis among extensive patient data depends on multiple variables such as the incidence and severity of hypoxia, medical history, personage, and overall health. Accurate diagnosis or best treatment for fetal hypoxia is challenging to identify. Existing technical requirements provide an accuracy of 99.85% better than the individual CTG classifier for hypoxic fetus classification. The study used a comprehensive approach in classifying fetal states and fetal sufferings—those are the initial stages of hypoxic fetuses that are valuable for our research and physicians to make better bioinformatics predictions. Process speed after the inclusion of more features is a model constraint that needs improvement. Materials and methods: Research, integrated unstructured, and structured collected the information from the clinical database from 24,877 pregnancies between 2010 and 2015 from the InfoSaude framework to decide how DNN-KER techniques might better assist in the hazard evaluation of unsuccessful labor all through gestation. Primary information covering the vast majority of the segment and clinical history of pre-gestation were joined with supplementary unstructured data slice into this utilization case, which was removed from brief history notes of clinical conditions, sensitivities, and illnesses. The clinical information from material science is confined to 50–100 characters. Essential standard articulations could remove the most predominant realities and language signals for potential invalidations.

At last, for around 2.5% of the references in every one of the medication and disease sets considered, the ensemble supervised likeness. The AI calculation was utilized to recognize and combine positive and physically tried misspelling. Gestation diseases are a typical reason for horribleness and mortality among moms, babies and children, prompting early termination, preterm births or fetal passings, and fetal distortions, and development imperatives. Contaminations may have indications like those of non-pregnant ladies that are asymptomatic or show, and their likelihood of turning out to be pregnant relies upon elements, for example, (a) financial and social factors, (b) populace predominance of disease, and (c) activities looking for wellbeing and wellbeing. Notwithstanding, we found no systematic method to gather information on an assortment of variables considered in this investigation, for example, the historical backdrop of contaminations among the populace examined, of which just 2.5% of pregnancies had a background marked by disease-related with their separate EHR.

3.1 Research Gap for Gestation Related Processes

In this inspecting analysis, it has been perceived that AI has been usable to an extensive degree of gestation connected intervals. The producers have agreed to isolate 18 percent of the results as part of the motherly/fetal achievement (M/F prospering) meeting, where no unique period has been tended to or pronounced. The primary clarification behind the current was to enhance maternal/fetal prosperity. In 12.2% of studies, fetal status has been cultivated to be monitored by GDM delivery surrenders, preterm birth, fetal new growth, toxemia, death, blood pressure complications, function and development, and enthusiastic flourishing.

Various cycles class is outlined by inspects tending to press insufficiency, placental issues deliberate finish of gestation (VIP), postnatal anxiety bothers each; unique sclerosis unforeseen work, HELLP issue, blood glucose, diabetes mellitus and head lupus erythematosus (SLE) each. To have zeroed in more than one gestation measure:

Preterm birth and unforeseen fetal development
Blood pressure issues
Pre-eclampsia and toxemia
Energetic prosperity.

Curiously, most of the evaluated considered separated genuine thriving related issues, while just 5.1% of findings completed appraisal identified with eager success issues, such as sadness or stress. In going with subsections, every gestation participation gathering will be inspected.

Fetal condition: The maximum of AI implementations in mentioning the fetal condition and flourishing was fantastically differentiated by results in this course of action. We see strategies that can assess maternal and fetal prosperity and efficiency, as may also be used as average fetal outcomes (for example, abnormalities revelation). ML has been practicing in most of the findings, trailed by CI, DM, IDSS, NLP, and VIS. Stores as information foundation have been portrayed by 78% of results. Publications inside this social event have offered clarification to operate CTG stories. The documents were collects from the educational collection of the "UCI ML Registry CTG", which contains 2126 FHR and uterine pressure factor assessments. Tests in this illuminating combination are excessive. Meanwhile, it comprises 70% evaluations of normal fetal condition, 20% accept the situation, and 10% unstable condition.

Inside this request, considers applied a type of information strategy: join choice, SMOTE, and discharge of boisterous information. One evaluation gathered CTG information from the Cardiotocography Databank, comprising aggregate accounts and applied part affirmation techniques for information arrangement. Data were collected from the Daisy educational list as fetal ECG stories were gathered from the instructive assortment as maternal stomach ECG accounts. Regulated learning demand assignments have been performed by all articles in this social event, and different existing works moreover applied execution learning as DR procedures.

Gathering procedures (additionally, solo learning) have been addressed. NLP frameworks have been functional to explore patient's ideas and responses on pre-birth tests (noticeable and non-meddlesome). The information has been amassed as client posts from online media. As of late referred to takes a gander, detailed wellsprings of knowledge are viewed as isolated since the information has been recorded at an earlier second. Regular information gathering has been addressed considers. Regardless of anything else, utilized for far away perception (home checking) of the fetal state and flourishing, joining the course framework and the fetal heartbeat.

Furthermore, the suspicion structure (part of the e-flourishing framework) utilized information amassed from clinical staff. The versatile presentation (also part of the e-success network), proposed to be used through patients and clinical advantages subject matter experts, amassed ceaseless information directly from human data. Finally, for fetal ECG accounts, continuous cumulative knowledge from PDAs and sensors was registered. A 16.6% of this class's results referred to the possibility that the predicted outcome could be used by the end constant (e-flourishing framework), by subject matter specialists (structure) for therapeutic benefits, or both (e-thriving framework).

Genetic flaws: Between 9% of findings that measured labor absconds, the accentuation is resolved to aneuploidy revelation, a gauge of typical blemishes and assumption. More minor examinations watched out for hypothesis for appraisal of the association among poisons and macrosomia, fetal heartbeat course of action, assessment of birth absconds giving insights about online media and portrayal of drugs prosperity in gestation. In addition to one AI use, many evaluations from this class deliberated for their inspirations, and ML was usable in various examinations. DM, CI, ace structure, VIS, and NLP are the other AI requests found. Most tests presented gathering activities, and two investigations introduced grouping criteria. Projected things are prototypes except for prototypes that provide an expert framework for modeling natural distortions in live births, similar to a work area framework consisting of experts in clinical benefits. The overview of counts is provided with all-out; LR and RF are among the most executed figures in this class at any rate. Diverse sources of data grouping have been used. More than one foundation was included in 42.9% of the findings. Clinical records, thought around, prosperity foundations, vaults, clinical material, electronic media and data generated by PC aggregate knowledge. Human data have been assembled by methods for overviews in 2 assessments, from which accumulated data continuously. 35.7% of findings uncovered using imbalanced instructive records. K-suggests figuring (solo getting the hang of, grouping technique) was represented to be used for diminishing the number of occupants in the more significant part class, and over-under looking at systems have been used.

Gestation-induced diabetes: A 8.3% of all assessments included have guided GDM analysis, providing the goals: hypothesis and observation. In this class, most of the evaluations made prototypes for GDM notion, followed by judgment very predictable partnership for GDM seeing from home and an expert framework for early attestation. One idea assessment of a wearable gadget could be found among the remaining results engineered as others, in the same route proposed for GDM seeing from home and one display focus for testing purposes. Inquisitively isolating and other gestation control orders, 38.4% of assessments in this class have provided information through a GUI on the possible use of the proposed contraptions by patients and clinical points of interest specialists. The approach is an extraordinary undertaking among the assessments in this class, and packing strategies have been applied in two of the accounting considerations. ML techniques were used in most evaluations, followed by IDSS, CI, KRR, MAS and master plan. DT, LR, RF, BN, and SVM are the most striking procedure appraisals. As for the wellspring of data used, clinical records think about accumulated data. For glucose evaluations, perceiving contraptions were used. Perceiving contraptions have been used appropriately as wearable devices for follow-up activity and telephone photographs of the patient's food verification. Other sources of data declared are: organized data, enlightening record from the Public Diabetes and Stomach Related and Kidney Illnesses Foundation (NIDDK), clinical equipment (for blood tests), understanding data from an approaching office-based birth partner evaluation called the early life plan and threat factors depicted by experts, and thorough examinations, beneficial application, and web application, and the ideal approach to managing the collection of this data was: 23% of the results reported for casual observation on continuing data collection.

Premature labor: An 8.3% of results were seen to take preterm births into account. In the screened forming, being organized by and significant to preterm birth gauge and affirmation of essential parts, a broad homogeneity is found in the screened forming, in addition to 2 evaluations plan to establish the relationship between preterm birth and openness to contamination, in the meantime specialists expect to see EHG accounts acquired during work from EHG obtained during standard gestation action. For all the evaluations, ML prototypes have been applied and transmitted. A web application focused on clinical benefits experts was suggested, which zeroed in on selecting the highlights possibly responsible for a high-preterm birth rate. In the assessments, composite learning design and hypostatization attempts were perceived. At any rate, the more frequently referred to are RF, DT and SVM, the overall outline of the recognized evaluations. It is fascinating to see that 30.7% of the findings used a similar enlightening rundown, including EHG accounts from the instructive collection of the term-preterm EHG. Information from clinical procedures, accumulated by external assessments and flourishing establishments, were used in the particular case excess assessments, which gathered data from human data through outline and clinical equipment techniques. In general, preterm transport considerations did not accumulate consistent information but recorded information. Most of the findings inside this plan have performed learning assignments utilizing imbalanced instructive combinations. Oversampling and examining strategies to change the class spread have been acted in various appraisals. A highlight choice cycle has been applied in 69.2% of findings.

Child development: Fetal improvement has been inspected in 7.7% of findings. In this class, things essentially introduced ML prototypes for supposition for birth results, check of fetal weight, the presumption for huge for pregnancy age or petite for birth age, suspicion for fetal progression variations from the norm, the figure of birth weight, worry for evaluation of head limit (HC), guess of fetal HC, and examination of the relationship existing between harms openness and low weight after entering the world. By far, most of the findings detailed utilizing ML methods, alongside in which DM frameworks were made. 75% of results finished arrangement assignments, by then lose faith was addressed in one appraisal. The hands' undertaking was to envision the infant kid's weight after entering the world (steady worth). It legitimizes alluding to how all inspections introduced prototypes, and none of the assessments utilized information accumulated persistently. Information source was clinical records, stores, clinical hardware as ultrasound scanners, topic specialists, study, thriving affiliation and human data through investigation. Most of the findings announced information organizing measures. In absent or inadequate information was denied. Meanwhile, missing attributes were supplanted with the remainder's focal point of the saw qualities.

Blood harming AND BLOOD PRESSURE Issues: Both toxemia and blood pressure issues have been watched out for in assessments, zeroed in on both. This course of action watches out for 11.5% of findings. As for eclampsia, most reviews will focus on its figure on all things considered, while the reason for assessments on blood pressure issues is altered: control and presumption, mortality relationship and adverse effect on gestation and unforeseen fetal development. The approach is the significant errand performed for this request by the reviewed reviews. Despite how prototypes are now the most suggested result in 66.67% of findings, enduring evaluations suggested powerful associations, flexible applications, and e-flourishing framework choices. 44.4% of the conclusions of this class amassed information from clinical records. In 22.2% of results, sensors were used to acquire knowledge (BP evaluations). In 11.1% of findings, by maternal inquiries and PDA use, information from human evidence was obtained. 16.6% of results utilized layout information, and 11.1% of findings utilized clinical stuff. Specialists' information was being used in 11.1% of findings. Enduring assessments utilized story from annals and conclusions. In 22.2% of the investigated considers utilization of an information organizing measure was alluded to 3 estimates detailed working with missing data. A diverse credit system has been utilized, single-attached attribution with mean worth was applied, and satisfaction with a standard evaluation of information. Just a single appraisal used part choice procedures. 22.2% recommended usable structures from all assessments in this representation. For toxemia figure and maternal notion, a sum of IDSS was implemented nearby three phenomenal applications for each job (remote or tablet application for patients and clinical advantages trained professionals, a web application for clinical advantages subject matter experts and a work zone application for clinical thought directors). A universal application was addressed toxemia gauge and home checking—a flexible application to screen pregnant ladies' success status enduring blood pressure issues. The two patients and clinical thought trained professionals could utilize the flexible application. An e-flourishing design proposed for hypertension affirmation could be utilized through a web application by clinical advantages subject matter experts. Alluded to assessments, BP detecting gadgets were utilized by the prenatal lady.

Mortality: Findings investigating mortality identified with gestation zeroed exclusively on the forecast. The prediction of extreme maternal bleakness (EMM) was taken into account in the prototypes of ML (arrangement). Neonatal mortality was concentrated. An IDSS was suggested in the main report, which also tended toward maternal and baby mortality. Using ML and CI techniques, a structure was developed, and ML, DM, and IDSS joined to create an e-wellbeing platform. It is worth noting that the three previously listed considered instruments made with GUIs (versatile or web applications) focusing on medical care experts or managers as end customers. Perinatal mortality has been tended to in (stillbirth), utilizing ML strategies. Blueprint attempts have been applied all through the three assessments. Additionally, proposed dimensionality decreased and assembling methods, by then, spatial apostatize prototypes were utilized by then. 55.5% of findings used clinical records for their information and considers utilized storeroom information. The data was collected from DATASUS, a public information document about baby mortality and live birth, and several instructive files are stored. Data accumulated through an outline has been used. Most itemized computations in this characterization are vital to backslide, discretionary forest areas and Bayesian associations. Most assessments (n = 5) showed using data pre-planning: incorporate decision. Besides, the underlying two estimates expected to oversee imbalanced educational lists: data sub-tried and self-assertive investigated, separately.

4 Proposed Knowledge-Based Graph Embedding Representation with DNN (KGER-DNN)

The deep learning model trains the input and represents the learned model as a pattern by visualization. The information graph concatenating prototypes take the triple form (h, t, r) as the triple validity's validity as input and output. A three-component architecture can be used as the general model: (1) Embedding lookup: linear translation of single-hot vectors to embedded vectors. A single-hot vector is a sparsely discrete, discrete input vector, e.g., the first entity can be defined as [1, 0, 0.0.0.0., 0]. A trio may be represented as (h, t, r), containing three single-hot vectors. (2) Techniques of interaction: modeling the interaction between vectors to establish a triple matching ranking. The central part of the model is this. (3) Analyzing: use the matching score to predict each triple's validity. A higher score means that it is most probable that the triple is right. (4) Categorization: The information graph embedding model falls into one of three groups, based on the modeling of the second part, respectively translation-based, neural-network-based, or trilinear-based, as mentioned below.

Translation-based: These prototypes translate the head entity's embedding by summarizing the vector relationship's embedding, then measuring the distance between the images of the translated head entity and the tail entity's embedding, usually at a distance of L 1 or L 2. Where (h, t, r), for distances of L 1 or L 2, are the embedding vectors of (h, t, r), p is 1 or 2, respectively, D is the embedding scale, and d is the dimension for which the scalar entries are HD, td, and rd. The first model of this kind was Trans A, with the score function the same as the equation above. The linear transformation of entities into a relation-specific space before translation makes many extensions. Such prototypes are both simple and efficient. However, due to over-strong expectations about translation using relationship embedding, their modeling capacity is typically weak. Consequently, it is not feasible to model those types of data. Knowledge-based information graphs (KGs) are commonly used representations of multi-dimensional information consisting of entities consider as (nodes) along with relationships (edges) that give a versatile hierarchical algorithm suitable for domain-specific knowledge common to all bases. Methods of concatenation strategies are useful for (a) understanding and operating on the latent attribute representation and the semantic relationship of KG constituents; (b) Data sparsity and inconsistency are effectively overcome, such as incomplete or multiple inconsistent 'one-to-one' relationship values; (c) improving subsequent deep learning implementations. France is well-known methods of translations that use simple assumptions to produce results that have proved to be an effective and reliable embedding model and are substantially accurate and scalable. To address the supposed inadequacies of Trans An in reflecting 'many-to-many' connections, a few improved prototypes (for example, Trans H Trans R, rascal, opening, and complex) were recommended. These procedures are planned to improve the adequacy of the connection forecast benchmark challenge. Trans A with a more unpredictable relationship-explicit portrayal (for example, projection lattices) of different information cardinalities (otherwise called information chart culmination). Nonetheless, we have appeared in past work that these prototypes don't give a decent implanting portrayal in which indistinguishable substances should be situated in little groups along with the subsequent inserting space. All in all, implanting approaches appear to report lacklustre showing. Besides, we have discovered that other notable best in class prototypes, for example, opening and complex, can occupy more Processor assets to direct open-space benchmark task preparing, albeit these prototypes' capacity to appropriately implant area explicit data portrayal stays muddled. Contrasting these prototypes, the actualized result showed that even in the wake of expanding the preparation interaction past the normal learning cycles, the standard inserting appraisal procedure shows low exactness for thick clinical KGsIn contrast, traditional installing frameworks are intended to address the assessment issue as opposed to picking implanting consistency, and bunch elements will, in general, utilize the subsequent implanting portrayal in every relationship as heads or tails rather than semantic ones in every relationship. DKGHTRATO has built up a translational inserting technique that joins Trans A with various ontological imperatives to learn portrayals of sorted multi-social information, initially planned to fuse biomedical and clinically applicable datasets, considering the perceived deficiencies of translational prototypes and their limits on the utilization of more wide area explicit datasets. DKGHTRATO upgrades Trans A translational installing and other improved prototypes, accomplishing high productivity even in extremely low without explicitly actualizing complex builds of model preparing stage portrayal, for example, those utilized in improved prototypes dependent on Trans A. Nonetheless, we evaluated whether the precision of the subsequent multi-social information installing is satisfactorily reflected by LP, showing that the nature of inserting isn't reflected by more unpredictable implanting portrayal approaches used to expand KG culmination. In this manner, to mirror improved Trans A prototypes utilizing projection grids, we broadened DKGHTRATO with extra capacities, while holding utilizing a bunch of individual hyperspaces connected to the task and substance of a similar kind. Likewise, we have built up an implanting stage that empowers many installing portrayal strategies to be applied and contrasted. We have utilized this strategy to recreate and mimic the majority of the strategies that upgrade the utilization of Trans A as an inserting procedure. Associate the vectors coming about because of every portrayal of Trans A communications to projection frameworks pointed toward improving common benchmark dataset's precision.

The proposed system consists of 3 modules extracting the features, training the Dataset, data classification. The structural design for the proposed methodology is determined in Fig. 4.1. The dataset has been collected through various sources, and it is stored as the main database for further processing. Hence, the requirement of optimal outputs has been done using this database by the machine learning system. When there are numerous data from the medical database, then machine learning outcomes will also be optimized. The classifier has classified the trained Medical y data, and it is estimated by various performance measures. The four classes have been trained in the deep learning architecture to get the trained model, and in our experiments, the four approaches taken into account are defined as follows: Trans A: the original Trans A solution for each connection using vector representation; Trans A+: a projection matrix is implemented as a technique to each contact concatenated with the neighbor as a vector representation, imitating some improved Trans A approaches (e.g., Trans H and Trans R); • KRAL: this is the original DKGHTRATO form, where different hyperspaces are used for each type of object and vector representation is used similar to Trans A for each relationship; • KRAL+: a projection matrix is used to embed each position meaning similar to Trans A. Max. (Ext.).

5 Deep Neural Network-Based

These systems use a nonlinear neural network to measure the similarity score for a triple network: where h, t, r are the embedding vectors of h, t, and r, respectively, NN is the neural network used to evaluate the score. Entity pairs are known as relationships of inputs and outputs. More precisely, the embeddings of the entity pairs $[h, t]$ are considered inputs that are randomly initialized at the starting and the weights. KGER-DNN optimizes entities' weights and inclusions based on their loss of function during learning. Network output weights are embedded relationships, and all entities and relationships share hidden layer weights, as shown in Fig. 1.

Given that KGER-DNN uses the embedding of pairs of entities as data, via a particular variable, it learns to embed each human entity. This contrasts with those approaches to matrix factorization that lose information in the form of entity-or entity-relationships by linking vectors. The network's output weights are the embedded relationships, and all entities and associations share the hidden layer weights, as seen in Fig. 1. KGER-DNN: Hidden layer mapping, which according to NN theory, is universal, is shared between definitions and relationships. A single-output node is

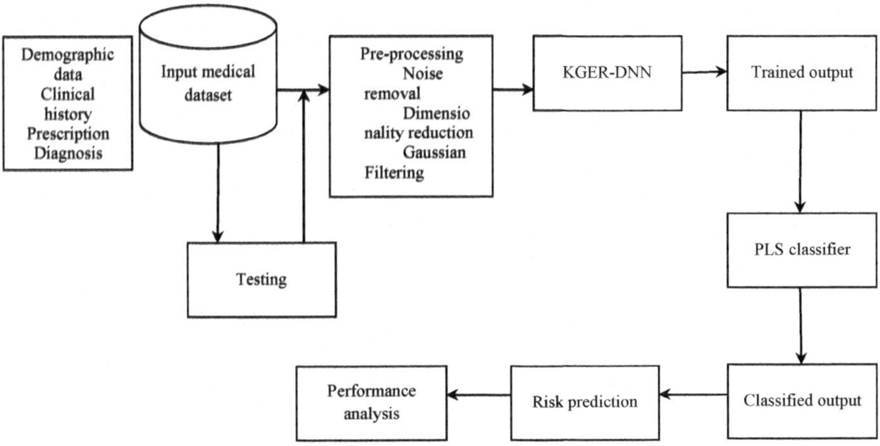

Fig. 1 Proposed architecture of the risk assessment prediction by applying deep learning

connected with each connection. The triple given score function (h, r, t) is known as f r (h, t) or, more appropriately, f r h, t. To show theoretical KGER-DNN capabilities, we use a single-hidden NN layer without a lack of generality and to characterize its score as:

L is the number of hidden layer nodes, wi $\in R$ $2d$ and β $r \in R$ is the hidden node's input and output weights. β $r = [\beta$ r 1 to. T, βr $L]$ T are the network's output weights that embed relationships. This is because the linear function acts as an activation feature in the last layer. φh, t $(wi, bi) = \varphi(hwi, [h, t] + bii)$ is the outcome of the ith hidden node and Φh, $t = [\varphi h$, t $(w1, b1), \ldots, \varphi h$, t (wL, bL)]T is feature mapping of the hidden layer of the network which is shared between all relations. h, $t \in R$ d is the embedding vectors of the head and tail, and d is the embedding dimension. As a consequence, wi, $[h, t] \in$.

R $2d$. Finally, $\varphi(.)$ is a function for activation, and h. the inner product is. i. KGER-DNN is competitive in space complexity due to the sharing of hidden layers in the architecture. The model's spatial complexity is O(Ned + NrL), where Ne, Nr are the respective number of entities and relationships. As stated above, if a model is not entirely expressive, a law that is unable to learn may be wrongly expected to be understood. It is, therefore, necessary to study the theories corresponding to an embedding model's expressiveness. Consequently, we now demonstrate that KGER-DNN is entirely descriptive, i.e., reflecting some fundamental truth about KGER relationships between entities.

6 Risk Assessment

The linked investigation of every gestation neighborhood is determined to acquire a danger score for every pregnancy. The connecting point is resolved as the info layer in the Profound learning KGER-DNN. It is dimensional of about 128 × 128 space with a range of 1.0. The number of neighbors considered positive for unsuccessful labor should be determined to identify the included information (32 novel qualities in contending). We utilize large numbers of the most excellent L2-standard radii that range from 0.125 to 0.55. On the record of acquiring a danger score for every incubation, eventually, no neighbor would discover tiny radii. Simultaneously, too many would think about enormous radii so that the subsequent extent of positive cases in the whole dataset will be around the absolute level of premature delivery. We found that by utilizing a span of 0.321025 in our execution, the danger assessment accomplished the best F1 evaluations. For unnatural birth cycle hazard assessment, we used two baselines. At first, 'Irregular' hazard esteem is translation created act the central standard. The populace-based methodology utilizes the incubation highlights in our outcomes to incorporate the deterministic positioning given as ' Both upheld by negligible # cases are considered by. Addresses the probability of an objective imprint (unsuccessful labor in this case) when the $f \in F$ work estimates $v \in \underline{V}(F)$. Addresses the likelihood of an accurate impression (in this occurrence, a premature delivery) happening when the capacity $f \in F$ has a worth $v \in V(F)$. E.g., P(Age Years) is the opportunity of early delivery occurring in a patient over 45-years old. However, $P(P)$ is the opportunity of an unnatural birth cycle happening in a drug quiet. For the 20,201 cases preparing populace and 5.91% of cases named premature deliveries, highlights upheld by at least 86 points are thought of, which is the base example size expected to arrive at a certainty level of 95% when the subsequent score is inside ± 5% of the deliberate/studied worth. For every gestation, to give a last danger appraisal positioning, the probabilities for every single indicated pair (f, v) fitting the past condition are normal.

7 Performance Analysis

7.1 Dataset Description

Table 1 describes the training and test set values for determining the risk prediction by collecting the dataset values during the gestation.

Demographic data: year at the beginning of gestation, year at the preceding date of marital status, level of education, occupation (36.7%), country of birth, last menstrual period (LMP), caste, level of education, occupation (36.7%) and occupation (7.1%), motherland, and local health office.

Table 1 Training figures and evaluation sets

Stats	Training set	Test set
Years	2010–2014	2015
Pregnancies	20, 2014	4676
Demographics	166,436	37,266
Clinical history	63,745	14,376
Prescriptions	103,010	20,882
Diagnoses	143,667	31,669
Procedures	54,520	13,385
Weeks 01–08	107,870	25,380
Weeks 09–16	197,831	45,403
Weeks 17–24	191,133	45,226

- Clinical history:

{HIV, bronchitis, candidiasis, hepatitis, pyelonephritis, syphilis, toxoplasmosis, urinary tract, vaginitis, vaginosis}, LMP, the most common diseases identified (2.5%), clinical history: weight (39.5%), height (34.3%) and BMI (25.6%), penicillin, plasil, sulfa}, the most common documented allergies to drugs (5.1%) {AAS, iodine, acetaminophen, amoxicillin, ampicillin, benzetacil, Buscopan, diclof}, (12.2%) {alcohol abuse, smoking, anemia, hypertension} and all clinical conditions identified.

- Prescriptions: Each medicine is known as a generic medicine.
- Diagnosis: For each diagnosis, the corresponding ICD-10 code, together with the accompanying type of appointment service (administrative term used in the InfoSaude system) and the medical specialty of the doctor, are given.
- Procedures: With procedure is associated with the medical specialty of the corresponding nurse or doctor.

The performance analysis of proposed method is illustrated below. The parameter to be considered for evaluation is accuracy, precision, recall, F1 score, and then AUC. By using the classified output, the various performance metrics have been calculated. Datasets to evaluate the projected methodology, clinical dataset is estimated. The performance of the model is analyzed by choosing the test data arbitrarily from the dataset as outcome data.

Accuracy: This shows correctly classified instances percentage in course of classification. It is evaluated as

$$\text{Accuracy rate} = \frac{\text{True Positive} + \text{True Negative}}{\text{Total Instances}} * 100$$

Precision: It measures gives what proportion of data that transmit to the network, actually had intrusion. The predicted positives (Network predicted as intrusion is TP and FP) and the network actually having an intrusion are TP. This is used to measure the quality and exactness of the classifier as shown below:

$$\text{Precision} = \frac{\text{True Positive}}{\text{True Positive} + \text{False Positive}}$$

Recall: Recall is the ratio real positives which are correct predicted positive and is defined as

$$\text{Recall} = \frac{\text{True Positive}}{\text{True Positive} + \text{False Negative}}$$

F1 Score: F1-score is simply the average value of recall and precision. The statistical calculation is also used in the F1-score for the results of the individual FN and FP classifiers. Definition of precision is judgment of accuracy, whereas recall is detecting the sample instance based on the attribute called faulty or non-faulty.

$$F1 - \text{Measure} = \frac{2 \times \text{Precision} \times \text{Recall}}{\text{Precision} + \text{Recall}}$$

Table 2 shows some observation of statistics of training and test sets, the outcome of the classifier has been estimated from the statistics of training and test sets datasets instances, then classifying the instances with the same observation, then the performance measures of various techniques of random forest, neural networks, KER is compared with the proposed techniques proposed KGER-DNN. Table 3 shows the comparison of performance in accuracy, precision, recall, F1-score, and AUC. It has been analyzed from the actual and predicted value from the objective of classes in confusion matrix, and it is represented in percentage.

In terms of accuracy, Fig. 1 indicates the contrast of different approaches. It is an accuracy comparison for clinical datasets between existing and proposed techniques. As shown in above figure, the Proposed_KGER-DNN achieves accuracy with a maximum percentage than existing techniques. Whereas random forest, neural network, KER approach have resulted in the worst performance by furnishing a minimum of accuracy value of about 78.9%, 80.1%, 84.2%. Finally, the Proposed_KGER-DNN technique operates more efficiently when compared with other prototypes by acquiring the maximum accuracy value of 93.5%.

In terms of recall, Fig. 2, illustrates the contrast between different approaches. It is a recall comparison for clinical datasets between existing and proposed techniques. As shown in above figure, the Proposed_KGER-DNN achieves recall with

Table 2 Comparison of performance of proposed (FDNN-GD system and existing algorithm

S. No	Techniques	Random forest	Neural networks	KER	Proposed_KGER-DNN
1	Accuracy	78.9	80.1	84.2	93.5
2	Precision	50.0	60.0	100.0	100.0
3	Recall	25.0	25.3	25.1	33.3
4	F1-Score	33.3	35.0	40.0	50.0
5	AUC	31.7	43.0	51.34	75.0

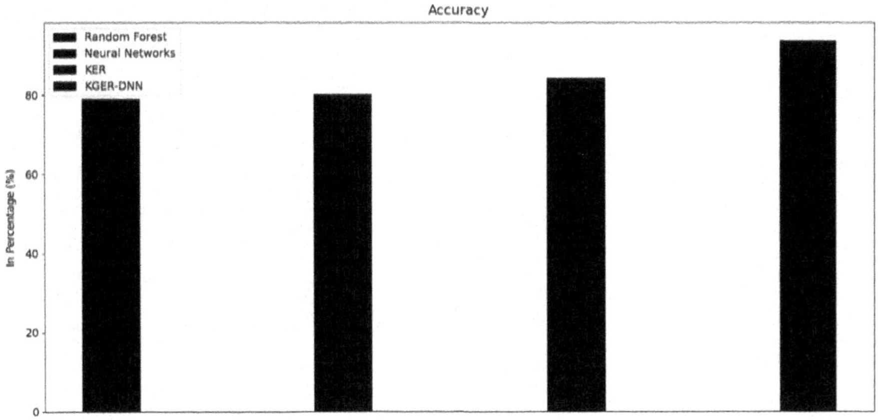

Fig. 1 Comparison of accuracy of the proposed and the existing techniques

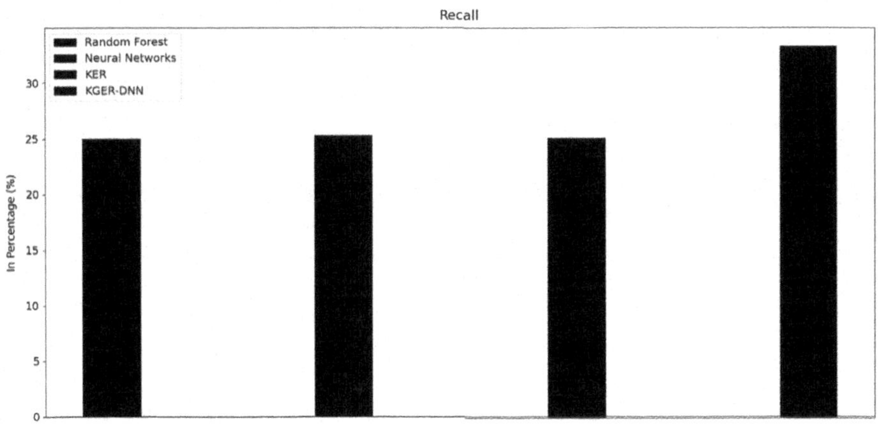

Fig. 2 Comparison of recall of the proposed and the existing techniques

a maximum p ercentage than existing techniques. Whereas random forest, neural network approach have resulted in the worst performance by furnishing a minimum of precision value of about 50%, 60%. Whereas KER gradually increases the recall value of about 100% than the other existing techniques. Finally, the proposed Proposed_KGER-DNN technique operates more efficiently when compared with other prototypes by acquiring the maximum recall value of 100%.

In terms of AUC, Fig. 3 indicates the contrast of different approaches. It is an AUC comparison for clinical datasets between existing and proposed techniques. As shown in above figure, the Proposed_KGER-DNN achieves AUC with a maximum percentage than existing techniques. Whereas random forest, neural network, approach have resulted in the worst performance by furnishing a minimum of AUC value of about 31.7%, 43.0%. Whereas KER gradually increases the AUC

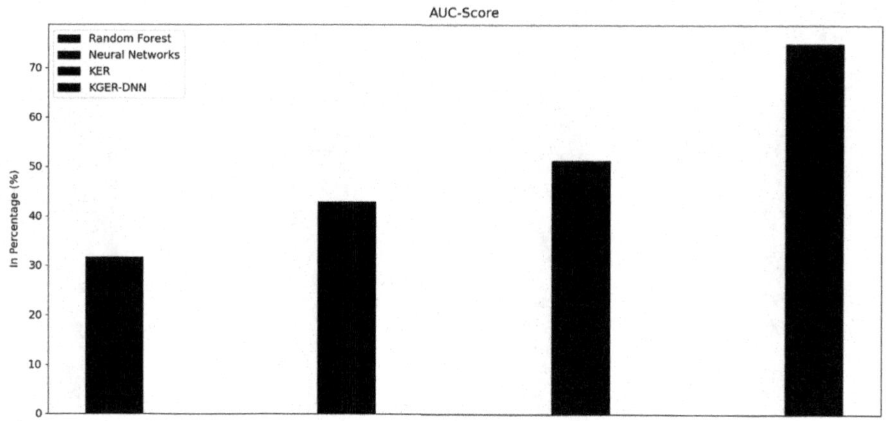

Fig. 3 Comparison of AUC Score of the proposed and the existing techniques

value by about 51.34% than the other existing techniques. Finally, the proposed Proposed_KGER-DNN technique operates more efficiently when compared with other prototypes by acquiring the maximum AUC value of 75.0%.

In terms of precision, Fig. 4 illustrates the contrast of different approaches. It is a precision comparison for clinical datasets between existing and proposed techniques. As shown in above figure, the Proposed_KGER-DNN achieves precision with a maximum percentage than existing techniques. Whereas random forest, neural network approach have resulted in the worst performance by furnishing a minimum of precision value of about 50%, 60%. Whereas KER gradually increases the precision value of about 100% than the other existing techniques. Finally, the proposed KGER-DNN technique performs more effectively compared to other prototypes by acquiring a maximum precision value of cent percent.

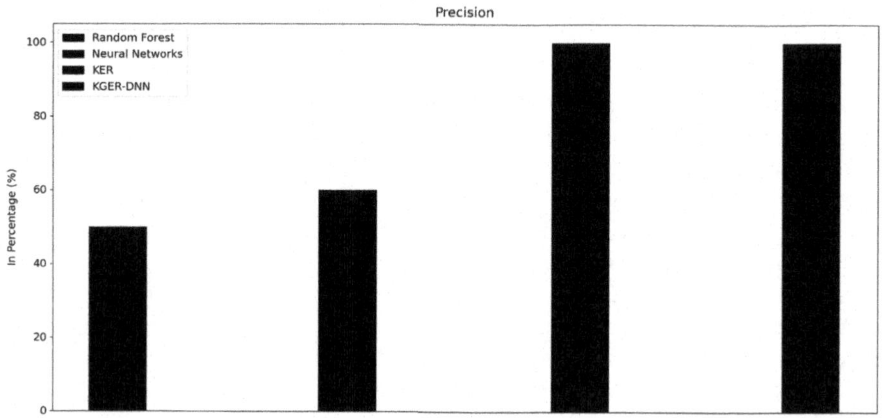

Fig. 4 Comparison of precision of the proposed and the existing techniques

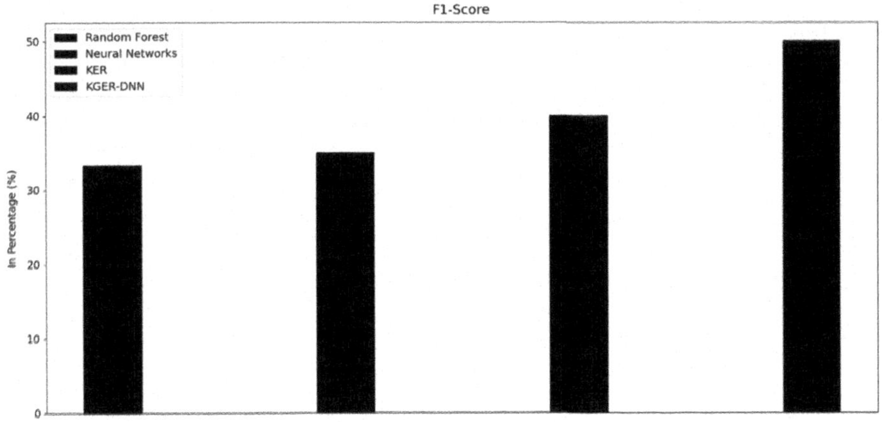

Fig. 5 Comparison of accuracy of the proposed and the existing techniques

For the F1-score, the comparison of different approaches is shown in Fig. 5. It is an F1-score comparison for clinical datasets between existing and proposed techniques. As shown in above figure, the Proposed_KGER-DNN achieves F1-score with a maximum percentage than existing techniques. Whereas random forest, neural network approach have resulted in the worst performance by furnishing a minimum of F1-score value of about 33.3%, 35.0%. Whereas KER gradually increases the F1-score value of about 40.6% than the other existing techniques. Finally, the proposed Proposed_KGER-DNN technique operates more efficiently when compared with other prototypes by acquiring the maximum F1-score value of 50.0%.

8 Conclusion

Thus, in this paper, we analyzed the different predictive techniques used to predict the hazards and complications of gestation. The ML techniques have provided a good accuracy for each of the problems identified in gestation, though there were certain drawbacks. The image analytics and deep learning techniques when employed with the prediction of complications can make antenatal care a highly safe period for women. These predictions help to prevent all complications and can provide a better insight to the physician. Thus, the framework can serve as a decision support system for the medical practitioners.

References

1. Fahrudin, T. M., Syarif, I., & Barakbah, A. R. (2017). Data mining approach for breast cancer patient recovery. *EMITTER International Journal of Engineering Technology., 5*(1), 36–71.
2. Moreira, M. W., Rodrigues, J. J., Oliveira, A. M., Ramos, R. F., & Saleem, K. (2016). A preeclampsia diagnosis approach using bayesian networks. In *Communications (ICC), 2016 IEEE International Conference on 2016 May 22* (pp. 1–5). IEEE.
3. Moreira, M. W., Rodrigues, J. J., Oliveira, A. M., Saleem, K., & Neto, A. V. (2016). An inference mechanism using bayes-based classifiers in gestation care. In *Ine-health networking, applications and services (Healthcom), 2016 IEEE 18th international conference on 2016 Sep 14* (pp. 1–5). IEEE.
4. Nagendra, V., et al. (2017). Evaluation of support vector machines and random forest classifiers in a real-time fetal monitoring system based on cardiotocography data. In *2017 IEEE conference on computational intelligence in bioinformatics and computational biology (CIBCB)*. IEEE.
5. Permanasari, A. E., & Nurlayli, A. (2017). Decision tree to analyze the cardiotocogram data for fetal distress determination. In *2017 international conference on sustainable information engineering and technology (SIET)*. IEEE.
6. Wicaksono, A. P., Badriyah, T., & Basuki, A. (2016). Comparison of the data mining methods in predicting the risk level of diabetes. *EMITTER International Journal of Engineering Technology., 4*(1), 164–178.
7. Zhang, Y., & Zhao, Z. (2017). Fetal state assessment based on cardiotocography parameters using PCA and AdaBoost. In *2017 10th international congress on image and signal processing, BioMedical engineering and informatics (CISP-BMEI)*. IEEE.
8. Hoodbhoy, Z., et al. (2019). Use of machine learning algorithms for prediction of fetal risk using cardiotocographic data. *International Journal of Applied and Basic Medical Research*, 9(4), 226.
9. Bhatnagar, D., & Maheshwari, P. (2016). Classification of cardiotocography data with WEKA. *International Journal of Computer Science and Network-IJCSN*, 5(2).
10. Tang, H., et al. (2018). The design and implementation of cardiotocography signals classification algorithm based on neural network. *Computational and Mathematical Methods in Medicine.*
11. Lakshmi, B. N., Indumathi, T. S., & Ravi, N. (2016). An hybrid approach for prediction based health monitoring in pregnant women. *Procedia Technology*, 24, 1635–1642.

Smart Healthcare System: Interface to COVID-19 Prevention Using Dual-Layer Security

Neetu Faujdar, Reeya Agrawal, Neeraj Varshney, and Mohommad Zubair Khan

1 Introduction

A family of viruses called as coronaviruses can lead mild to severe illnesses like common cold, pneumonia, severe acute respiratory syndrome (SARS), and Middle East respiratory syndrome (MERS). The novel coronavirus disease (COVID-19) was first spotted in Wuhan, China, in December 2019 [1]. It was considered to be cases of pneumonia without any etiology. By January 3, a total of 44 patients with similar conditions were reported by China to the WHO. Major symptoms that were reported were flu-like symptoms such as fever, cough, and cold. Few of the patients also faced difficulty in breathing or lung complications. This virus was named as severe acute respiratory syndrome 2 [2]. It was proclaimed as a pandemic by the World Health Organization on March 11, 2020 [3]. Coronavirus outbreak has caused a serious harm on the life and property of many people around the globe. It has led to serious chaos and deep worries in people's mind because of its potential harm, severity, and the ability to spread at a very high rate [4]. In most cases, people contaminated with the COVID-19 infection will develop mild to moderate symptoms like dry cough, mild fever, tiredness, sore throat, diarrhea, headache, or loss of taste and smell [5]. Elderly people or people having medical problems like diabetes, obesity, cardiovascular malady, severe respiratory ailments, and cancer have a greater risk of

N. Faujdar (✉) · R. Agrawal · N. Varshney
GLA University, Mathura, U.P., India
e-mail: neetu.faujdar@gla.ac.in

R. Agrawal
e-mail: reeya.agrawal@gla.ac.in

N. Varshney
e-mail: neeraj.varshney@gla.ac.in

M. Z. Khan
Taibah University, Madinah, Saudi Arabia
e-mail: mkhanb@taibahu.edu.sa

A. K. Tyagi et al. (eds.), *Intelligent Interactive Multimedia Systems for e-Healthcare Applications*, https://doi.org/10.1007/978-981-16-6542-4_8

developing severe symptoms like pain in chest, difficulty in breathing, and shortness of breath [6].

We aim to elucidate the effectiveness and advantageousness of the dual-layer security and access system in multiple avenues where existing solutions fail in some capacity [7]. This illustrates how this system is better than traditional systems such as biometric or keypad-based systems [8]. This system is especially beneficial for physically challenged people. The system is built from the ground up with a singular focus on privacy. It will prevent leakage or hacks of sensitive user biometric data such as fingerprints [9]. It also enables a much higher level of flexibility concerning security, as making a system extremely secure has its tradeoffs [10].

Human brain–computer interface works on the principle of first convening the EEG waves from the brain into digital signals and then into meaningful information that can be parsed and processed by the computer [11].

There are various different types of security systems used all around the world in areas ranging from mobile phones to microwaves and from suitcases to nuclear submarines [12]. The various SS such as physical keypads, fingerprint-based biometrics, or simple lock and key systems have their own advantages and disadvantages. For example, let us take a simple lock and physical key-based system [13]. The biggest utility of such a system is in its sheer simplicity, and the ease of operation. Such systems are cheap to create and require no maintenance [14]. They have stood the test of time and are extremely reliable. While they have their own drawbacks such as the possibility of the key being misplaced due to an accident [15]. They also have a major flaw in terms of their secureness due to the possibility of foul play because of the key getting cloned, copied, or stolen by nefarious elements [16].

After the preliminary stage of Facial recognition, the password authentication is done by using a non-invasive method of brain–computer interface using either earphones or a heads-up display [17]. The dual-layer security system is extremely future proof as it can be enhanced with only software updates without requiring any updated hardware thus increasing the efficiency and conserving resources considerably [18]. The brain–computer interface can also be used as an input mechanism to enter data and select options which is illustrated in Fig. 1. [19].

Password hashing technique called RIG can be used for client independent systems. This provides flexibility for choosing between memory and the number of iterations [21]. RIG is useful for systems with limited resources [22]. This chapter shows the vital importance of linking biometric information with individuals and using this data to prevent attacks on national security from anarchists and terrorists [23]. This chapter shows that users do not know how to properly protect their passwords and shows various techniques to prevent brute force attacks [24]. The implementation is known as password multiplier is available for all to use. Biometrics enhances security but still, there are problems. The problems can be solved by fusion and multimodal systems [25]. This chapter leads us to the conclusion that Eigen faces algorithms work better in 2D and fisher faces algorithms work better in 3D [26]. This chapter shows that the biometric systems contain flaws, and they should not be used without proper analysis and multilayer biometric systems are better [27]. This chapter demonstrates that the facial recognition techniques used by

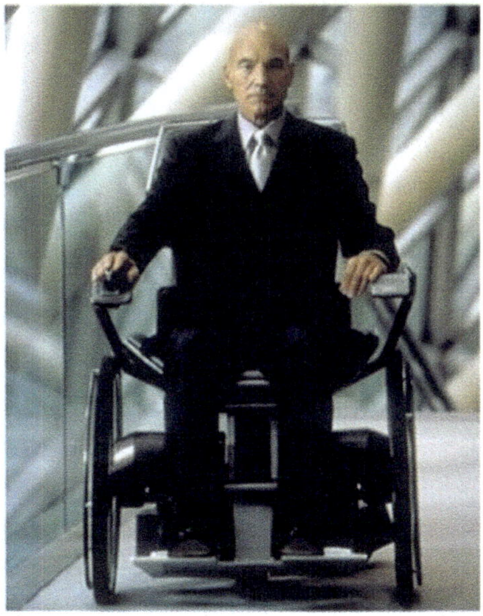

Fig. 1 Future application potential of brain–computer interface [20]

major companies are not secure and put the users at risk. The chapter shows that it is better to store data in the cloud because it is more scalable and provides greater performance [28]. It shows that cloud storage has a lower cost and can have better security than traditional methods. This chapter shows that the BCI system can be created using low power and low cost [29]. It shows how Bluetooth can be used to transfer data to the computer for processing and to progress to the final layer of the system [30]. This chapter shows that BCI has enormous potential in other areas such as video games along with virtual reality to make the experience immersive [31]. This chapter concludes that facial recognition is a new technology, and it is only a tool and not a perfect or final solution, and before using it, we need to study the constitutional and legal implications [32]. This chapter shows the growth in the field of the brain–computer interface and mentions the future potential of the system. It also shows the various challenges that we face [33]. This chapter shows how a low-cost brain–computer interface can be created to better the lives of people and allow them to live more independent lives. Virtual keyboards can be based on EOG and EMG signals [34]. This study shows the usage of the brain–computer interface using only one intracranial electrode. It allows users to type letters using EEG waves [35]. This chapter shows that physically disabled people such as those with paralysis can be able to move cursors on a virtual screen by using a brain–computer interface [36]. Facial recognition has emerged as the single most useful tool in the arsenal of law enforcement to ensure that guilty people are punished and innocent people are spared [37]. Coronavirus is a very deadly disease that can kill millions of people around the world and can wreck the world and can wreck the world economy [38]. It can become the biggest problem that has been faced by humankind since the world war.

Research suggests that coronavirus can kill up to 2 to 3% of the affected population [39]. It is a very deadly and uniquely horrible virus that needs to be very serious. It has already killed more than 150,000 people by the mid of April of 2020 [40]. If we do not act by changing the infrastructure for a post-COVID world, then we are committing a big mistake. Research suggests that coronavirus can survive on surfaces such as metal for more than 2 to 3 days [41]. It can survive on different surfaces for different durations. The survival strength of the virus depends on the humidity and the temperature of the environment [42]. This chapter shows us steps that can be taken to curtail the spread of the virus. This chapter has shown that coronavirus can last on surfaces for different durations [43]. The relative humidity and temperature of the environment in which the surface in question is present is the biggest factor that can affect how long the virus can last on it [44]. This shows the potential for using our computers in a way that allows us to be freed from constraints and allows the transfer of thoughts directly to the computer [45]. This type of interface can have tremendous implications for the world of software and computer science [46]. Research suggests that masks prevent the spread of coronavirus by the means of droplets, and this can lead to a decrease in the number of those infected and subsequently will reduce the number of deaths. Masks are very effective in stopping the spread of the coronavirus [47]. The current expert opinion along with the mandated guidelines by the various governments of the world suggests that mask-wearing is most effective when a large percentage of the population is compliant [48]. Masks should be worn for the greater good along with rational self-interest [49]. Brain–computer interfaces can be used to authenticate users in some types of computer networks, and this can be done by the means of some sort of electrophysiological signals in reaction to specific inputs [50].

2 Methodology and Approach

The dual-layer security and access system use a Bluetooth-based system that is an advanced headset that contains an EEG sensor that can read the activity of the brain and communicate to the computer via wireless means. The other component is a webcam-based system and a computer system running the code based in MATLAB.

Steps to be taken for the development of the dual-layer security and access system: Formulate a plan as well as a structure for strategizing and executing the algorithm with the purpose of use as an application for the same.

- Research plan
- Resource plan
- Workflow
- Structure ideation
- Documentation ideation.

Do an extensive review of the existing literature to know about how the ideas can be implemented. Research on the existent algorithms, models, strategies, and any other resource available. Gather data, models, techniques, as well as all resources which may be required. Decide upon the technology to be used to acquire the EEG sensing device brain sense learn about the workings of brain sense decide the hardware and algorithms for facial recognition decide and design the system for the dual-layer security and access system. Implement the code in MATLAB and OpenCV to complete the documentation [51]. Think about the future application and ways in which the project can be extended. The dual-layer security and access system works on the principle of screening first and verifying later the first preliminary layer involves facial recognition using a very fast algorithm that uses minimal resources and does not require any special equipment such as infrared sensors, apart from a basic camera. The final layer of verification involves brain–computer interface [52]. The user is required to wear a specialized headset that can detect changes in the EEG waves produced by the brain, and these waves show a noticeable difference when the user performs a specified action such as blinking or sleeping. Figure 2 illustrated face recognition technique.

The brain–computer interface software can be trained to recognize the times when a user blinks, and register the response along with the associated time stamp instantaneously. This phenomenon can be utilized to authenticate a numeric password. The password can be relayed through audio via headphones into the ears of the user. The user needs to blink when they hear the correct digit on the headphones. Let us take an example where the pass code is 321 [55]. Now the numbers start being played in the headphones and as soon as the first digit of the pass code appears, the user needs to blink, and the response is registered. This means that the user should blink after hearing the first digit, i.e., "3," then the next digit, i.e., "2," and then the next and final digit, i.e., "1." As soon as the pass code is correctly authenticated, the login process is successful and the user can access the physical space or data. Explanation of how brain sense works is shown in Fig. 3.

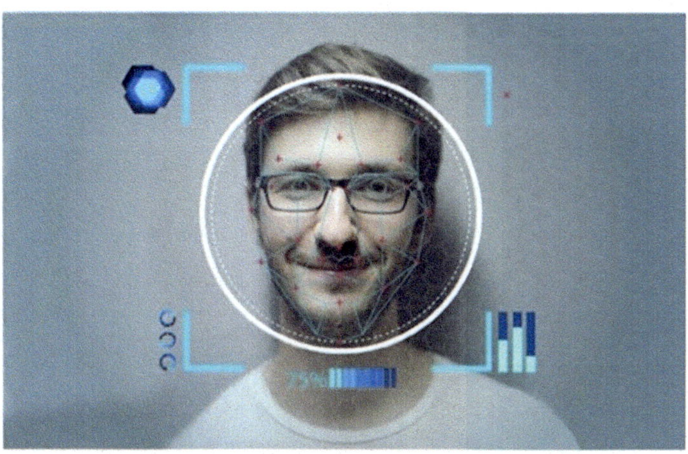

Fig. 2 Example of facial recognition technique [53]

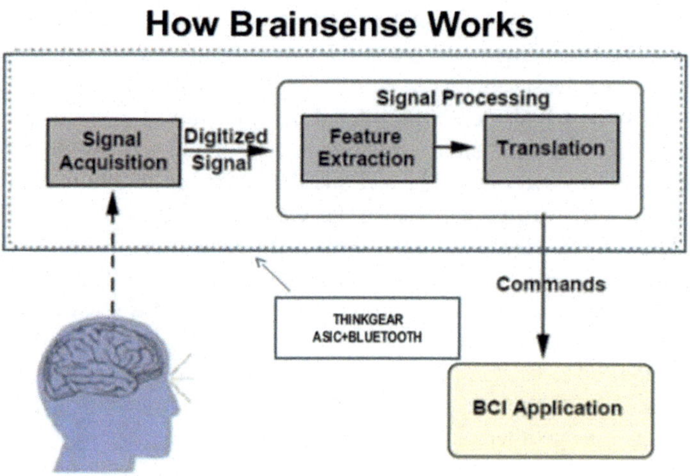

Fig. 3 Explanation of how brain sense works [54]

There are a vast number of steps that can be taken to ensure enhanced security. The first step that can be taken is to ensure that the numbers relayed in the headphones for authentication appear in a random order, so that nefarious elements are unable to interpret the passcode by calculating the time elapsed between blinks. Figure 4 shows the class diagram of facial recognition system, and Fig. 5 shows the real-life image of brain sense device [56].

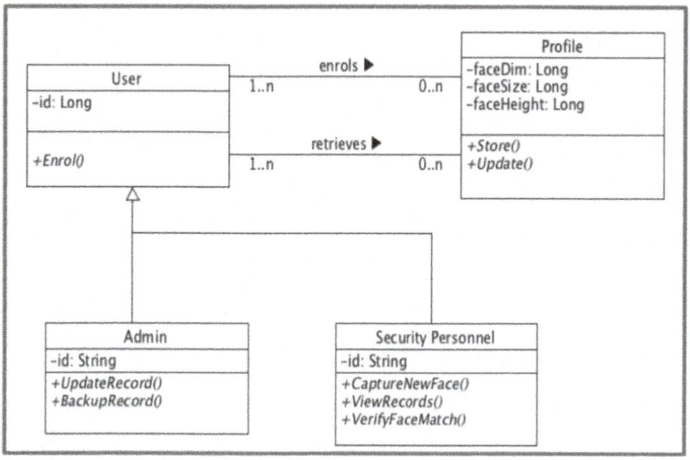

Fig. 4 Class diagram of facial recognition system

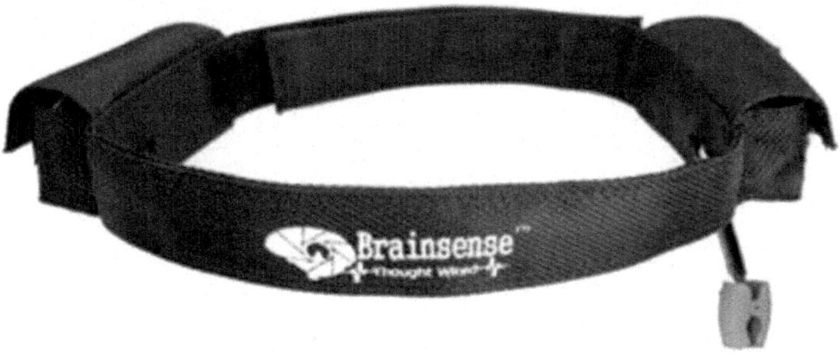

Fig. 5 Real-life image of brain sense device [57]

3 Methodology

There are various different types of security systems used all around the world in areas ranging from mobile phones to microwaves and from suitcases to nuclear submarines. The various SS such as physical keypads, fingerprint-based biometrics, or simple lock and key systems have their own advantages and disadvantages. For example, let us take a simple lock and physical key-based system. The biggest utility of such a system is in its sheer simplicity, and the ease of operation. Such systems are cheap to create and require no maintenance.

They have stood the test of time and are extremely reliable. They also have a major flaw in terms of their secureness due to the possibility of foul play because of the key getting cloned, copied, or stolen by nefarious elements. Brain–computer interface-based security and access system has a multitude of features that make the system the best option for a variety of avenues. The dual-layer security and access system is especially useful for providing physically disabled people with the means to access utilities such as lockers. If blind person has to use traditional lock systems such as those based on fingerprint biometrics or entering pass codes through a keypad, they face enormous difficulties which might be insurmountable at times. The problems can arise from being unable to locate the key hole to lack of security in entering the pass code in plain sight of nefarious elements. Figure 6 shows the brain sense device system.

The dual-layer security and access system is especially useful in areas where privacy and extreme security are the major concerns. The dual-layer security and access system can be used for allowing physically challenged people who suffer disabilities such as blindness, paralysis, and loss of limbs to operate terminals such as ATM systems, bank lockers, and home security systems with ease. The dual-layer security and access system allows them to enter their authentication details just by thinking. A brain sense device is illustrated in Fig. 7.

The dual-layer security and access system is highly secure and can be used in places such as defense installations, and other places where security is paramount. The dual-layer security and access system is better than traditional systems used for ATMs access as the traditional systems have the possibilities of fraud and theft. ATM

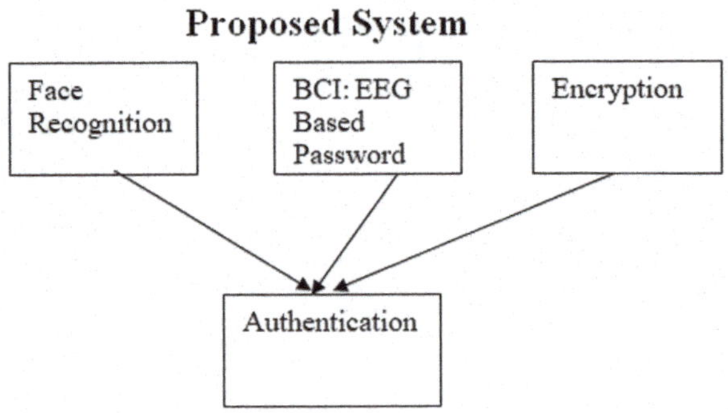

Fig. 6 Brain sense device system

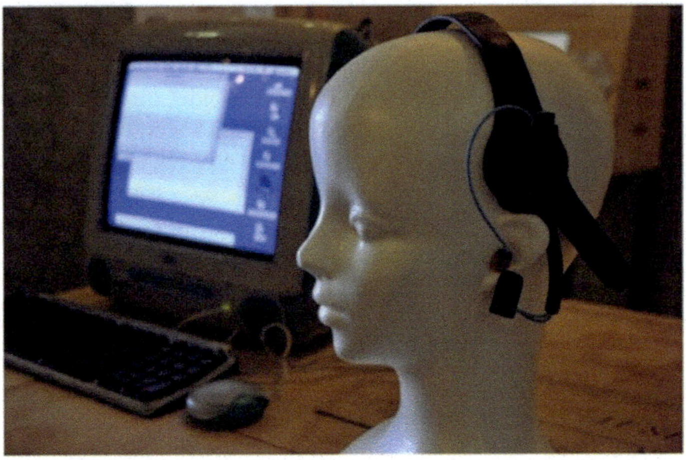

Fig. 7 Brain sense device [40]

cards can be cloned or stolen. The process of entering the password is also not secure as when the user enters the password into the terminal, there is no privacy, and all nefarious elements can find out the password by using hidden cameras or binoculars.

The dual-layer security and access system solves all these issues by requiring a dual layer of security in a way in which no one can guess or find out the password. The dual-layer security and access system is also designed with the possibility of forced access of security systems in mind. In cases when thieves force a user to open a lock for an ATM, home locker, household door locks, or any other such lock or access system, then the user is helpless and has to provide the thief with access. Example of brain–computer interface is shown in Fig. 8. In the dual-layer security and access system, the user will have a special password that will unlock the lock, but will alert the authorities and send the GPS coordinates of the location to the police for prevention of the crime. This makes the dual-layer security and access system

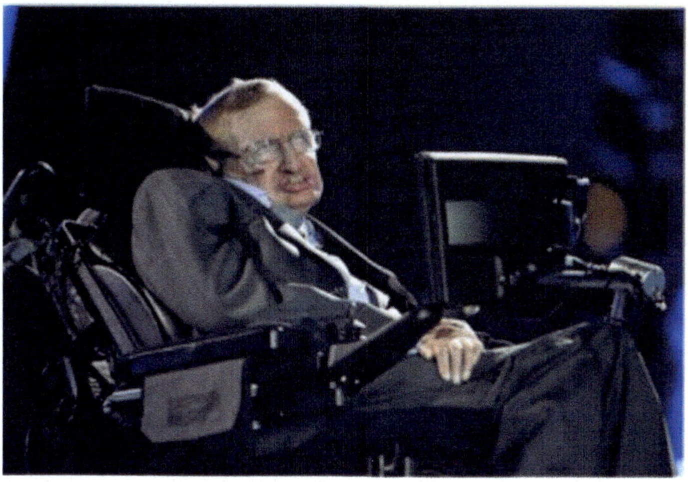

Fig. 8 Example of brain–computer interface [58]

unique in giving the user the physical security when in positions of coercion while at the same time keeping the data or the physical valuables secure.

There are various types of security systems exists, like primitive as lock and key and voice signature-based system. A biometric system is one that uses characteristics that uses one or more than one of the physical or behavioral features of the individual such as fingerprint, retina, iris car, voice, gait, palm-print, and others. These unique features of an individual arc known as traits, modalities, indicators, or identifiers.

Unimodal biometric systems, such as those using only as single physical trait are not successful in all cases as they suffer from numerous setbacks such as lack of universality, acceptability, and a the problem of theirs not being distinct enough. Such biometric systems, henceforth referred to as unimodal biometric systems, lack accuracy and are not as operationally efficient in tends of performance. Figure 9 depicted the demonstration of ATM card cloning.

Absolute accuracy is desired in biometric systems, but it cannot be achieved, but we can get close to perfection. Absolute accuracy is much harder to achieve in systems that arc unimodal because of issues of intra-class variations, spoof attacks, lack of universality, interoperability issues, noise in the sensor data, inter-class similarities, and other issues. Biometric systems can have varying levels of accuracy, and this can be calculated by the usage of two distinct rates known as FRR and FRR. FAR refers to the false acceptance rate. FRR refers to the false rejection rate. Multimodal biometric systems minimize FAR and increase the FRR, but this is a trade-off that we have to be willing to make [60].

The perfect biometric system is one that is secure, permanent, universal, distinct, and is highly acceptable. There is no current biometric system that meets all of the specified requirements at the same time. It has been found after lots of research that there might not be a single trait that can satisfy our requirements, but a combination

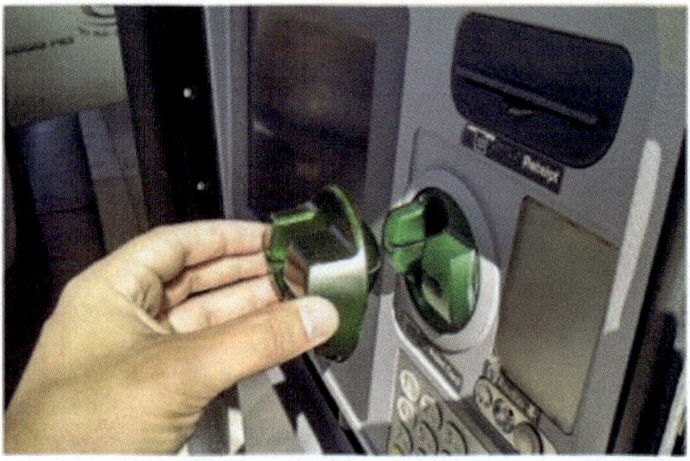

Fig. 9 Demonstration of ATM card cloning [59]

of different traits is capable of doing the job. This means that multimodal biometric systems arc successful at this while unimodal biometric systems fail at this. The key is to make aggregate data from unimodal biometric systems and use intelligent decision making on them to reach a correct decision [61].

Multimodal biometric systems have emerged as a new and unique solution to the problems faced by security systems of earlier times. It is a very highly promising approach that uses the evidence of various biometric traits to create a final decision that has a nearly certain chance of being the correct decision. Due to their high reliability, multimodal systems have evolved in the last few years and are considered a better option as compared to unimodal systems. While unimodal biometric systems work only based on one single trait like fingerprint or retina, multimodal systems work by combining various traits such as using both fingerprint and retina at the same time. This allows the system to use the better features from each individual biometric [62].

There are multiple avenues in life where a security system needs to be highly secure. There are also many security systems that are a high value target in the eyes of the highly capable thieves and forgers. ATM systems are an intersection of both of these and need the latest technology to stay safe from unwanted and nefarious elements. As attacks on ATMs have taken an upward trajectory due to the coining of new means of hacking and cloning. ATMs can be compromised by eavesdropping attacks that involve the thief watching the person entering the PIN into the machine. They can be cracked by spoofing where a copy of the card is created. Malware and shimming attacks are also a constant source of worry for bank and security officials.

4 Result and Discussion

4.1 Face Detection Recognition System

For face detection recognition system, suppose that we are having an input face image V which is to be verified, after we found the mean mass vector Ω and Vth mass image vector of the same the distance then to be calculated is Euclidean distance which can be calculated by formula.

$$\varepsilon V = |\Omega - \Omega 2| \tag{1}$$

In case, the distance is lower than energy theta (θ), then the entered image is said to be known image, and if it is greater, then the entered image is termed as unknown image. In this process, total of 180 images were used in which 90 were authentic and 90 were unauthentic. All the coordinates of authentic images were grouped in four and were in the set of learning, and then the distance of every member was found and checked. In this process of face detection, accuracy was found to be more than 95%, and it was more than some previous face detectors which we had reviewed. This type of face detection technique was developed using nulled and ranged space of class within the parameters of face area. In this technique, amalgamation was attempted in two different ways.

- Level which is featured;
- Level which has to be decided.

Consolidating data at choice level requires the development of classifiers exclusively on invalid space and ranged space. At that point, these two classifiers are joined utilizing three choice combination methodologies. Alongside two old style choices combination strategies sum regulations and item rule; we utilize our own choice combination method which imperializes each classifier space independently to upgrade consolidated execution. Our method of choice combination utilizes linear discriminant analysis (LDA) and nonparametric LDA on classifier's reaction to upgrade class detachability at classifier yield space. Figure 10 shows the sample

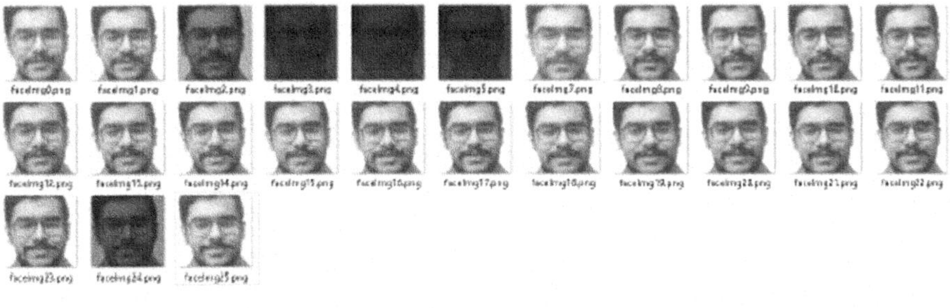

Fig. 10 Sample for face detection technique

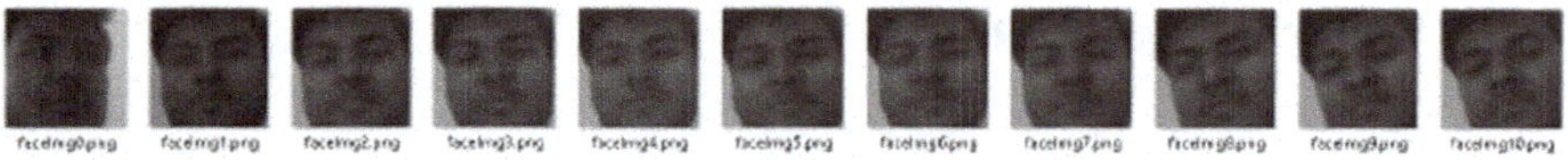

Fig. 11 After fusion level

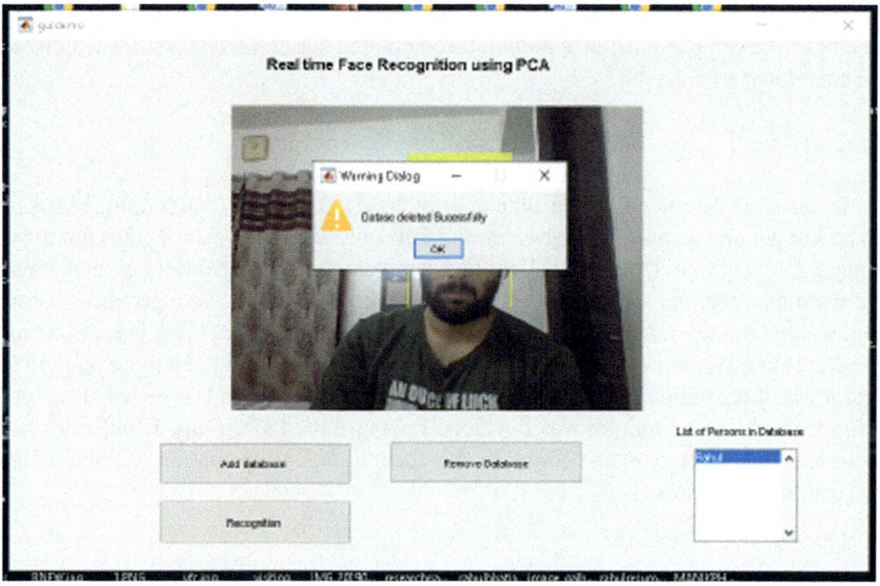

Fig. 12 After adding in database successfully

for face detection technique, and Fig. 11 shows the sample after fusion level. Sample after adding in database successfully is illustrated in Fig. 12.

4.2 Image Enhancement

A perfect high-pass channel is utilized for picture improvement to make a picture honing. These channels underline fine subtleties in the picture and the nature of a picture profoundly debases when the high frequencies are weakened or totally expelled. Conversely, upgrading the high-recurrence parts of a picture prompts an improvement in the picture quality. For instance, on the off chance that the face picture is given as information, at that point, the channel work for a perfect high-pass channel is communicated as Eq. (2)

$$(u, v) = \begin{cases} 0 \ \text{if}(u, v) \leq Do \\ 1 \ \text{if}(u, v) > Do \end{cases} \tag{2}$$

where (u, v) is the separation between focal point of the recurrence square shape and JF(u, Xv) is the improved picture. So also, the iris and palm pictures are improved by this channel, and it is communicated as (u, v) and JP (u, v) separately.

4.3 FEP-RSA-MM Testing

Picture acquisition is a procedure to catch the natural info picture. The wedged contribution image is improved by the high-passing channels. Improved image emphasize esteems are removed by the BEMD. From that point forward, the element esteems are intertwined by the combination method. At last, the melded highlight esteems are given for coordinating. At that point, the figure writings of facial and singular unscrambled in the FEP-RSA-MM testing by RSA decoding. The private key of RSA unscrambling got from the key age calculation. RSA operation is shown in Fig. 13.

RSA Decryption Algorithm

Input: The collector's private key (d) and they got scrambled figure content.

Output: The original plain text.

Step 1: Subsequent to completing the RSA unscrambling.

Step 2: the prepared component esteems from the information base and the info picture from the testing is given as the contribution to the relationship-based coordinating.

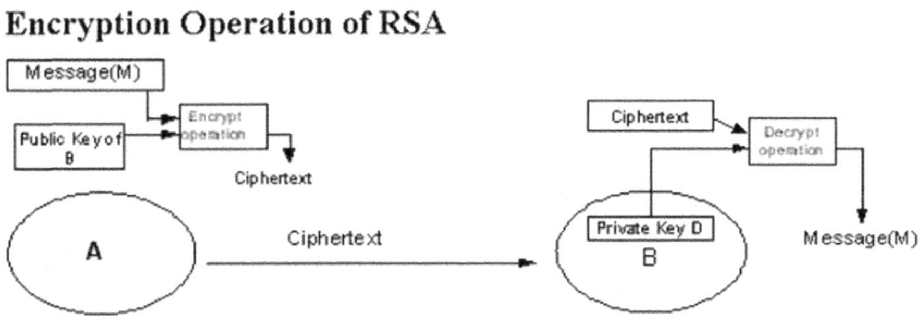

Fig. 13 RSA operation

4.4 Correlation-Based Matching

In the FFP-RSA-MA connection-based coordinating, segment is the most significant procedure, which is handled by two information, includes values: database highlight esteems and info picture highlight esteems. A coordinating method predicts the choice of people dependent on the relationship among the highlights. At that point, the picture-based biometric confirmation (e.g., facial and fingular) got by this relationship-based encoding. The prepared picture melded include vector and info coordinating picture intertwined highlight vector speaks to as (x, ay) and g (x, ay) at position (x, y) individually. The size of the prepared picture is a $Wf \times Hf1$, and the information coordinating picture is

$$1Wg2 \times 1Hg$$

where $1Wf1 < 1Wg$ and $1Hf1 < 1Hg$.

Multimodal biometric system assumes a significant job in acknowledgment frameworks. Right now, are three sorts of biometric segments, for example, facial and fingular are considered while playing out the confirmation procedure. Presently a day, programmers took person's biometric qualities for getting to the client's information. In view of this issue, the biometric highlights melded by the FLA so as to upgrade the security of client's information. Moreover, the RSA cryptography utilized for scrambling the melded vector to improve the strength of this framework. Table 1 explains the risk analysis factor during compilation.

To evaluate the impact of higher subjects of learning sample performance on nulled and ranged space, we evaluate the detection accuracies for various number of learning samples images. The accuracies are evaluated for number of learning sample as per level ranging from two to nine. From Table 2, it can be said that performance of nulled area is lessening with a greater number of samples and provides only fifty percent accuracy rate when highest number of learning samples are taken. This shows that it has negative effect on nulled area when number of learning samples is higher. Little increment in nulled area sample improves the performance of nulled area. While in ranged area, performance betters with a greater number of learning sample up to a limit, but the performance shows decrement when limit is crosses.

From the table, it is clear enough that nulled area lessens with higher number of sample while ranged area increases up to a limit but again lessens. Face recognition by PCP is shown in Figs. 14, and 15 is depicted the original, null, and ranged comparison.

4.5 Combined Face Recognition, EEG, and RSA

We have amalgamated face, finger, and RSA at level of decision. We took the entire sample from stored database and found the distribution per subject according to various parameters like test, learning, and authentication. The distribution to each

Table 1 Risk analysis

Compile error	Low	Unlikely	Ensure that the code is correct and does not have errors
Error in input of data from brain sense	High	Somewhat likely	Make sure that the device is calibrated properly and that it has been worn properly on the head
Problem in data transfer from brain sense to processing computer	High	Unlikely	Ensure that the wireless connection made via Bluetooth is strong, and it does not get disturbed
Change of facial structure	Medium	Unlikely	In cases when the person's face undergoes a rapid and drastic change, the system can adapt by requiring the longer full password
Privacy issues	Low	Unlikely	Make sure that the data gathered from the sensors is stored using state-of-the-art hashing techniques in secure clouds
Security access	Medium	Unlikely	Use random order of numbers which are to be played in the earpiece for authentication using brain–computer interface
Processing issues	Medium	Somewhat likely	Ensure that the algorithms and programs behind the dual-layer security and access system have enough data to reach the correct results
Run-time errors	High	Unlikely	Check that all the data is accessible and all the code does not contain any compilation errors, while also ensuring that the data transfer and data gathering stages do not encounter any glitches
Technology obsoletion	Low	Unlikely	Use latest hardware that is of a modular nature, so that it can be updated in the future without changing the whole setup

segment was done according to sample distribution done individually for each segment. Tables 3 and 4, respectively, show the segment division for each parameter.

Table 2 Performance of nulled area

No. of learning samples	Nulled area	Ranged area
Two	96.11	66.12
Three	92.34	75.43
Four	88.75	82.89
Five	83.12	78.22
Six	76.23	67.21
Seven	76.34	64.22
Eight	61.49	59.21
Nine	50.00	56.78

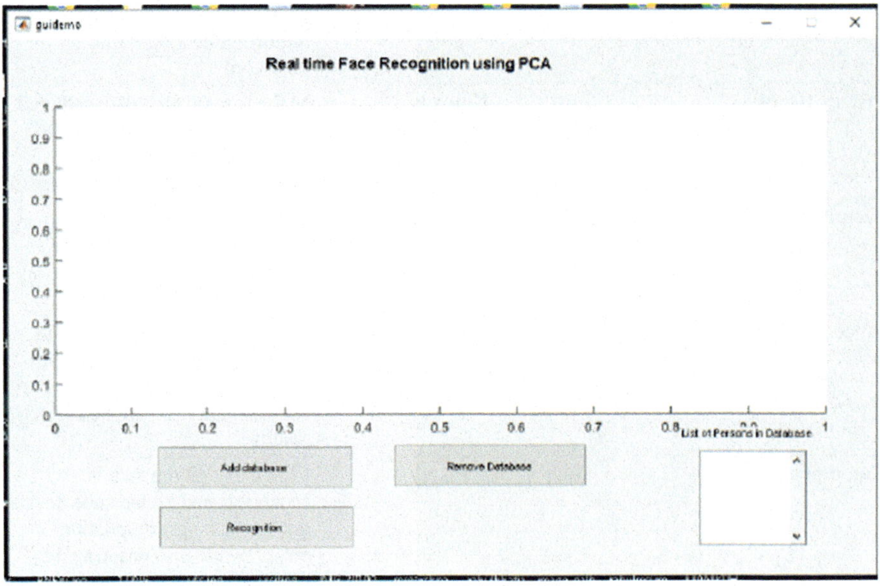

Fig. 14 Face recognition by PCP

5 Conclusion and Future Work

The results of the dual layer security system are successful. We can see that the facial recognition and the EEG sensor work along with the RSA encryption to provide a superlative experience to the user. We get enhanced security compared to other existing security systems, and we get even better results than we would have gotten if we had just used a single type of security apparatus. We find that authentication using brain sense is successful the vast majority of the times, and failure is only associated with either hardware problems or incorrect parsing of data. The dual-layer security and access system has been created by using brain sense, and

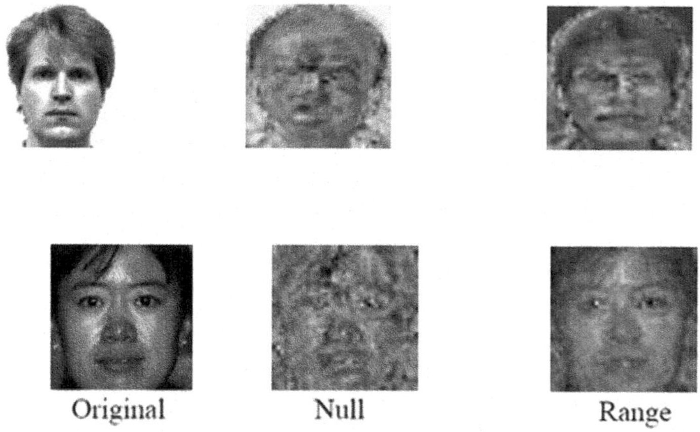

Fig. 15 Original, null, and ranged comparison

Table 3 Sample division for facial database

	PID		ORB	
	First trial	Second trial	First trial	Second trial
Train	5	5	2	2
Authentication	5	5	3	3
Evaluation	70	70	5	5

Table 4 Sample division for finger database

	XKa and XKb			
	First trial	Second trial	First trial	Second trial
Train	3	2	2	1
Authentication	1	2	2	3
Evaluation	4	4	4	4

implementing the algorithms in MATLAB and OpenCV. The other supporting hardware required is a Bluetooth-enabled computer, computer-connected camera, input and output devices, and a network connection. The dual-layer security and access system is successful and is deployed on a system where it can be used to enhance security and safety. The dual-layer security and access system also provides help and assistance to the physically challenged to enable them to access services and unlock systems. The biggest potential benefit of the dual-layer security and access system can be in reducing the spread of coronavirus and in helping humanity to fight this disease. Coronavirus can be spread by touching the same surfaces in situations like ATM machines, and coronavirus can remain on the machine. If the dual-layer security and access system is used, then we can eliminate all problems of touching

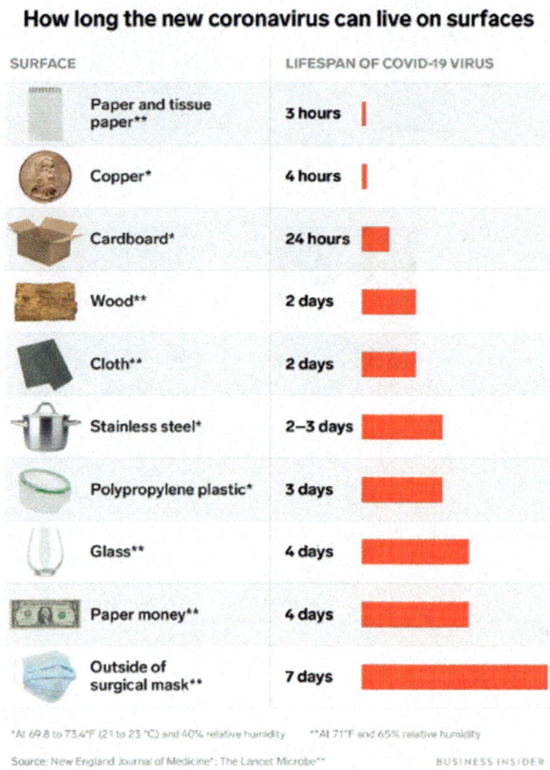

Fig. 16 How long the new coronavirus can live

surfaces for entering codes in ATMs or buildings. This will be a helpful boost in humanity's fight against the menace of coronavirus. Figure 16 shows about how long the new coronavirus can live.

The dual-layer security and access system has huge benefits for user privacy by not storing details of biometrics that can be compromised. The dual-layer security and access system can also be used in the future for national security purposes by enabling a centralized and highly secure database to access and process the facial data recorded by the cameras and to use this data for preventive and predictive purposes. The dual-layer security and access system can be used for both, forward and backward reasoning. The dual-layer security and access system can be used for interacting with computers by simply thinking of what we want to do and the computer understanding it. The modular nature of the dual-layer security and access system allows constant upgradation without changing the whole system and also allows remote software updates to enhance capabilities. In the future, the dual-layer security and access system will enable us to live in the world of science fiction.

References

1. WHO? (2020). WHO Director-General's opening remarks at the media briefing on COVID-19 - 11 March 2020. Available: WHO. (2020). WHO Director-General's opening remarks at the media briefing on COVID-19 - 11 March 2020. Available.
2. La Marca, A., Capuzzo, M., Paglia, T., Roli, L., Trenti, T., Nelson, S. M.
3. Reprod Biomed Online. *41*(3), 483–499, (2020). Published online 2020 Jun 14. 10. 1016/j.rbmo.2020.06.001https://www.ncbi.nlm.nih.gov/pmc/articles/PMC7293848/.
4. Corman, V. M., Landt, O., Kaiser, M., Molenkamp, R., Meijer, A., Chu, D. K. Detection of 2019 novel coronavirus (2019-nCoV) by real-time RT-PCR. *Euro Surveill.* (2020). https://doi. org/10.2807/1560-7917.ES.2020.25.3.2000045.
5. Wang, W., et al. (2020). Detection of SARS-CoV-2 in different types of clinical specimens (in eng). JAMA, 2020/03//2020.
6. Kong, W., & Agarwal, P. P. (2020). Chest imaging appearance of COVID-19 infection. *Radiology: Cardiothoracic Imaging, 2*(1), e200028.
7. Bernheim, A., & Mei, X. (2020). Chest CT findings in coronavirus disease-19 (COVID-19): Relationship to duration of infection. *Radiology*. https://doi.org/10.1148/radiol.2020200463
8. Lee, E. Y. P., Ng, M. Y., & Khong, P. L. (2020). COVID-19 pneumonia: What has CT taught us? *The Lancet Infectious Diseases, 20*(4), 384–385. https://doi.org/10.1016/S1473-3099(20)301 34-1
9. Shi, H., Han, X., Jiang, N., et al. (2020). Radiological findings from 81 patients with COVID-19 pneumonia in Wuhan, China: A descriptive study. *The Lancet Infectious Diseases, 20*(4), 425–434. https://doi.org/10.1016/S1473-3099(20)30086-4
10. Minaee, S., Kafieh, R., Sonka, M., Yazdani, S., & Soufi, G. J. (2020). Deep-COVID: Predicting COVID-19 from chest X-ray images using deep transfer learning. *Medical Image Analysis, 65*, 101794.
11. Wang, C., Horby, P. W., Hayden, F. G., & Gao, G. F. (2020). A novel coronavirus outbreak of global health concern. *Lancet, S0140–6736*(20), 30185. 2020 Jan 24.
12. Cohen, J. P., et al. (2020). Covid-19 image data collection: Prospective predictions are the future. arXiv preprint arXiv:2006.11988 (2020).
13. Chest X-Ray Images published by Paul Mooney. https://www.kaggle.com/paultimothym ooney/chest-xray-pneumonia.
14. Kathiresan, S., et al. (2020). Automated detection and classification of fundus diabetic retinopathy images using synergic deep learning model. *Pattern Recognition Letters*.
15. Gautam, C., et al. (2020). Minimum variance-embedded deep kernel regularized least squares method for one-class classification and its applications to biomedical data. *Neural Networks, 123*, 191–216.
16. Umer, S., et al. (2020). Person identification using fusion of iris and periocular deep features. *Neural Network, 122*, 407–419.
17. Saraswat, S., Awasthi, U., & Faujdar, N. (2017). Malarial parasites detection in RBC using image processing. In *2017 6th international conference on reliability*. Infocom Technologies and Optimization (Trends and Future Directions) (ICRITO).
18. Altamash, M., Avinashwar, N. F., & Saraswat, S. (2019). Video based facial detection & recognition. *Identity*.
19. Bobrov, P., et al. (2011). Brain-computer interface based on generation of visual images. *PloS one, 6*(6), e20674.
20. Kaufmann, T., et al. (2011). Flashing characters with famous faces improves ERP-based brain–computer interface performance. *Journal of Neural Engineering, 8*(5).
21. Lance, B. J., et al. (2012). Brain–computer interface technologies in the coming decades. In *Proceedings of the IEEE 100. special centennial issue* (pp.1585–1599).
22. Wang, Y., & Jung, T. P. (2011). BA collaborative brain-computer interface for improving human performance. *PLoS ONE, 6*(5), e20422.

23. Liao, L. -D., Lin, C. -T. , McDowell, K., Wickenden, A. E., Gramann, K., Jung, T. -P., Ko, L. W., & Chang, J. -Y. (2012). In *Proceeding of the IEEE BBiosensor technologies for augmented brain-computer interfaces in the next decades* (pp. 100).
24. Nishimoto, S., Vu, A. T., Naselaris, T., Benjamini, Y., Yu, B., & Gallant, J. L. (2011). BReconstructing visual experiences from brain activity evoked by natural movies. *Current Biology, 21*(19), 1641–1646.
25. Bilalic´, M., Langner, R., Ulrich, R., & Grodd, W. (2011). BMany faces of expertise: Fusiform face area in chess experts and novices. *Journal of Neuroscience, 31*(28), 10206–10214.
26. Kerick, S., Ries, A., Oie, K., Jung, T. P., Duann, J., Chou, J. C., Dai, L., & McDowell, K. (2011). B2010 neuroscience director's strategic initiative. *Army Research Laboratory Technical Report*, ARL-TR-5457.
27. Iandola, F. N., Han, S., Moskewicz, M. W., Ashraf, K., Dally, W. J., & Keutzer, K. (2016). SqueezeNet: AlexNet-level accuracy with 50x fewer parameters and¡ 0.5 MB model size. arXiv preprint arXiv:1602.07360.
28. Huang, G., Liu, Z., Van Der Maaten, L., & Weinberger, K. Q. (2017). Densely connected convolutional networks. In *Proceedings of the IEEE conference on computer vision and pattern recognition* (pp. 4700–4708).
29. Badrinarayanan, V., Kendall, A., & Cipolla, R. (2017). Segnet: A deep convolutional encoder-decoder architecture for image segmentation. *IEEE Transactions on Pattern Analysis and Machine Intelligence*, 39(12), 2481–2495.
30. Ren, S., He, K., Girshick, R., & Sun, J. (2015). Faster r-cnn: Towards realtime object detection with region proposal networks. In *Advances in neural information processing systems.*
31. Dong, C., et al. (2014). Learning a deep convolutional network for image super-resolution. In *European conference on computer vision.* Springer.
32. Zeiler, M., Fergus, R. (2014). Visualizing and understanding convolutional networks. In *European conference on computer vision.* Springer.
33. Al-Nafjan, A., et al. (2017). Review and classification of emotion recognition based on EEG brain-computer interface system research: a systematic review. *Applied Sciences, 7*(12), 1239.
34. Komlosi, S., Csukly, G., Stefanics, G., Czigler, I., Bitter, I., & Czobor, P. (2013). Fearful face recognition in schizophrenia: An electrophysiological study. *Schizophrenia Research, 149*, 135–140.
35. Mehmood, R. M., & Lee, H. J. (2016). A novel feature extraction method based on late positive potential for emotion recognition in human brain signal patterns. *Computers & Electrical Engineering, 53*, 444–457.
36. Degabriele, R., Lagopoulos, J., & Malhi, G. (2011). Neural correlates of emotional face processing in bipolar disorder: An event-related potential study. *Journal of Affective Disorders, 133*, 212–220.
37. Kashif, N., Ag, A. A. I., Lifen, W., Abzetdin, A., Jamal, D. M. (2016). Smart home for elderly living using wireless sensor networks and an android application. In *IEEE 10th international conference on application of information and communication technologies.* AICT.
38. Garrett, W., Christopher, P., Nisha, R., Gabriel de la, C., Shivam, G., Sepehr, N., Bryan, M., Maureen, S. -E., Matthew, T. E., & Diane, C. J. (2018). Robot-enabled support of daily activities in smart home environments. *Cognitive Systems Research*, 58–72.
39. Rozita, T., Salah, A. A., Kok, C. W., Mok, H. V. (2013). Smart GSM based home automation system. In *IEEE conference on systems, process & control (ICSPC2013).*
40. Hamed, B. (2012). Design & implementation of smart house control using LabVIEW. *International Journal of Soft Computing and Engineering, 1*(6), 98–106.
41. Himanshu, S., Vishal, P., Vedant, K., & Venkanna, U. (2018). IoT based smart home automation system using sensor node. In *4th international conference on recent advances in information technology.* RAIT.
42. Ghosh, S. (2020). Police in China, Dubai, and Italy are using these surveillance helmets to scan people for COVID-19 fever as they walk past, and it may be our future regular. *Business Insider.*

43. Ruktanonchai, N. W., Ruktanonchai, C. W., Floyd, J. R., & Tatem, A. J. (2018). Using google location history data to quantify fine-scale human mobility. *International Journal of Health Geographics, 17*(1), 28.
44. Mohammed, M. N., Syamsudin, H., Al-Zubaidi, S., AKS, R. R., & Yusuf, E. (2020). Novel COVID-19 detection and diagnosis system using IOT based smart helmet. *International Journal of Psychosocial Rehabilitation*, 24(7).
45. Mohammed, M. N., Hazairin, N. A., Al-Zubaidi, S., AK, S., Mustapha, S., & Yusuf, E. (2020). Toward a novel design for coronavirus detection and diagnosis system using IoT based drone technology. *International Journal of Psychosocial Rehabilitation, 24*(7), 2287–2295.
46. Mohammed, M. N., Hazairin, N. A., Syamsudin, H., Al-Zubaidi, S., Sairah, A. K., Mustapha, S., & Yusuf, E. (2020). Novel coronavirus disease (Covid-19): Detection and diagnosis system using IoT based smart glasses. *International Journal of Advanced Science and Technology, 29*(7), 2019.
47. Syed, L., Jabeen, S., & Manimala, S. (2018). Telemammography: a novel approach for early detection of breast cancer through wavelet-based image processing and machine learning techniques. In *Advances in soft computing and machine learning in image processing* (pp. 149–183). Springer.
48. Kunnakorntammanop, S., Thepwuttisathaphon, N., & Thaicharoen, S. (2019). An experience report on building a big data analytics framework using Cloudera CDH and RapidMiner Radoop with a cluster of commodity computers. In *International conference on soft computing in data science* (pp. 208–222). Springer.
49. Adebiyi, M., Famuyiwa, B., Mosaku, A., Ogundokun, R., Arowolo, O., Akande, N., & Adebiyi, E. Computational investigation of consistency and performance of the biochemical network of the Malaria Parasite, plasmodium falciparum. In *International conference on computational science and its applications* (pp. 231–241). Springer.
50. Oladele, T. O., Ogundokun, R. O., Awotunde, J. B., Adebiyi, M. O., & Adeniyi, Diagmal, J. K. (2020). A malaria coactive neuro-fuzzy expert system. In *Computational science and its applications–ICCSA 2020: 20th international conference, Cagliari, Italy, July 1–4, 2020, Proceedings, Part VI 20* (pp. 428–441). Springer International Publishing.
51. Strohbach, M., Ziekow, H., Gazis, V., & Akiva, N. (2015). Towards a big data analytics framework for IoT and smart city applications. In *Modelling and processing for next-generation big-data technologies* (pp. 257–282). Springer.
52. Vidal-García, J., Vidal, M., & Barros, R. H. (2019). Computational business intelligence, big data, and their role in business decisions in the age of the internet of things. In *Web services: Concepts, methodologies, tools, and applications* (pp. 1048–1067). IGI Global.
53. Velez, F. J., Chávez-Santiago, R., Borges, L. M., Barroca, N., Balasingham, I., & Derogarian, F. (2019). Scenarios and applications for wearable technologies and WBSNs with energy harvesting. *Wearable Technologies and Wireless Body Sensor Networks for Healthcare, 11*, 31.
54. Panigrahy, S. K., Dash, B. P., Korra, S. B., Turuk, A. K., & Jena, S. K. (2019). Comparative study of ECG-based key agreement schemes in wireless body sensor networks. In *Recent findings in intelligent computing techniques* (pp. 151–161). Springer.
55. Yousefi, M. H. N., Kavian, Y. S., & Mahmoudi, A. (2019). On the processing architecture in wireless video sensor networks: Node and networklevel performance evaluation. *Multimedia Tools and Applications, 78*(17), 24789–24807.
56. Deng, Z., Wu, Q., Lv, X., Zhu, B., Xu, S., & Wang, X. (2019). Application analysis of wireless sensor networks in nuclear power plant. In *International symposium on software reliability, industrial safety, cyber security, and physical protection for nuclear power plant* (pp. 135–148). Springer.
57. Sodhro, A. H., Zongwei, L., Pirbhulal, S., Sangaiah, A. K., Lohano, S., & Sodhro, G. H. (2020). Power-management strategies for medical information transmission in wireless body sensor networks. *IEEE Consumer Electronics Magazine, 9*(2), 47–51.
58. Swayamsiddha, S., & Mohanty, C. (2020). Application of cognitive internet of medical things for COVID-19 pandemic. *Diabetes & Metabolic Syndrome: Clinical Research & Reviews.*

59. Rodrigues, J. J., Segundo, D. B. D. R., Junqueira, H. A., Sabino, M. H., Prince, R. M., Al-Muhtadi, J., & De Albuquerque, V. H. C. (2018). Enabling technologies for the internet of health things. *IEEE Access, 6*, 13129–13141.
60. Singh, R. P., Javaid, M., Haleem, A., Vaishya, R., & Al, S. (2020). Internet of medical things (IoMT) for orthopaedic in COVID-19 pandemic: Roles, challenges, and applications. *Journal of Clinical Orthopaedics and Trauma.*
61. Alassaf, N., Gutub, A., Parah, S. A., & Al Ghamdi, M. (2019). Enhancing the speed of SIMON: A light-weight-cryptographic algorithm for IoT applications. *Multimedia Tools and Applications, 78*(23), 32633–32657.
62. Qadri, Y. A., Nauman, A., Zikria, Y. B., Vasilakos, A. V., & Kim, S. W. (2020). The future of healthcare internet of things: A survey of emerging technologies. *IEEE Communications Surveys & Tutorials, 22*(2), 1121–1167.

Pregnancy Women—Smart Care Intelligent Systems: Patient Condition Screening, Visualization and Monitoring with Multimedia Technology

S. Usharani, P. Manju Bala, R. Rajmohan, T. Ananth Kumar, and S. Arunmozhi Selvi

1 Introduction

It is a nation's duty to provide the following important things to their people such as proper healthy diet for pregnant woman, awareness education about child health and adequate medical facilities. Satisfying these will pledge successful efforts for the growth of the nation through human resources. Most of the maternal death (around 99%) occurs in the developing countries. Around 850 women die each day due to pregnancy. Exchange of knowledge between health care industries are not organized in most developing countries or in smart cities. A survey says out of 100 pregnant women, 55 of them have not done their consistent checkup at the beginning of pregnancy, which leads to a higher child and maternal death rate in rural areas. Because of these complications, the population is facing a major medical crisis. Proper health care facilities should be provided by government from starting period of pregnancy with appropriate health assistance will reduce the maternal death and result in the birth of healthy children. Pregnant women in rural areas lack proper awareness of medical and technological advancements to mitigate maternal fatality risks. In the course of pregnancy, at least two ultrasound scans are needed to monitor the fetal health at regular intervals. Proper and timely checkups can result in safe delivery. The cost of the medical checkups are also high and unaffordable.

In the proposed system, sensors are attached to monitor the important parameters like heartbeat, temperature and kicking. The readings are accessible through mobile device. In the new era, many researches are ongoing to improve the quality of life, new inventions of reducible cost and storage are used to increase the smart medical care. In particular, because of the increase in population and decrease in the ratio of doctor to people, smart healthcare is in high demand, and some people are busy

S. Usharani (✉) · P. M. Bala · R. Rajmohan · T. A. Kumar
Computer Science and Engineering, IFET College of Engineering, Villupuram, Tamilnadu, India

S. A. Selvi
School of Computer Science & IT, DMI St. John the Bapist University, Lilongwe, Malawi

A. K. Tyagi et al. (eds.), *Intelligent Interactive Multimedia Systems for e-Healthcare Applications*, https://doi.org/10.1007/978-981-16-6542-4_9

travelling for treatment to a specialist hospital. Over the next several years, the smart healthcare market is expected to be over numerous trillion dollars. There are many criteria needed for an effective smart healthcare system, including low cost, high precision, ease of use medical sensors, the pervasive design of the structure and reducible time delay in decision making. While attempts have been made over the past several years, even though many researches are ongoing for the past several years, these criteria cannot be fulfilled in a single system. The usability of the sensor directly depends on the invasiveness; the complexity of installation and monitoring signals determine the high cost precision rest on the sensitivity of the sensors and the implanted software algorithms; and time period of delay totally hinge on the number of signal characteristics. Numerous smart healthcare models from various viewpoints have already been suggested. Some existing systems try to solve issues in smart cities by evaluation of voice, identification of feelings and patient's state acknowledgement.

A signal capturing technique is used to analyze and store the signals from the operators. Heart beat and movement of fetal are two different signals captured for analysis. These signals are transferred from mobile devices to the cloud-based server for processing and the cloud-based server shares the processed result back to the doctor. For example, in a smart healthcare framework in Fig. 1 shows a smart home installed with various sensors to get various data such as fetal movements and heartbeat rate, mother's blood pressure and diabetes results, and then, these data are forwarded to the cloud server for processing. The processed result such as heart beat signal is shared with the doctors and hospital, who will examine the results. Depending up on the accuracy of the result, patient may be called in person or prescription will be sent.

To ensure the health as well as wellbeing of a pregnant mother and her infant child, monitoring of pregnancy is important. Actually, at routine visits of maternity care

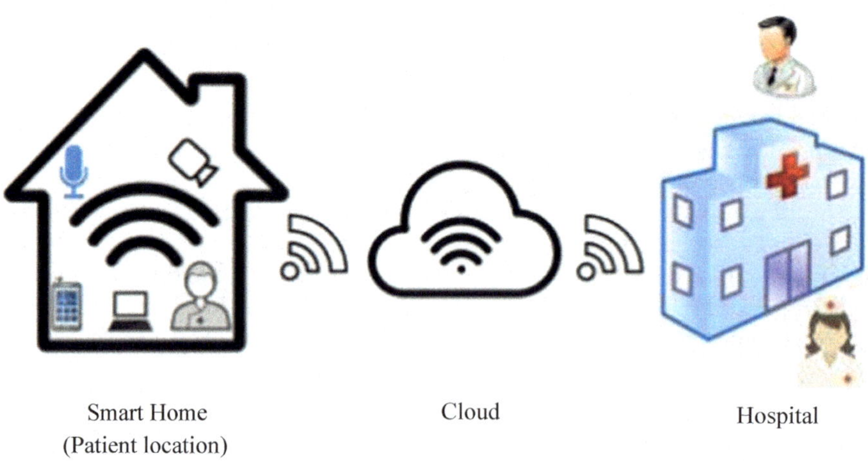

Fig. 1 Smart health care monitoring system

centers, health care workers conduct this tracking. With the help of new technology like the Internet of things (IoT), it is become feasible to constantly control, map and distribute personal medical measurements in near real-time in more effective manners than it has ever been. This advancement has also greatly contributed to maternity care possibilities, as IoT securely links sensors (such as smart wristbands) to servers, allowing tracking and data analysis from everywhere at any time via Internet Web applications. It has been well understood that when applying to healthcare services, IoT applications have not achieved their maximum potential.

In pregnant women, monitoring technology is shown to facilitate health variables. Optimally, self-controlled supervision will involve pregnant women more now than ever before in their health care. This could conserve maternity care money by, for example, minimizing the number of appointments or finding potential complications. Another potential use of this technology was its detection of measures of health promotion and assessment of high-risk mothers as well as those with an elevated risk of pre-diabetes. Health data collected will allow health care workers to check through on their clients and construct recommendations about individualized care. The monitored information could also be used for extra checkups or treatments to automatically identify high-risk patients. Health care workers and the testing community also require practicable, accurate and reliable measuring instruments.

Wearable allow the constant tracing, in normal life, of individual physical exercise and behaviors as well as biochemical and physiological factors. Dynamic signs such as body temperature, heart rate and BP (blood pressure), and also blood respiratory rate, position and physical exercise with the use of ballisto-cardiograms (BCG), electrocardiograms (ECG) and other devices are the most broadly measured information. Wearable photograph or cinematographic schemes may hypothetically have additional medical information. It is probable to support transferable devices to sneakers, eyewear, bracelet, clothes, jackets and jewelry. Wearable gadgets can go into skin appendable devices also. Sensors will be installed throughout the room like beds, high chairs and comforters. Usually, a smartphone is being used to capture information and send it for storing and processing to a Web server. For researching movement patterns, there have been two main types of smart technology which are used. Some instruments, such as the gyroscope, multi-angle recording devices and accelerometer, have been created by health care professionals to track activity habits. Other gadgets, such as on fitness trackers and smart phone applications and add-ons, were established for wellness users. Wearable sensors and data processing techniques are most often used together during multiple situations to execute posture evaluation tasks.

Innovative alternatives to health crises could be wearable devices. The research analysis of smart wearable implementations in healthcare is momentarily explained in this chapter. Any uses of wearable devices are developed for patient safety and quality management, such as weight controlling and monitoring of physical movement. For patient management and health management, smart systems are also used. Wearable apps may have a direct effect on professional decision making. Some assume that wearable devices, such as patient rehabilitation elsewhere in hospitals, may decrease the quality of health treatment while lower the amount of care. Wearable technology has immense promise in prenatal care, such as smart bracelets, but it also faces obstacles. Maintaining the long-term dedication of patients with this new technology is one of the main challenges. It is important to consider the desires and obstacles of the target audience to address this obstacle so that system viability and appropriateness can be assessed in an authentic sense. IoT systems are typically tested with functionality testing and expert opinions at present, but health care viability analysis is seldom done. In maternity services, the introduction of wearable devices, such as smart bracelets, includes an appreciation of the opinions of mothers and commitment to methods. For researchers who could really add additional Ml algorithms to the datasets, the big data produced by smart technology is both an obstacle and an opportunity.

The remaining structure of the chapter is organized as follows: Sect. 2 describes the related work carried over in the diagnosis of pregnant women using intelligent systems. Section 3 summarizes the various smart devices for monitoring pregnant women and fetal movements. Section 4 elucidates the importance of biosignal analysis in monitoring the heartbeat rate of pregnant women and fetal. Section 5 demonstrates the efficiency of using smart wrist bands for continual monitoring of pregnant women health parameters such as heart beat, blood pressure, glucose level and diabetes risk.

2 Related Work

As a smartphone application, Android Java-DSP that communicates with sensors and allows simulation. This has also aided in the development of signals analysis. Firstly, in this framework, an interface was designed between these external sensors as well as on device sensors to track the physiological signals of humans. It also investigated the mobile sensing pattern and applied it to improve digital signal processing by developing medical sensor frameworks including external sensors. It is a small interface with low-power wireless sensors which can capture and relay real-time kinematic and physiological data. The downside to this method is that the patient who is hospitalized is monitored [1–3]. The certain proof shown that cardiovascular diseases is the main cause of older people's hospitalization. If the elderly undergo care in an hour, there are further chances of recovery. It has been built as well. To recognize a dropping of the carrier, an Android mobile phone with a sensor is used, but this Android phone is recognized as a health device. Through using the TCP/IP protocol over Wi-Fi, the Android device would then be attached to the monitoring device. Because of this scheme, people who are aged and critically ill may live in their own home safely and comfortable in the awareness that they are being watched. The downside to this method is that it recognizes elderly persons when they are most likely to have unexpected outbreaks such as heart disease and stroke [4–6]. The image-based device obtains the ECG signal from a digital camera; such data is processed and saved in the memory on a tool such as MATLAB and data transfer across the public Internet. Then, via Android phones, the original picture is made available to the doctor. The objective of this system is to provide the intensive care unit surveillance system with vital signs and criteria and to render these data accessible to doctors who may not have been in hospital or in the world. The doctor is notified in the event of any irregularity by sending a message to his mobile device from the server. The downside to this report is that the results will not be sent to the geographically based doctor because of the poor Internet access. The picture is taken by the sensor, which has to be HD and costs a lot [7–9]. Creation and deployment of the wireless wearable component with a mobile phone for significant health tracking. Smart shirts are made with ECG sensors in this device and can be used by every type of patient to track his or her status in real time to get the necessary treatment or medication. This programs are primarily built with elderly individuals in mind when they live in certain homes alone. Therefore, this device essentially tracks the aged for the goal of self. The consequence of this method was that the method was able to track and identify the cardiac problems of patients in real time while they were wearing a sports jersey with an ECG sensor. In comparison to this, with background tracking software and an automated 108 call device, the system also delivers visual information to the patient to receive the appropriate care in time. The downside of the machine is that it mainly works on older people and requires a shirt that costs a lot [10–12].

Wireless universal healthcare on multiple mobile platforms through sensor connectivity, data collection, data visualization, etc. There is a single wireless wellness device controller. Modules for individual mobile devices have been developed to incorporate health care on multiple platforms. UTMS and CDMA provide more functionality than Wi-Fi and Bluetooth, and smartphone platforms endorse all this wireless connectivity. They began by analyzing the right health care mobile phone model, then defining the source code for the mobile device platform and eventually designing the mobile career development for that specific platform. For multiple systems, they have different and improved debugging environments. The downside of this article is that they really do not show the actual library of mobile heath applications [13]. The physiological characteristics of the patient, such as the patient's blood pressure and pulse rate, are constantly observed. In order to monitor the health condition, this device is primarily useful for pregnant women to monitor different metrics such as blood pressure, heart rhythm and lethal activity. This machine needs to track upwards of one patient at a time and to be able to quickly detect patients' heart rate and heart rhythm. There is a sensorimotor connected to the person's blood in this device to calculate signals from the remote monitoring and transmit those signals to the server. This device will monitor the patient's unusual behaviors, lift the patient's alarm and give the physician and SMS/email for medication. The primary benefit of this scheme is to expand the right to improve the quality of life of patients. The disadvantage of this method is that patients must be hospitalized in order to monitor the physiological conditions of the patient constantly. If the amount of patients in the hospital is admitted above the prescribed limit, this WSN becomes difficult [14]. The patient tracks his or her personal health via smart phones, providing additional details such as the user's location and providing protection and continuity. For this reason, modern technology is employed. They choose a wireless system called near field communication technology that communicates with electromagnetic radio fields in order to preserve protection [15]. To view patient records, NFC technology has been used, and this data are stored in the EMR database of the hospital. All the data would be moved from EMR to NFC tag while the patient is discharged. The downside to this article is that this method relies solely on the preservation of the database instead of delivering resources such as the closest hospital directory and alerting family members [16].

3 Health Monitoring Based on IoT System

Rural women lack the awareness of appropriate medicine whenever is necessary. They even deem medical costs prohibitively expensive. Therefore, certain critical parameters such as pulse, pressure, and fetal moving are determined in this device. Warning processes are indicators of our software. It helps to obtain information on health status of pregnant women in remote areas and provides a handheld mobile medical system that enables to accurately diagnose unplanned miscarriage, thus helping to minimize the risk of prenatal and maternal death. Figure 2. shows the system architecture for health monitoring system based on IoT.

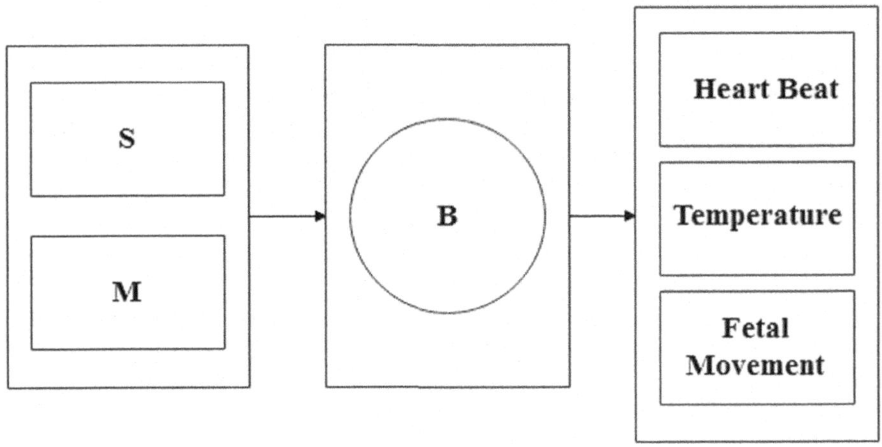

Fig. 2 System architecture for health monitoring system based on IoT

3.1 Heartbeat Measurement

Using the heartbeat monitor, the fetal heart rhythm is determined. A modulation amplification uses the inputs from the electrode and is then converted to the appropriate frequency range. The output is supplied as the Atmega input reaches a certain threshold. For fetal pulse rate measurement, a pulse rate sensor is available in the system.

3.2 Temperature Measurement

Temperature sensors from the LM35 series are precision interconnected temperature sensors. The output is linearly proportional to the temperature of the Celsius. The temperature sensor is being used to calculate the mother's temperature and transfers it to Breadboard is indeed a microcontroller that takes these signals as parameters and is programmed to have the desired output using Arduino software. The Arduino receives feedback from a piezoelectric buzzer and alarms any time if the value is beyond the thresholds. Figure 3 shows the block diagram of temperature measurement.

3.3 Fetal Movements

When the first movements of the fetus, called "Fetal Movement," between pregnancy weeks 16 and 25. Some females tend to experience movements very early as 13 weeks during pregnancy. When they are in a quiet spot, either seated or falling asleep, pregnancy women are inclined to feel the baby shifting. The motions of the baby are characterized by pregnant women as birds, anxious or a skidding motion. It can be complicated at first to know whether the baby has moved. In separating those first infant motions from energy, food cravings and other internal movements, second and third time mothers are much more expert. For certain hours of the day, babies seem to shift around as they switch between wakefulness and rest. Typically, they are most active around 9 p.m. to 1 a.m. as if to seek to get in to sleep. This rise in movement is attributed to varying levels of blood sugar. Babies can also adapt to noises or contact, and if they do not settle in relaxed places, they can also push their moms. Table 1. shows the measurement of fetal moves.

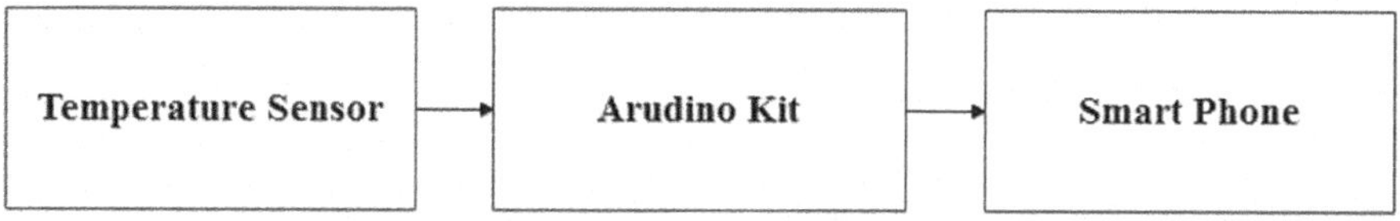

Fig. 3 Temperature measurement

Table 1 Fetal movement measurement

Period (in h)	Normal movements of fetal	Abnormal movements of fetal
1	>4	<2
2	>7	<5
24	>15	<8

3.4 Hardware Setup

Different types of sensors were used for the system application to measure critical factors such as temperature, pulse rate, maternal blood pressure and fetal activity. Sensors are connected to the device, so it allows to read and display it. Increasingly, IoT allows the convergence of applications capable of linking to the Web, delivering personal medical information and providing real-time information to clinicians who support it. It uses the following sensors.

3.4.1 Accelerometer Sensor

The measurement instrument sensor is one of the most popular mechanical occurrence detectors. Accelerometers are accessible that can calculate one, two or three analogous axis acceleration. The gestures of the fetus are largely due to the uterine vascular condition of placental abruption. These gestures are referred to as "Fetal Movements." The infant will begin moving from the fifth quarter onwards, but the mothers will not notice it. Physicians may be able to accurately predict the infant state and growth by monitoring the fetal activity.

Ultrasound screening tracks fetal movement, although this is costly. It uses an accelerometer sensor. The ADXL335 is a lightweight, slim and low-power sensor with signal-conditioned voltage outputs and has three axes. An acceleration with a minimal broad spectrum of ± 3 g would be measured. Three output voltage pins, namely AOUT, BOUT and COUT, have an accelerometer sensor. Bandwidths with a scale of 0.5–1600 Hz for both the X and Y axes and a scale of 0.5–550 Hz for the Z-axis can be chosen to accommodate the application. The ADXL335 is offered in a 16 lead, plastics lead times flip chip kit with a thin, low profile. The accelerometer sensor is wirelessly designed to measure fetal motion. The data from the accelerometer sensor is sent to the Arduino controller using the RF transmitter and receiver modules. Table 1 describes the fetus kicking count as normal or irregular. The fetus count continues from the fifth quarter onwards, but the mother does not follow it. The motion of the baby can first be detected in the fifth month by the mother. It is known to be a significant occurrence of fetal hypoxia if the diminished fetal activity is fewer than ten times every 12 h. Therefore, urgent steps must be taken to prevent these problems.

3.4.2 Temperature Sensor

Temperature sensors are primarily used for the measurement of maternal body temperature. It will more precisely calculate temperature than to use a thermistor. During pregnancy, it is normal for a woman's body temperature to rise. The woman's body produces extra heat throughout pregnancy due to accelerated digestion, high hormone production such as progestin, high turnover on the woman's body due to the extra weight as the pregnancy continues as well as the collection and processing of infant nutrition and slides beneath. Around the same time, the female has enhanced peripheral circulation, which contributes to heat dissipation from the body. The LM35 sensor runs between 4 and 30 V. It occupies the spectrum between −55 °C and + 150 °C.

3.4.3 Heart Rate Sensor

The heart rate sensor kit could be used for maternal heart rate control. Pulse waves, which are variations in the volume of a circulatory system that happen as the heart pumps, are determined by an optical heart rate monitor. By calculating the gap in volume using an optical sensor as well as a green LED, pulse waves are observed. The adoption of a pulse wave detector optimized optical filter throughout the sensor block reduces the influence of artificial light like red and near-infrared rays. This makes the acquisition of pulse signals of high quality, also outdoors. Furthermore, the use of optical sensor technologies developed over several years enabled ROHM to improve the responsiveness of the sensor block drastically. Help for low brightness lower VF LEDs enables a low voltage optical blood pressure tracking device to be accomplished without any need for additional circuitry. This leads to prolonged running times in wearables with reduced battery life.

3.4.4 Blood Pressure Sensor

For any human being, blood pressure is a serious issue. It is the strain exerted on the walls of arteries by the flowing blood. The ratio of pulse rate to diastolic pressure is defined in terms of blood pressure. The mercury sphygmomanometer can be used for blood pressure tests. The level of the column of mercury is taken into account of this calculation of blood pressure. For automatic blood pressure, the oscillometric procedure is used. One of the significant heart rate is blood pressure (BP). Blood pressure can begin to vary significantly for a pregnant woman over the span of ten months. During pregnancy, that is what makes them sound dizzy. Blood pressure control is very important as the difference of blood pressure may influence the oxygen delivery to the infant. Usually, elevated blood pressure throughout pregnancy does not lead to significant issues. Hypertension, though, will become existence for both mom and baby if it gets out of control. There will be risks if elevated blood pressure persists beyond 20 weeks of pregnancy. They may experience preeclampsia. This

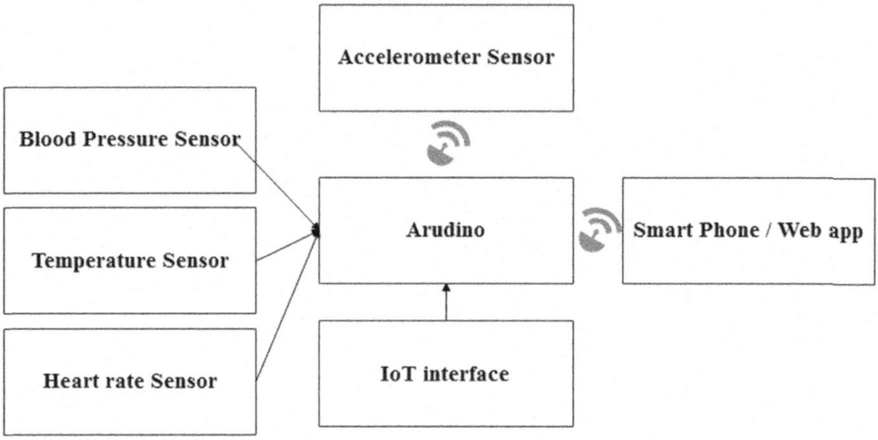

Fig. 4 Framework for IoT system

disorder will lead the organs, including the kidney and brain, to suffer significant damage. Preeclampsia is also known as depression caused by toxemia or pregnancy. It is also very necessary for maternal blood pressure to be detected.

3.4.5 Methodology

Figure 4 shows the framework for IoT system. The temperature sensor, heart rate sensor, blood pressure sensor and accelerometer sensor are operated by an Arduino controller using this technique. This controller analyzes the data from the sensors and the effects are simulated. IoT relates to specific machines' inter-networking. Without involving human to-human and human-to-computer interaction, IoT may transmit information over a public. The IoT that is used in this technology would be able to transmit long-distance data. A microcontroller board based on the ATmega328 is the Arduino UNO. It has 14 optical pins for input/output, 6 analog inputs, a 16 MHz crystal oscillator, a USB, an ICSP header, a power port and a reset button. This can be connected directly to the analogue input pin as the value detected from sensor is from an analog form. Before any more step can be completed, ADC can transform to digital signal in this Arduino microcontroller. The Arduino will interpret the signal as well as the output would be in the voltage form of the digital signal.

3.5 Experimentation and Result

In this section, the simulation results and analysis for the proposed approach regarding the health care monitoring system is discussed in the following section. Also, the results for various evaluation measures such as accuracy, precision, recall,

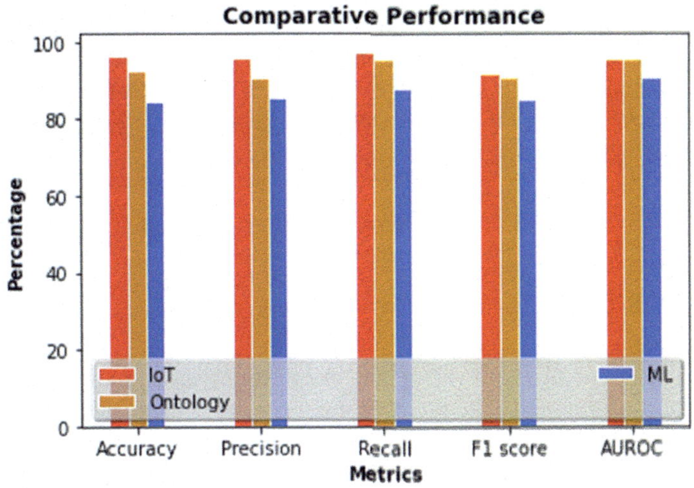

Fig. 5 Performance evaluation of IoT system

F1 score and AUROC are shown in the Fig. 5. The experimental analysis for the proposed approach is implemented under the simulation platform of Cooja. An event driving node communication and discrete platforms are used to run the program.

The experimental analysis reveals that the performance metrics such accuracy, precision, recall, F1 score and AUROC of the IoT-based health monitoring approach provides very efficient monitoring than other approaches.

4 Health Monitoring System Based on Biosignal Analysis

Through new developments in signal processing techniques and wireless communications, researchers were currently investigating the modern technologies for continual healthcare applications in a very stable, cost-effective and accessible space. One way to achieve this mission is to return to the fundamentals and to develop a communication interface for wearable sensors using devices like the Arduino MKRZero panel. In addition, the basis of such an induction system is dependent on machine learning and deep neural networks. These are some of the highest suitable methods to generate diagnostic accuracy is to use a mixture of convolutional neural network (CNN) and swarm intelligence (SI) as of now. While we have concentrated more on implementing a simple specialized maternity monitoring system in this study, we plan to progressively turn our attention to big data in the development to empower our system that is capable to identify almost all potential issues via machine learning and artificial neural networks dependent on heart rates variability. Coefficient is a very significant aspect that should be gotten rid of when any medical complications are diagnosed. Our suggested framework uses elements from the presence of a high connection between the patient's present status and the environmental circumstances under which it lives and the likelihood of some health issue that could arise through pregnancy in the context. Similarly, the flourishing field of analysis intends to use ontology to relate the features, disorders and therapies of pregnant mothers.

4.1 Biosignal

A body that may be at the level of the liver, cell layer or molecular threshold absorbs sensor information. There are different sensing signals, including the electroencephalogram (EEG), which is the brain's electrical activity; the electrocardiogram (ECG), which is the heart's electrical activity; the electromyogram (EMG), which is the muscle sound signal's electrical activity; the electroneurogram; the eye's good reading habits. The Photoplethysmogram, often refers to as PPG, tests the de-coloration of a skin during each pulse as blood peruses through blood vessels and veins. By evaluating light propagation or reflex ion over the skin, it tests the dynamic environments in the blood at the surface of microvascular membrane. One of the key benefits is that PPG sensors provide a less disruptive way to measure heart beat results. Therefore, for heart rate measurements, this device investigates PPG data. In order to identify or track particular clinical or pathological disorders, biomedical indicators are mainly used. In particular, the study of biological processes in healthcare uses these indicators. Signal thresholding, accurate identification of the signal design through evaluation, extraction of features and dimensionality reduction for definitive function or malfunction and prediction of possible functional or dysfunctional activities by the use of machine learning strategies are the goals of data interpretation.

4.2 Dataset

For analysis, Physionet's BIDMC PPG and respiration repository are used. Within this repository, there are 55 videos, each with its own length of 8 min, each containing:

- 126 Hz PPG signal analyzed.
- Biological variables, such as heart rate (HR), respiratory rate (RR), and saturation level of blood oxygen (SpO2). At 1 Hz these are tested.
- Fixed conditions, for example, age and sex.
- Direct breath descriptions.

The file formats which are included are in the form of a CSV format (semi-colon value). Statistics belonging to pregnant women were extracted out of all 55 recordings for analysis in order to remain in the nearest proximity of pregnancy symptoms.

4.3 Preprocessing

The first goal is to identify PPG signal diastolic pressure levels to measure the heartbeat. The status reports must be planned before they are fed into the information environments framework to improve this. Signals from one of the sample samples collected after noise reduction. For this design, the different preprocessing steps being taken are described as follows.

(1) Removal of Noise: To extract excessive noise from of the signals, an integrated feature called bacon and fitful from Python's scipy collection has been used.
(2) Peak up-sampling: Only inside the frequency sensor field being used can a signal be detected. If the pulse persists beyond the limits of the sensor, at those stages, the peaks identified appear smooth. In this scenario, to identify (nearly) smooth sections of the signals close to its limit, a sampling feature is being used and a spherical spline is used to estimate the transmission peak.
(3) Peak advancement: For study, the data is normalized to stay around 0 and 1024. The information is lifted to a power of 2 after it has been viewed as a numpy sequence. The goal is to allow the spikes more apparent by improving the frequency ratio.

4.4 Analysis

The biggest difficulty when measuring heart rate lies in the precision of the peak position labelling being used. The peak locations are critical when measuring heart rate changeability (HRC) measurements. RMSSD (root mean square of the successive differences), which is the basic formula for measuring heart rate, is used to measure peaks.

$$\text{RMSSD} = \sqrt{\frac{1}{m-2}\sum_{j=0}^{m-2}\left((R-R)_j - (R-R)_{j+1}\right)^2} \quad (1)$$

In order to classify specific heart rate and chart the peaks, a simple moving or rolling mean is determined. For this, on both halves of each data point, a key length of 0.80 s is set. These segments are filled with the median signal for the aspect of the signal that goes well beyond sliding window, and no linear equation is produced for these parts. The regions of interest (ROI) are then defined as two critical regions where the signal is larger than the rolling average. The range per second for beating is calculated as:

$$60 \leq \text{BPM} \leq 180 \quad (2)$$

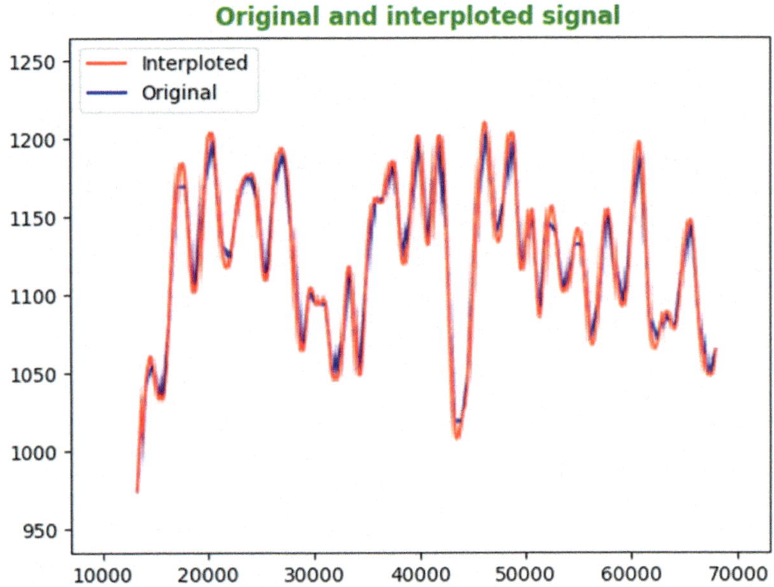

Fig. 6 Preprocessing signal

All the peaks observed are placed in a numbered series. Use the numpy.diff() method to create a new array (R_l list) (Eq. 3) that contains the feature extraction from the heights

$$R_l = \left(\frac{\text{diff(peak)}}{\text{samplerate}}\right) * 1000 \tag{3}$$

Now, all that remains is to obtain from such a list that necessary variable (i.e.,R_l list). The R-R interval is given by the average R_l list. The fast Fourier transformation is used for generating spatial frequency variables, such as HF and LF. In normal spatial frequency calculations, i.e., HF (0.17–0.6 Hz), LF, the complete power range is measured (0.05–0.15 Hz). In spite of phase and voltage, the elements LF and HF were assessed. Figure 6. shows the signal after preprocessing.

4.5 Experimentation and Result

The conceptual design of the process is related to the optical pulse detectors sold by the company. In order to guarantee the precision of the data analysis with a time span of one minute, observations were made three times. You can see the collected records of vital signs. The heart rate analysis from an electronic device would be recorded on the data collection form that was analyzed to summarize all the gathered information.

The outcomes of capturing IoT-based heartbeat information with a high reliability rate are in the 76–98 BPM levels. The data collected from the heartbeat is always listed as usual since it is in the 60–100 BPM level. These findings suggest that the architecture suggested is working properly. The outcome of heartbeat information is shown in Tables 2 and 3. Figures 7 and 8 shows the visualization of heart rate monitoring for women and fetal.

Table 2 Heart rate (BPM) for pregnancy women

Id	Original	Interpolated	Accuracy (%)
WOO1	75	77	97.40
WOO2	79	78	98.73
WOO3	81	82	98.78
WOO4	78	80	97.50
WOO5	82	81	98.78
WOO6	73	75	97.33
WOO7	70	69	98.57

Table 3 Heart rate (BPM) for fetal

Id	Original	Interpolated	Accuracy (%)
COO1	84	85	98.82
COO2	88	86	97.73
COO3	79	81	97.53
COO4	90	88	97.78
COO5	92	91	98.91
COO6	85	86	98.84
COO7	86	85	98.84

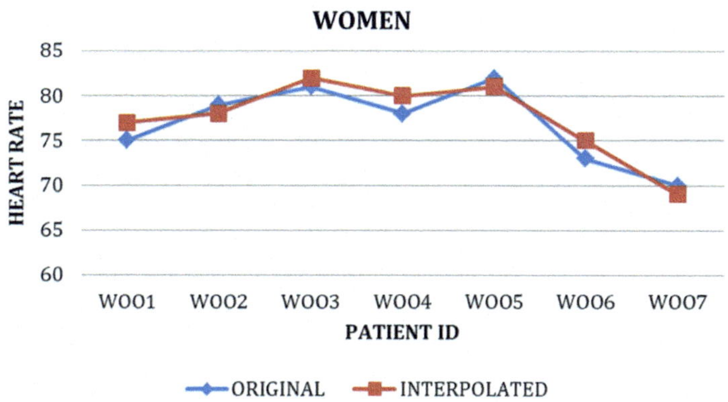

Fig. 7 Pregnancy women heart rate monitoring

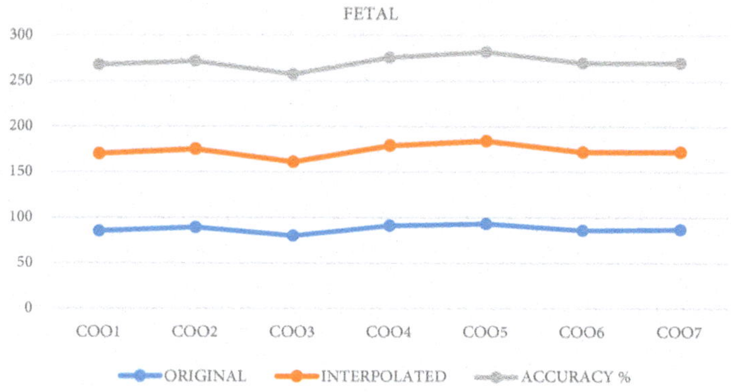

Fig. 8 Fetal heart rate monitoring

5 Health Monitoring Based on Smart Wearable Devices

Wearable devices, smart fabrics and other advances in health apps (mHealth) offer promising new possibilities to improve pregnancy health detection, clinical tracking and leadership beyond conventional care environments. Rapid technological developments in wearable technologies are now expanding medical health care tracking functionality and have tremendous enhancing early diagnosis of disorders of pregnancy. Pregnancy is a stage of life that requires rapid physiological and behavioral changes, and more careful therapeutic supervision may help some greater risk females. Smart technologies has also been used in in the field of maternal issues to facilitate weight loss, increase patient adherence in the treatment of chronic diseases, including obesity, heart failure, breast cancer and heart disease and to enhance general health.

There are currently a range of consumer-based mobile devices that track strength training and other environmental behavior improvements as well as control physiological variables (e.g., blood pressure) on an ongoing basis, but none targeting pregnant ladies. Far less findings have analyzed the views of the patient and practitioner about the feasibility of using these software solutions to track maternal health and atmospheric factors constantly and the resulting effects on medical decision.

In the early diagnosis of serious adverse outcomes related to pregnancy, wearable sensors and other intelligent devices may play a significant role along with encouraging change in patient and physician experiences for successful pregnancy health care system. In the clinically significant stage of an undesirable pregnancy result wearable sensor devices produce extensive, complex databases that can be used to classify existence, climate and developmental health risks. A new analysis used mobile sensors to monitor fluctuations in blood pressure in high-risk pregnant mothers with hypertension and showed a reasonably high reliability of forecast.

In order to promote patient compliance to prescription drugs, wearable tools and other intelligent electronic gadgets are now used; hence, digital sniper nests also have the capacity to wireless communication sync with the smartphones of a patient to deliver constant stories, monitor the usage of prescription and geo-location. By introducing major changes in the way investigators enroll, receive approval, gather data and engage with patients, Apple's Research Kit is dramatically improving the way clinical research is conducted. Research Kit, for instance, is now used to explain why some women experience post pregnancy depression (PPD) and some do not engage in a clinical analysis by approaching women all over the world. Using a variety of wearable detectors cloud computing, AI algorithms, and smartphones, investigators can now monitor the mental state of a woman after birth to promote accurate intervention of PPD. Although a major problem remains to incorporate high amounts of interconnected clinical and health data to educate intelligent decision support systems and identify clinical anomalies, computer programmer's work with doctors to improve pattern detection of pregnancy complications caused by pregnancy by the use of digital health information and developments in functional disabilities.

The aim of this analysis was to determine the desires, degree of convenience and possible issues of health care professionals and their clinicians in the use of wearable devices in a rural, clinically underutilized hospital in Southern Appalachia to track pregnancy care. We also examined the potential advantages and limitations of wearable medical technology and the kinds of data that clients and clinicians would really like to see collected during pregnancy for health and environmental tracking. This study will resolve a major disparity between the pregnant community and their clinicians in the expectations and acceptance of integrating wearable and smart mobile devices technology into fertility treatments.

The current study aims to recognize how intelligent digital technologies (e.g., mobile applications (apps), wearable devices) are currently being used by pregnant women and the healthcare professionals in the rural South and their expectations of integrating these intelligent tools to track pregnancy care. The aim of this study was to determine the desires, degree of convenience and possible issues of health care professionals and their clinicians in the use of wearable technology in a remote, underserved community's clinic in Southern Appalachia to track maternity care. This study will resolve a substantial disparity between the pregnant community and their clinicians in understanding and acceptance of integrating portable and smart digital device technologies into fertility treatments.

5.1 Methodology

In a hypothetical experimental feasibility study with neutral pregnant women, the efficacy of smart armbands was checked. During their first weeks of pregnancy diagnostic tests 16 pregnant primiparous women were trained at two pregnancy clinics in Southwest Finland. (a) $\geq$ 18 years of age, (b) $\leq$ 15 gwks, and (c) singleton pregnancy were specific criteria for candidates. Women who did not really understand Hungarian were disqualified or who did not have smartphones or computers that were equipped with the smart bracelet. It was suggested that fifteen participants were able to determine the viability of everyday exercises in the target community as well as to calculate the sample group.

Original written and verbal knowledge about the experiment was given by the health care workers at the pregnancy clinics. All qualified women (N = 16) were concerned in taking part in the study and interacted by telephone with the analysis team. The researcher presented more specific details about the analysis during each phone conversation, and a facial appointment was scheduled if the woman was able to attend. According to work-related prohibitions towards carrying a smart bracelet, two women refused to engage after obtaining the study data over the phone. The investigator was met the thirty women and given formal, medical intervention. At the session, the attendees were given smart armbands and guidance for using them. From training to 1 month pregnancy, the women were told to wear the armbands constantly, as eliminating the bracelet raises the risk of failing to be used.

5.2 Smart Wristband as a Measurement Tool

The choice of a smart bracelet for a long-term menstrual monitoring analysis is affected by many factors. Firstly, a wristband's weight, scale and level of support play key functions in growing wear time. In addition, the participants may be motivated to wear the device through an effective social interaction, such as an onboard monitor and an integrated smartphone framework. In allowing longer periods between system charging and data synchronization, adequate battery energy and internal file storage are also critical. Due to its low cost, smooth design on bands, wearable device and capacity to calculate steps and heart rate, smart bracelet was selected from the accessible, affordable cost devices. It combines a biosensor and a consumer-available behavior monitor. This smart bracelet, compact (21 mm × 12.3 mm) and light (29.6 g), measures movement, range (based on movement), energy used, heart beat climbing stairs, physical exercise speed and overall sleep. The data is constantly obtained and synchronized to the website or the app. On a single occasion, the battery charger will last up to several days. The device needs two hours to charge. Various variables can shorten the battery life among charging (e.g., display intensity and movement warnings). In the stable non-pregnant community, when worn through relatively slow walking speed and pulse failure in sleep, it has shown strong accuracy in calculating step counts, but it overestimates the pulse rate when activity frequency advances.

5.3 Data Collection and Outcomes

The primary result was the regular usage (crack period) over an eight month follow-up duration during pregnancy and the postpartum period of the smart bracelet. In an IoT-based framework where many sensing, interaction and computing capabilities have been utilized, the smart armbands were used. The information gathered by the bracelet was transferred through a transit unit, which was a mobile or tablet, to the computers. Once a day or during wearing the intelligent armbands, the respondents were requested to synchronize the information. Throughout the analysis, the information was available to investigators and respondents via different sensors. The device's wear period was assumed to be usable in the server. Both respondents answered a checklist for personal data before they were selected. The observations of the respondents with the smart bracelet (fulfilment, demonstrated interest and personality changes in behavior) were examined through telephone interviews performed by the research assistants. During the analysis, each respondent was questioned ten times; frequently after the first data processing month; and once a month afterwards. A voicemail has been sent to ask for a time suitable for a follow-up call if a respondent was not reached for comment. Multiple-choice and open questionnaire were used in the telephone interview. In fact, pregnancy and infancy information were obtained from the participant electronic record.

5.4 *Data Analysis*

Adjusted thresholds, trust ranges, median and scope were used as dependent variables to define and summarize the context data of the respondents and the wear time of the handsets, and measures with fractions were used for propositional factors. By measuring Cohen's kappa factor, cross compatibility between the empirical wear period and the personality wearing period was investigated. For this, for each weeks of pregnancy and postpartum cycle, the target wear time was categorized (All the time: 7 days/week $\geq$20 h/day; some days/week: $\geq$3 days/week; Once a week: $\geq$1 1 day/week; Not at all: 0 h/week). The processing of data comprised 24 h of the day. In addition, the sum of appropriate peak time information was evaluated for a minimum of four days a week with the standard of 10 h of phase count data at peak period per day.

To consider the practical use of the intelligent bracelet in greater detail, we examined whether the days of pregnancy were correlated with the device's wear period. We therefore used a clustered linear mixed system with multiple steps which include one inside-factor calculation (time as categorical). The design of conditional symmetry variable has been used for some time. Analyses were conducted both regularly and on the basis of pregnancy weeks of pregnancy. All experiments were conducted with the context of the two-tailed test set at 0.05.

5.5 Experimentation and Result

In the research, 16 pregnant women enrolled. The average participation age of respondents was 24 years (ranging from 18 to 37 years). The respondents' average pre-pregnancy body mass index (BMI) was 23.2 kg/m2. For all of the respondents, the follow-up stayed until one quarter after birth attendee features are illustrated in the Table 4, Pregnancy women characteristics.

During their pregnancy weeks, the respondents used the equipment for thirty days, ranging from 8–14 weeks. This is resulting in a global average use over the seven-month postnatal cycle of 28 days per individual. The length of the gestation had an effect on the time of research. In the one month span, the daily average wear period was about 6 to 8 h. When the respondents were sleep, the gadgets have been used more; 75% of the wearing time was waking up period.

Few critical feedbacks were given by respondents on the efficacy of the initiatives. Eight respondents viewed the system as overestimating the sequence of iterations due to the finger's inactivity. The women often found that the moments of strength or the climbing of the staircase were not correctly recorded. The underestimation of time expended sleeping has been stated by some respondents. The heart rate calculation was found by one respondent to be inaccurate.

During the long follow-up era, problems in synchronizing the smart bracelet with their devices, laptops or desktops were very common ($n = 12$), even though the system would synchronize itself via Bluetooth at regular periods Software upgrades, abrupt power shutdowns and switching to a mobile phone or device were more technological problems. The respondents handled the difficulties on their own in most situations, while some mentioned requesting for assistance from their partners ($n = 5$) or from an investigator ($n = 2$).

Such real-time data obtained using wearable system sensors were combined with data from the UCI machine learning repository to predict the risk of heart disease, BP and diabetes problems. Such methods for the prediction of other diseases are generalized.

Table 4 Pregnancy women characteristics

Characteristic	Value
Age	20–28 yrs
Body mass index	23.2 kg/m^2
Gestation week	7–14 weeks
Employment	Working—6 Home Maker—10
Diabetes	Yes—4 No—12
Heart disease risk	Yes—2 No—14
Blood pressure	Yes—2 No—14

The characteristics listed in the input data are as shown in the Table 5. Class 1 shows the existence of heart failure, issues with BP and depression in the data collection and Class 0 demonstrates avoidance. The patient database is broken down into 80–20% as a learning and evaluation data. RNN, CNN and TCN algorithms are used to train the predictive models. Using efficiency indicators such as specificity, reliability, remember and f-score, the design was assessed.

In order to incorporate disease detection, such real-time data is analyzed. The findings of the estimation method are checked and accepted by the physician specialist and eventually aligned with the pregnancy women's actual medical condition.

The comparative analysis is given in Table 6 for different estimation techniques such as RNN, CNN and TCN algorithms Also, Fig. 9 shows the visualization of performance metrics of RNN, CNN and TCN. From the visualization, it states TCN produce better metrics than RNN and CNN.

Table 5 Confusion matrix of prediction

Prediction	Class 1	Class 0	Total
Class 1	4	7	10
Class 0	6	3	10
Total	10	10	20

Table 6 Performance analysis of wrist bands

Evaluation metrics	CNN	RNN	TCN
Accuracy	94.67	95.61	95.89
Precision	90.18	90.29	91.56
Recall	89.45	88.67	90.34
F-Measure	85.23	86.41	87.36

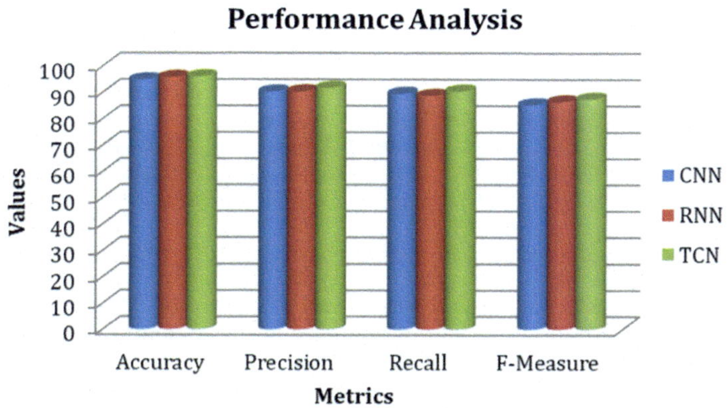

Fig. 9 Performance metric analysis

6 Conclusion

Most maternal deaths takes place at home in emerging and under developed countries. To avoid these problems in this chapter, we described health monitoring of the pregnancy woman in various methods such as IoT-based mobile or Web app, biosignal processing and wearable devices using IoT sensors. In the first method, a portable assistive device is designed to minimize these pregnancy risks, and critical parameters such as temperature, women's pain and fetal heart rate are monitored using various sensors. Even for minor gestures, the device is compact and extremely sensitive, and thus favored as a home surveillance device. Infant mortality is minimized by daily monitoring of the critical parameters of fetuses and women in rural areas. The parameters computed are passed via the IoT. It offers both fetuses and women with quality and efficient health assistance. The findings are shown on the cell phone with the IoT. In second method, a basic evidence of the idea of a device designed to carry out ongoing, noninvasive health surveillance of pregnant women utilizing their biosignals. In the last method, the practical used during the pregnancy of a smart wristband was considered to be fine. The wearing time, nevertheless, decreased significantly in the post-pregnancy era. A practicable probability is the constant recording, logging and transmission of personal health indicators in real time using armbands in maternity services. There is a need to carefully assess the design and comfort of this system. All the three methods are used to monitor the health of pregnancy woman to improve growth of the fetal to reduce complications and to avoid maternal death of woman or fetal. Performance evaluation of the proposed method reveals that engaging intelligent devices for pregnancy women health monitoring is efficient when compared to traditional methods. The future research work can be carried over in designing AI-based neuro-system and IoT devices for prediction of illness progression.

References

1. Grym, K., Niela-Vilén, H., Ekholm, E., Hamari, L., Azimi, I., Rahmani, A., Liljeberg, P., Löyttyniemi, E., & Axelin, A. (2019). Feasibility of smart wristbands for continuous monitoring during pregnancy and one month after birth. *BMC pregnancy and childbirth, 19*(1), 1–9.
2. Gupta, Y., Kumar, S., & Mago, V. (2019). Pregnancy health monitoring system based on biosignal analysis. In *2019 42nd international conference on telecommunications and signal processing (TSP)* (pp. 664–667). IEEE.
3. Alamri, A. (2018). Monitoring system for patients using multimedia for smart healthcare. *IEEE Access, 6*, 23271–23276.
4. Rajan, D., Spanias, A., Ranganath, S., Banavar, M. K., & Spanias, P. (2013). Health monitoring laboratories by interfacing physiological sensors to mobile android devices. In *2013 IEEE frontiers in education conference (FIE)* (pp. 1049–1055). IEEE.
5. Lee, J. -V., Chuah, Y. -D., & Chieng, K. T. H. (2013). Smart elderly home monitoring system with an android phone. *International Journal of Smart Home, 7*(3), 17–32.
6. Shusterman, L. (2002). *Remote patient monitoring system with garment and automated medication dispenser*. U.S. Patent 6,471,087, issued October 29, 2002.
7. Jeon, B., Lee, J., & Choi, J. (2013). Design and implementation of a wearable ECG system. *International Journal of Smart Home, 7*(2), 61–69.

8. Pavithra, M., Rajmohan, R., Ananth Kumar, T., & Ramya, R. (2021). Prediction and classification of breast cancer using discriminative learning models and techniques. *Machine Vision Inspection Systems, Volume 2: Machine Learning-Based Approaches,* 241–262.
9. Dhivya, S., Jayakumar, D., Pajany, M., & Rajmohan, R. (2018). Temperature and humidity monitoring from remote system using IOT with alert system for landslide. *International Journal of Pure and Applied Mathematics, 119*(14), 761–765.
10. Usharani, S., Manju Bala, P., & Balamurugan, R. (2020). Voice based form filling system for visually challenged people. In *2020 international conference on system, computation, automation and networking (ICSCAN)* (pp. 1–5). IEEE.
11. Usharani, S., Saravanan, D., & Parthiban, R. (2017). Resource allocation through energy in IoT network. *International Journal of Scientific Research in Computer Science, Engineering and Information Technology, 2,* 84–86.
12. John, A., Ananth Kumar, T., Adimoolam, M., & Blessy, A. (2020). Energy management and monitoring Using IoT with CupCarbon platform. In *Green computing in smart cities: Simulation and techniques* (pp. 189–206). Springer.
13. Woodbridge, J., Nahapetian, A., Noshadi, H., Sarrafzadeh, M., & Kaiser, W. (2009). Wireless health and the smart phone conundrum. *ACM SIGBED Review, 6*(2), 1–6.
14. Aminian, M., & Reza Naji, H. (2013). A hospital healthcare monitoring system using wireless sensor networks. *Journal of Health and Medical Informatics, 4*(02), 121.
15. Rajakumar, G., Kumar, T. A., Samuel, T. A., & Kumaran, E. M. (2018). Iot based milk monitoring system for detection of milk adulteration. *International Journal of Pure and Applied Mathematics, 118*(9), 21–32.
16. Devendran, A., Bhuvaneswari, T., & Krishnan, A. K. (2012). Mobile healthcare system using NFC technology. *International Journal of Computer Science Issues (IJCSI), 9*(3), 428.

Prediction of COVID-19 Outbreak with Current Substantiation Using Machine Learning Algorithms

N. Indumathi, M. Shanmuga Eswari, Ayodeji Olalekan Salau, R. Ramalakshmi, and R. Revathy

1 Introduction

Corona virus (COVID-19) is a viral infection that infects persons, birds, and mammals. For such an extremely novel pathogen such as COVID-19 especially one with high reproductive ability, this virus is harmful as it causes respiratory tract infections. This virus is a cluster of RNA viruses identified as 2019-nCoV virus [1]. They are classified into various subspecies, namely: alpha, delta, beta, and gamma, in which the first two cause infections in human beings. As at present, there are seven human corona virus varieties as Human corona virus 229E (HCoV-229E), Human corona virus OC43 (HCoV-OC43), SARS-CoV, Human COVID NL63(HCoV-NL63, New Heaven Corona virus), Human corona virus HKU, Middle East Respiratory Corona virus Syndrome (MERS-CoV) previously known as novel corona virus 2012 and HCoV-EMC, Novel corona virus (2019-nCoV) also identified as Wuhan pneumonia or Wuhan corona virus [2]. As a communicable disease, it is transferred from one person to another by direct communication and globules.

In January 2020, the SARS-CoV-2 virus was officially identified as the cause of COVID-19. COVID-19is derived from the SARS corona virus which causes severe respiratory disease, inflammation in the nose, nostrils, or upper throat. COVID-19 affects human beings with and without symptoms. Usually, the morality rate and

N. Indumathi · M. Shanmuga Eswari · R. Revathy
Department of Computer Applications, Kalasalingam Academy of Research and Education, Krishnankoil, Virudhunagar, Tamil Nadu 626126, India

A. O. Salau
Department of Electrical/Electronics and Computer Engineering, AfeBabalola University, Ado-Ekiti, Nigeria

R. Ramalakshmi (✉)
Department of Computer Science and Engineering, Kalasalingam Academy of Research and Education, Krishnankoil, Virudhunagar, Tamil Nadu 626126, India
e-mail: rama@klu.ac.in

A. K. Tyagi et al. (eds.), *Intelligent Interactive Multimedia Systems for e-Healthcare Applications*, https://doi.org/10.1007/978-981-16-6542-4_10

spread of disease of patients depend most times on the pre-medical conditions of the patient. The pandemic started at the time of mid December 2019 in Wuhan, China. Pneumonia was observed to be one of its symptoms and persons affected by SARS were usually observed to have difficulty in moving or talking. In January 2020, World Health Organization (WHO) announced that COVID-19 is treacherous to humans and is a public health emergency. Majority of countries have taken preventive measures to safeguard their people through wearing masks, social distancing, travel bans, border shutdown, travel restrictions, and lockdowns. This situation has slowed down the economic and life status of people [3]. The majority of corona viruses are not dangerous. Till now there is no specific vaccine for this but some of the drugs like chloroquine and hydroxyl chloroquine have been found to reduce its severity [4].

Although the outburst of this virus has been on the increase and has increased mortality rate among humans, the field of Machine Learning (ML), Artificial Intelligence (AI), Deep Learning (DL), and Statistics has provided various methods to predict this virus and also its outcomes [5, 6]. The aim of this study is to build up a prediction model and to make an expert system based on its decisions.

Sujath et al. [7] analysed the outcome of COVID-19 cases and proposed measures to reduce it in India. The authors used Kaggle data for predicting the efficiency of the model. Regression algorithm and regression auto vector machine learning algorithms were used to predict COVID-19 cases. The ANFIS and optimized swarm algorithm was used to predict the cases of infections in China and the USA. Al-Qaness et al. [8] used WHO official data to model a system to predict COVID-19. This model is able to predict the outcome of COVID-19 cases for a period of10days in China and the USA.

Elmousalami et al. [9] proposed a method for the determination of COVID-19cases. In this method, they used time series prediction and numerical correlation methods. Day level predictions were analysed based on active cases. Yang et al. [10] developed an AI model based on SARS dataset. They used dynamic Susceptible Exposed Infectious Recovered (SEIR) to forecast the infectious contagion apex and its sizes.

COVID-19 data set is an example of time series data. A number of studies have been conducted to develop more effective models and techniques to predict COVID-19occurrences. Yudistira [11] presented an LSTM model for capturing the pattern and dynamic graphs with RNN with the aim of predicting COVID-19. The results show that the number of COVID-19 cases increased until it reaches a certain peak curve in the graph. Tomar et al. [12] analysed the COVID-19 cases in India. A time series model was used to accomplish this. This model had challenges in the training phase. This led to many attempts to increase the memory size of the time series model using various algorithms. After optimizing this model, each time series was used as a node in a tree structure. In the early years of time series databases, it was easy to develop a system that could be used by a computer without a storage system, because computer storage capacities were low and there was no need for any system at all. Authors in [13] used deep learning to detect COVID-19. According to Li et al. [14], four classification models, namely, random forest, logistic regression, artificial neural network, and naïve bayes were used and then compared to predict COVID-19 disease and their performances were evaluated. The deep learning model was found to have the highest accuracy of 94% in detecting the disease. Among these four methods, random forest obtained high performance in classifying the disease.

Among an extensive range of ML algorithms, MLP, and ANFIS provided capable results in the prediction of COVID-19 outburst. The authors in [15] recommended that ML can act as an effective tool to enhance the novelty in future COVID-19 outbreak prediction.

The authors hope that the finding of this study will open a new paradigm in the field of medicine. The aim of the study is to design an efficient model which is capable of accurately predicting the clinical outcome of an individual diagnosed with COVID-19. This will help to enable the identification and timely intervention of those who are most at risk or suffering from this dreaded virus [16]. This chapter presents the implementation of C5.0 decision tree and deep learning model that achieves very high accuracy for the early diagnosis of COVID-19 prediction. However, we did not only apply ML algorithms but have also compared them with respect to rate of accuracy and error of predicting COVID-19 occurrence. The symptoms of COVID-19 are shown in Fig. 1.

In the detection of the fourth human corona virus, HCoV-NL63, identified in a 7-month-old baby with bronchiolitis and conjunctivitis, some authors have identified that corona virus causes tiredness, breathing difficulty, flu, cough, and severe headache. Since other infectious illnesses, including influenza and cold, have close symptoms to COVID-19. The fourth human coronavirus HCoV-NL63 can cause human corona virus-associated symptoms and infections. We also demonstrated that HCoV-NL63 can cause human corona virus-associated respiratory tract inflammation that is different from other coronavirus respiratory tract inflammations. The symptoms of patients are not easy to differentiate from other respiratory illnesses and this is one of the reasons there is a great deal of difficulty in tracking and identifying the number of cases of infected people in Saudi Arabia, Qatar, United Arab Emirates, and several European countries. Nearly 60% of the people with SARS developed fever, cough, headaches, muscle pains and a runny nose. These symptoms

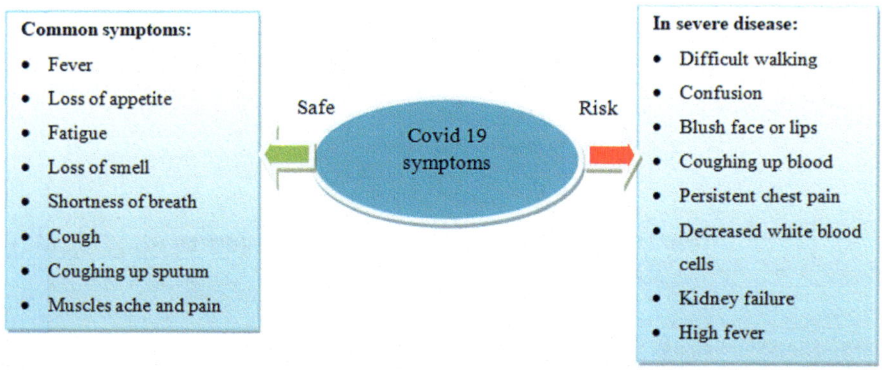

Fig. 1 Symptoms of covid-19

typically appear between 2 and 15 days after exposure to the disease. Other, milder, symptoms of SARS include fatigue and chills. SARS was first discovered in China in November 2002 and was responsible for more than 800 cases in that country before it was declared eradicated in April 2003.

Kumar et al. [17] designed a patient monitoring system that was used to monitor the heartbeat, temperature and respiration level of COVID-19 patients. To forecast time series data of the mortality rate, hybrid ANFIS and MLPICA (multi-layered perceptron-imperialist competitive algorithm) are proposed. With these models, the epidemic and overall mortality rate will be significantly reduced.

This virus which has no known cure has caused financial loss and low economic productivity in all the nations of the world. It has mercilessly halted everything in society on a fragile basis. ML is used to construct different predictive models, and their output is computed and evaluated [18, 19].

1.1 Study Area

To achieve the purpose of this study, the district of Virudhunagar was chosen as the case study. Figure 2 shows the Virudhunagar district which was created on 15 March 1985 on the deviates of the former Ramanathapuram district which was one of Tamilnadu's districts. The district of Virudhunagar lies between 9° 07 and 10° 22 North latitudes and longitudes of 77° 22 and 79° 25 East. The District is about 4222 square kilometres in area. It is bounded by the Western Ghats to the west, and by the north of Madurai, in northeast Sivagangai district, in east Ramanathapuram and in the south surrounded by Tuticorin district.

The district is divided into two divisions, namely: Aruppukkottai and Sivakasi. There are 32 panchayat towns, 294 panchayat unions, 3612 wards and 1098 wards in

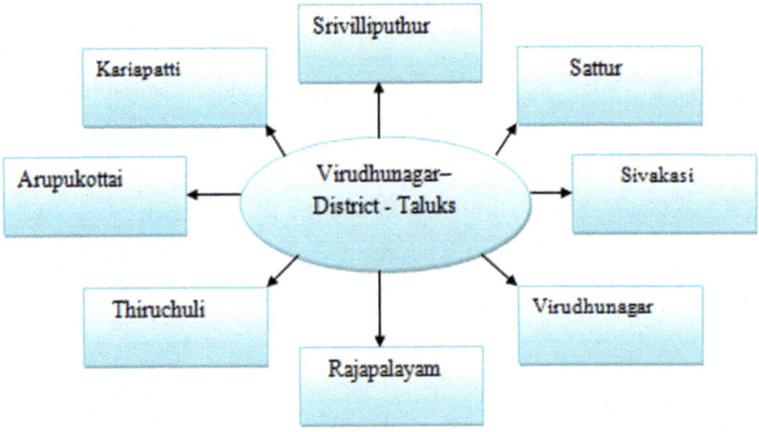

Fig. 2 Map of the study area

Table 1 Divisions, taluks and villages of Virudhunagar district

S. No	Revenue divisions	Revenue taluks	Revenue villages
1	Aruppukottai	Aruppukottai	83
		Kariapatti	107
		Tiruchuli	150
		Virudhunagar	61
2	Sivakasi	Sivakasi	45
		Srivilliputhur	50
		Rajapalayam	39
		Sattur	65
Total			**600**

Source District Revenue Administration Department in India

the district. In the past, this division was under the control of Virudhunagar, Trichy, and Madurai provinces of the erstwhile Madurai Nayak dynasty. In this paper, the taluks affected area was analysed and special focus was made on the critical zones in the Virudhunagar district. Overall, 600 villages and 8 taluks were investigated and presented in Table 1.

As per the census of Virudhunagar district, the district has a population of 1,942,288 as of 2011, of which 967,709 are male and 974,579 are female. The population of the Virudhunagar district in 2019/2020 is 2,052,365 (uidai.gov.in as of Feb 2019). Similarly, the total number of literates is 965,828 of which 689,829 are male and 696,616 are female. About 88.89% of the total population is urban.

1.2 Industrial Background

The district of Virudhunagar is famous for its industries. The places that are famous for their industries are Virudhunagar, Aruppukkottai, Kariapatti, Sivakasi, Sattur, and Rajapalayam. Sivakasi, the Kutti Japan, is well known throughout India as a place for printing, fireworks and matching industries. Although Sivakasi's two diametrically opposite sides have had to co-exist with each other over the last century, the people of this district never showed any animosity towards the people of the other side. Today, there are scores of parties in celebration of each other's festivals as well as each other's cultures. Sattur is famous for its Nib manufacture and for the manufacture of matches. Rajapalayam is known for manufacture of textiles, surgical cotton, bandages, woven cloths, nightwear, spinning and weaving mills and cotton markets. Cement and oil mills are located in and around Virudhunagar. Chatrapatti (Virudhunagar district) is a major producer of surgical cotton gauze and the nearby towns of Dhalavaipuram and Muhavoor manufacture women's nightwear. Handloom and power loom are concentrated in Aruppukkottai. Kariapatti is known for the production of nuts and bolts. This area is a crowded place because of the industries. So many people in these areas are not still aware of the Covid-19 pandemic and have not to keep maintaining social distancing and other precautions.

The town of Thiruchuli is synonymous with Sri Ramana Maharishi, and of the temple of Sri Ramana Ashrama, which is on the side of the hill. It is a wooden structure that is sometimes described as a hut with a tin roof, which has been built on the same spot where the sage came to the Ashrama, as devotees still speak. The hut is open to the public, and the shrine and grounds also include a museum dedicated to the guru.

Srivilliputhur is known for Andal temple. The temple's gateway tower stands 192 ft (59 m) tall and is thought to be the official emblem of the Tamil Nadu state. It is famous for its sweet Palkova manufacturing, agriculture, and wildlife forest. Majority of people are working in matches and firework industries. They are closely sitting and doing their work. So social distance is not possible in this region. This is the main reason why the COVID-19 virus is seen to spread faster in this area.

1.3 Virudhunagar District Covid-19 Cases

With 10,155 instances, Virudhunagar has now become the second district in the south to cross the five-digit mark after Madurai. The district has so far accumulated more than 9000 cases, after passing 1000 cases on 7th July, 2020. For instance, the district had reported more than 500 cases once every day, thrice more than 400 cases on 10 occasions, 300 or more cases, and seven days with more than 200 cases. While the towns of Sivakasi, Virudhunagar and Aruppukottai, and the adjacent rural areas, have more active cases, cases were seen to reduce in the other eight regions.

2 Material and Methods

2.1 Proposed System Procedure

The system tested using data from Virudhunagar, Tamilnadu, districts in India. The following steps were used to develop the proposed system.

1. Data collected
2. Datamining and deep learning techniques were used for classification of danger zone identification
3. Comparison of both techniques
4. Prevent the infection rate in and around Virudhunagar district.

2.2 Data Collection

The statistical dataset is collected from various sources like newspapers, web scraping, and local bodies. The dataset was collated from March 13 to July 26, 2020, in Virudhunagar district, Tamil Nadu, India. The dataset had the details of the infectious status of taluks in Virudhunagar. The algorithms help to classify these statistical data and separate the taluk into green, red, and yellow zones respectively.

2.3 Classification and Prediction Algorithm

The major intention of this study is to classify the COVID-19 data using classification and prediction algorithms with ML to forecast the affected regions into danger zone, moderate zone, and safe zone. This process involves three phases such as data pre-processing, building of models, and validation of the models. The classification model is shown in Fig. 3.

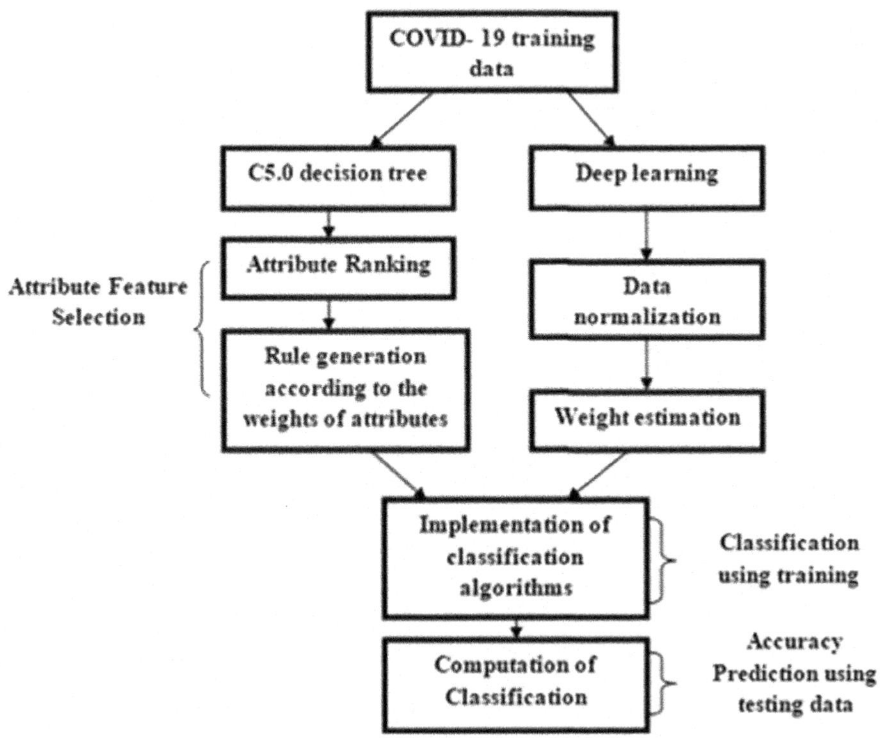

Fig. 3 Classification of COVID-19 data for prediction of COVID-19

2.3.1 C4.5 Algorithm Steps

Input: Virudhunagar dataset

Output: Decision classification tree

Pseudocode:

- Find normalized gain ratio of each input attributes
- Take maximized normalized gain
- Split the decision node
- Add child nodes.

This procedure helps in pruning and handling incomplete data sets. Therefore, all errors are treated as equal.

2.3.2 C5.0 Algorithm Steps

Input: Virudhunagar dataset

Output: Decision classification tree

- Obtain the maximum information gain for each attribute
- Segment the decision tree based on max. information gain
- Subset of former will be split afterwards.

This algorithm comparatively gives better results than that of C4.5 and is easy to implement. With options of cross validation and sampling of data, the proposed system achieved effective results with C5.0 algorithm which gave less variable misclassified costs.

As data pre-processing is significant before training the model, it increases the accuracy of the algorithm. C5.0 usually attributes ranking by estimating the weight of the attributes and by generating the rules according to its features. But for the neural network method, the data should be normalized before training the model.

Computation of various systems can be defined as a competition between various computations. In the context of an inference system, the computation refers to the calculation of probability that a particular conclusion is correct, while the competition refers to the computation by the system that comes closer to the truth.

Normalization is a method frequently used for the preparation of data using ML algorithms. The aim of data normalization is to transform the numeric values present in the dataset without modifying or losing its information. It helps improves the training speed of the neural network. To normalize data, data samples are divided into equal categories, and then frequencies (or clusters) of these categories are created. Normalization can be applied to both raw (unprocessed) data and fully filtered (transformed) data. It commonly speeds up the network learning since the data obtains a value close to 0. It is otherwise known as feature scaling, where the numeric values are reduced to a scale between 0 and 1. In data normalization method, linear transformation is carried out on the original data. Maximum and minimum values from the data are taken and each value is substituted using Eq. (1). This equation is used to scale the variable values between 0 and 1. The principle of min max normalization is defined as follows.

$$Z = \frac{X - \min(X)}{\max(X) - \min(X)} \tag{1}$$

X refers to variables that have to be normalized. The pre-processed data is then segregated into a training set (70% of COVID-19 data) and a testing set (30% of COVID-19 data) [18]. Classification algorithms are then applied using the training set of data, whereas the testing set helps in computation of categorization accuracy. The flow diagram is presented in the Fig. 3.

C5.0 is an advanced model of C4.5 technique. Both are referred to as classification methods and were introduced by Ross Quinlan in 1993. C5.0 builds as a decision tree by splitting the attributes recursively. In this study, we use COVID-19 dataset to classify the regions which are greatly affected by COVID-19 (danger) or moderate or safe. The C5.0 decision tree itself has built-in gain ratio attribute selection to select the relevant features from the COVID-19 dataset. The attributes that contain maximum weight are finally chosen as a splitting attribute [19]. After selecting the particular attributes from the complete dataset, the rules are generated to build a precise decision tree. The COVID-19 testing data is feed into the trained decision tree which predicts the accuracy of the C4.5 decision tree. When compared with other methods of producing decision trees or generating rule sets, C5.0 performs better than C4.5 in terms of execution speed, reminiscence occupation and good accuracy.

Deep learning models are artificial neural network algorithms that are supervised learning algorithms that derive the weights of the neuron through the gradient descent optimization method. These models help us understand complex data from data points by using different computational techniques. There are numerous applications of deep learning models such as image and text recognition, machine translation, spam filtering and categorization, NLP. Various challenges associated with deep learning are computationally intensive, low stability, limited processing power, high complexity, the number of parameters, and the so-called over-fitting which is when the algorithm outputs an output that is similar to the model it was trained on. This results in suboptimal accuracy of the model. For instance, training the neural network consists of thousands of artificial neurons linked together to perform a task. The model connects each neuron to the other. The learning process works in the same way by feeding the network with millions of images of various objects (e.g. cats) and other image contents (e.g. bird, dog). It gradually learns to recognize different patterns and to generate similar images by considering the different human viewing patterns. Deep learning model begins by training a network (actually a large group of non-linear neurons and their connections) using data and having that data used as input for the training process. The output layer obtains and delivers the processed information from the hidden layer of the model accordingly. Typically, the process of training involves assigning weights to neurons, so that they calculate a certain result given certain input data and through changing parameters in the program. There are four layers in neural network called convolution, deconvolution, recurrent and fully connected. Generally, input layers are known as visible layer and the second layer called as hidden layer which is between input and output layer of defined neural network. The last layer is known output layer which produces the output of given input.

Normally, deep learning consists of so many hidden layers and each layer is strongly organized by the next layers with weight. So, if weight is associated with a previous layer and if that previous layer is connected to layer n, layer n is associated with a weight of layer $n + 1$. So, the final hidden layer in layer n is much stronger than the initial hidden layer (and all other layers within this layer) it's just that the connections between the layers of the hidden layers are weak. The sum of weights is calculated at each layer by the gradient descent method, and after that, the function of activation is proliferated to the subsequent layer. The gradient descent sends out the values for fine-tuning the errors from output to the hidden layer. The learning rate is constantly adjusting itself by weighing the data by a certain parameter called the learning rate. As a result, the weight correction in each layer is effective and leads to complete convergence. Hence, the deep learning model applies hidden layer activation instead of applying input layer activation. The COVID-19 training data is passed to the input layer of the model and then the weights of the neuron are evaluated. If the data is well balanced with equal weights on different inputs, the net value of the neuron is 1. If the data, are not well balanced, the neuron with a lower activation value becomes active (denoted by -1 in the equation above) and a value of 1 is assigned to its weight. As a result, the model becomes symmetric. The input neurons also become symmetric in the case that they have both a low and high activation. Thus, the net value of the neuron is positive if the number of activated weights is large and positive if the number of activated weights is small. Thus, the number of active neurons equals the number of input neurons times the number of symmetric neuron weights. Once the model is trained, the network is tested for performance by computing the weights which indicate the relative importance of the neuron in performing a particular function. If the network learns that one neuron is more important than another, then the weight with a greater influence on the result is determined to be the one assigned to that neuron. The training pattern is, again and again, feed forwarded to the network until it gets the converged state of the network [17].

2.4 Neural Network Steps

Input: Virudhunagar district dataset with specified parameters

Output: Classification result of danger zones

Steps:

- Dataset is fed into the defined neural network input layer
- Then transferred into the hidden layers
- Random interconnections between layers with random input is performed
- Bias is added with input after weights are multiplied with them individually
- Activation function is calculated based on transfer of weighted sum
- Features are extracted from the activation function
- This is then transferred into output layer
- After this, weights are adjusted to minimize the error by using the cost function.

2.5 *Performance Testing*

After training of classification algorithms, the models are validated by using performance metrics such as accuracy prediction, error rate, precision, specificity, and sensitivity. The formulas for testing performances are given by Eqs. (3)–(7).

2.5.1 Accuracy Prediction

The prediction of accuracy in ML algorithms is an efficient way to measure how far the model classifies the data efficiently. The accuracy score is typically calculated by taking the log-likelihood proportions of the instances, separated by the accepted count of the model with the same accuracy. The accuracy score of the model is typically called the 'confidence interval of the accuracy', or 'error'. The better the accuracy score is, the more uncertain we are about the model prediction. As an example, the error between 4 and 5% could be the same as the accuracy score of the model. So, the bigger the uncertainty, the better we can say that there is uncertainty about the model prediction. Thus, for a given number of examples, the expected number of correct predictions for the classifier is determined. It is usually performed by means of a confusion matrix which is presented in Table 2. It is a clean and clear cut way of presenting the prediction outcome of the classification algorithm which is often called a contingency table. Classification accuracy is mainly proving the number of correctly classified data out of all the remaining data [19].

More accurately, it is specified as sum of true positives and true negative values which is divided by the sum of original valid values, original negative values, original positive values, and incorrect negative values. It is also simply referred to as the total of perfectly classified data separated by total number of data X 100. Basically, the

Table 2 Matrix representation

Status	Correct	Incorrect
P (Positive)	TP	FP
N (Negative)	FN	TN

null hypothesis is tested with the help of the computational model based on random sampling. Let's get back to the mathematical aspect of prediction. In order to evaluate the models, samples with the same random sampling distribution are considered. The model predictions with respect to data from different random samples are different because the sources of variation in data are different. The tests of significance can therefore be subjected to several types of refinements. For each of these types of refinements, the confidence intervals can be calculated and, for the simplest case, the test is considered to be significant (as calculated using the minimum α). The confidence interval can also be visualized by plotting the cumulative distribution function against the actual distribution for the observed data points.

The Confusion matrix can be visualized as a tree diagram with the missing data point represented as a node and the predicted values of the target variable represented as leaves. A node is a positive vector of data points. A leaf is a single data point for which the predicted value is the corresponding one. Each leaf represents one of the missing values and corresponds to one of the columns of the matrix. For each predicted value of the target variable that is missing from the matrix, the values of a tree point to an image of a dungeon. The connectedness of the values to each other indicates that they are more probable to be taken together than to be taken apart.

True positive (TP) means finding the correct values.

False positive (FP) means finding the incorrect values.

False negative (FN) means finding the correct values to incorrect values.

True negative (TN) correct values are predicted as false negative based on the confusion matrix calculation in Table 2. First, fed the test data, secondly, predict the result and calculate the predictions based outcomes.

2.5.2 Error Rate

The classification error rate is calculated from the misclassified instances over the entire testing set of instances. It is determined by the total number of misclassification instances that is divided by total number of instances. We can compute the classification error rate using the following code:

```
// [L] classifier.pl // [R] conf.rb
classifier = classifier :: binary_model .fit(c("c(1,0),c(0,1))).reduce(0)
classifier.resize(100)
 fn(result) -> usetuple(result).flatMap
{ |x| result[x.lower()][: 2] }
 classifier.grade_failures(result).count()
if result.count % 2 == 0 :
 for i in 1 .. 8 :
 print fn(result)
```

Prediction of classification accuracy alone is classically not adequate to compose the decision. Hence accuracy prediction along with misclassification error rate, precision, sensitivity and specificity obtain detailed information on how the MLmodel classifies the data. These three performance metrics describe the MLprediction through a contingency table.

2.5.3 Precision

Both precision and sensitivity are used to examine the efficiency of the ML model. Since the precision equation doesn't have both TN and FN, the precision value provides a biased result, especially for misclassified instances. In cases where a single classifier correctly identifies the misclassified instances, the number of false positives will be small. To avoid misclassification, one can use precision regression to generate a model that is intended to minimize false positives. However, this solution may not be feasible for low-latency applications.

$$\text{Precision} = \text{TP}/\text{TP} + \text{FP} \tag{2}$$

2.5.4 Sensitivity

Sensitivity is often termed recall. Sensitivity and specificity are the statistical performance measures of classification. It is a key testing method to test the ML algorithm. Sensitivity should be measured while learning the learned classifier. So, the test set should be provided to the algorithm without any patterns present to it. Try to find all the features for which the classification is not performed at the first stage, or the classifier is unable to discriminate between inputs. These are called dead classifiers. These are the inputs that the machine learning algorithm is unable to classify the class. Sensitivity usually determines the proportion of correct values that are rightly predictable.

2.5.5 Specificity

Specificity computes the ratio of negative values that are perfectly acceptable. Hence, it is also known as true negative value. Specificity is equal to the default logical negation of a (positive) value. The standard value of the false negative ratio is, all else being equal. This ratio gives importance to each degree of truthfulness. Since the specificity equation doesn't have both false negative and true positive, the specificity provides a biased result, especially for misclassified instances [20]. The testing performance formulas are given below,

$$\text{Accuracy Rate} = \frac{\text{Number of correctly classified instances}}{\text{Total number of instances}} \quad (3)$$

$$\text{Error Rate} = \frac{\text{Number of misclassification instances}}{\text{Total number of instances}} \quad (4)$$

$$\text{Precision} = \frac{\text{Number of true positives}}{\text{Number of true positives} + \text{Number of false positives}} \quad (5)$$

$$\text{Sensitivity} = \frac{\text{Number of true positives}}{\text{Number of true positives} + \text{Number of false negatives}} \quad (6)$$

$$\text{Specificity} = \frac{\text{Number of negatives}}{\text{Number of true negatives} + \text{Number of false positives}} \quad (7)$$

3 Results and Discussion

3.1 Age Group

Classification techniques were used to better understand how COVID-19 affects individuals, as well as to validate and predict recovery. Figure 4 shows the different age groups and percentages of cases based on the dataset. The figure shows that COVID-19 is most likely to infect people between the ages of 20 and 50. The graph was used to examine the characteristics and construct classification representation for an evaluation of the performance.

Fig. 4 Age group affected ratio

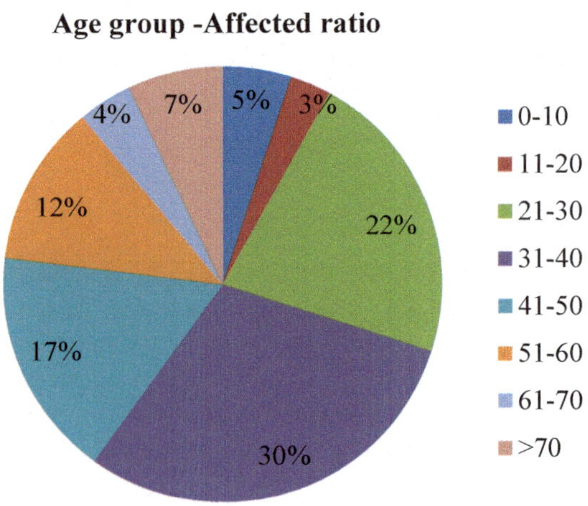

In order to classify the COVID-19 data, we employed effective methods such as C5.0 decision tree and neural network model to envisage the future incidences of COVID-19. The C5.0 decision tree decomposes the occurrence of COVID into a number of related categories, representing the probable scenarios: (1) potentially respiratory causing; (2) not respiratory causing; (3) unclear; (4) possibly causing; (5) affected incident; and (6) not incident. We then utilized a neural network to identify the statistical significance in the occurrence of cancer for the six posterior categories. The work was carried out using a java based programming tool called 'R', which is flexible since it supports many packages and functions. The proposed models are designed and classified into different classes such as safe, moderate, and dangerous for the period of March 2020 to July 2020. Both of these algorithms work efficiently according to their individual capabilities.

3.2 *Analysis of Regions*

Figure 5 shows the results of the statistical analysis of COVID-19 in Virudhunagar district from March 2020 to July 2020. The results show high COVID infection rate between 9 and 26th of July as compared to 8–28th of March. In these periods, high number of COVID cases occurred, the active cases, discharge cases and death cases are graphically presented in Fig. 6. Among these regions, Sivakasi, Virudhunagar and the unknown region reach the highest occurrences of COVID- 19.

3.3 *Classification of COVID 19*

Figures 7 and 8 show the extent to the classes of the COVID-19 zones are classified into safe zone and moderate zone. Safe zone symbolizes green (death < 2), yellow (death > 2 and < 8), and red (death > 8 and above). The COVID-19 cases are classified and predicted roughly 75% both safe or moderate zone and 25% red zone. When

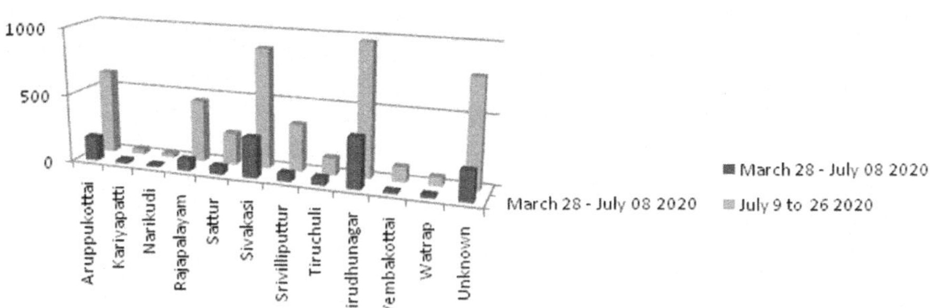

Fig. 5 Statistical analysis of COVID-19 in Virudhunagar district

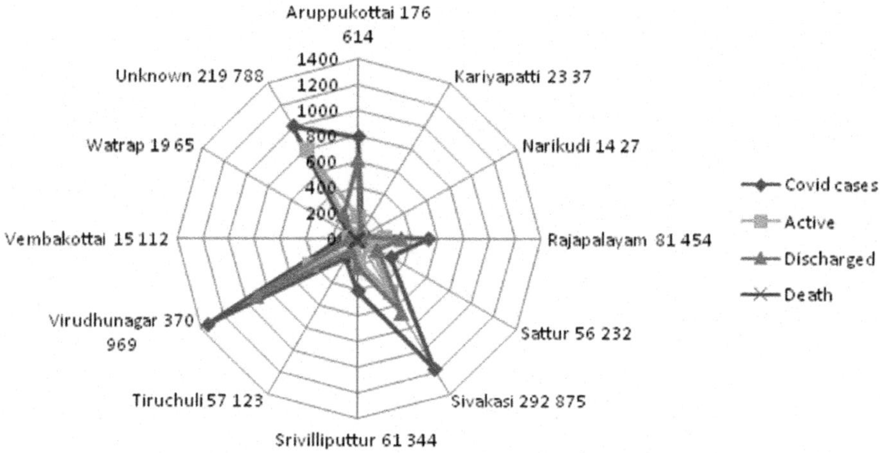

Fig. 6 Region wise status of COVID-19 during March 2020–July 2020

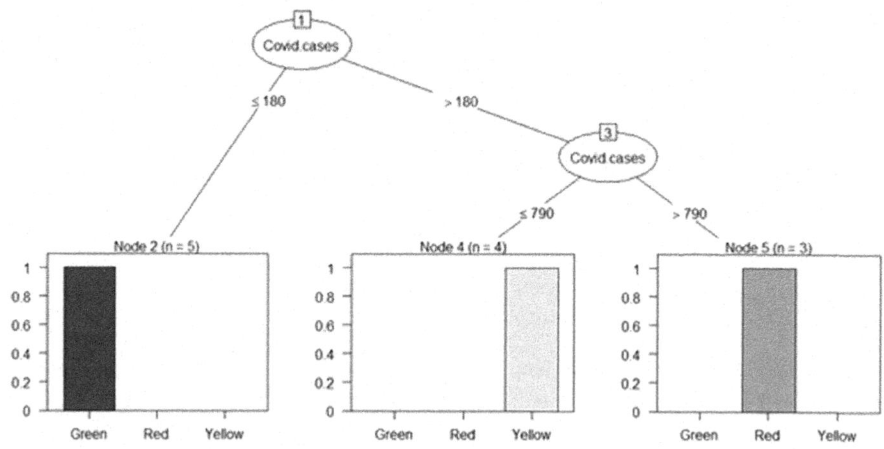

Fig. 7 Classification of COVID-19 data using C5.0 decision tree model

compared with the deep learning model, the accuracy of classification is better than the decision tree model. The classification was possible on a few images even when the subjective classification accuracy ranged from 95 to 96%. The operational cost of the training was substantially lower than that of deep learning models.

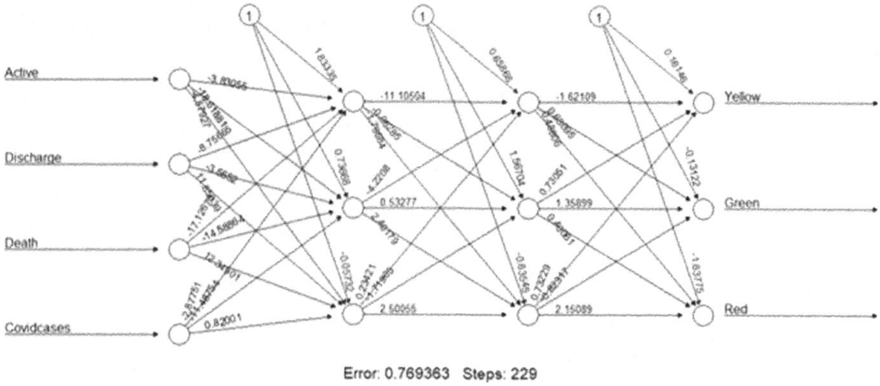

Fig. 8 Classification of COVID-19 data using deep learning model

Table 3 Performance of C5.0 and neural network model for COVID-19 data

Classification algorithms	Accuracy rate (%)	Error rate (%)	Precision (%)	Sensitivity (%)	Specificity (%)
C5.0	95.92	4.08	98	96	97
Deep learning (NN)	98.06	1.94	99	99	99

3.4 Performance Metrics

The performance of classification models is determined using accuracy, error, precision value, and other performances which are presented in Table 3. From the classification results, the deep learning model achieved a high accuracy rate, precision value, sensitivity, and specificity along with low error rate as compared with C5.0 decision tree model. The model offers an error rate of 0.24% and sensitivity of 0.83% which is significantly less than the C5.0 decision tree model that has an error rate of 4.08% and a sensitivity of 96%. The accuracy of the model indicates how well the algorithm has classified the target set. This can be considered an assessment of the accuracy of a machine learning model and its predictive ability over the existing decision tree method.

3.5 Research Opportunities and Emerging Trends

The corona outbreak has resulted in numerous new research opportunities for present and future epidemics. For example, researchers may be able to use the model to get a better understanding of how rabies outbreaks spread in a community or whether insect-borne diseases can be traced to one or more species. The following are some of the most influential study opportunities.

- Other variables should be included to improve the accuracy of the prediction, such as population size, demographic characteristics, person and community trends, quality of facilities available, virus strain type and infectivity, and so on.
- Predicting CoV-2 protein structure: Artificial intelligence can be used to find the formation and function of different CoV-2 proteins, as well as their interactions with human proteins and the cellular environment. Accumulation of resistance genes in flu vaccines is an epidemic. Despite decades of research, vaccines containing traces of live flu virus often only cover about 60–70% of circulating flu viruses. Because researchers know little about the genes that turn harmless flu proteins into infectious viruses, it is hard to predict the regions of a vaccine that would be most effective. Developing effective algorithms will help determine the role of different socioeconomic variables that decide the epidemic's vulnerability, spread, and progression. This will aid in the effective distribution of resources in large countries with insufficient healthcare resources.
- Using AI to analyse social media data: We may also use AI to know and analyse social media data for real-time epidemiological data collection specific to COVID-19 for disease surveillance. We would also use machine learning and AI to analyse the social media data and provide real-time updated information on the onset, presentation, incidence and outcomes of disease outbreaks in rural [21]. Robotic-based contactless care and drug distribution: AI-based Robots may be used to conduct contactless service and remote treatments, thus reducing the need for medical personnel to come into contact with infected persons. Furthermore, COVID-19-enforced lockdowns have output in specific variations in air essence around the world.
- Climate Change: COVID19 enforced lockdowns have resulted in noteworthy revolution in the quality of air around the world. However, there is a widespread belief that these lockdowns result in retaliation emissions [22]. Future research will provide a more in-depth analysis of the age and population distribution with other characteristics.
- Risk assessment: Artificial intelligence algorithms can predict the risk of serious disease linked to COVID-19 of people of various ages. Such algorithms may be used to take preventive steps to avoid virus spread to vulnerable groups in society.

4 Conclusion

The mortal rate due to COVID-19 is increasing rapidly every day; thus, proactive steps need to be taken to alleviate or completely eradicate the virus. As researchers are working on this problem to obtain the solution, a number of predictive models are implemented to serve as an early detection method. Based on this predictive model, the health department can take preventive measures before controlling the infection rate. This also helps the public will get aware of the current situation.

Therefore, this study presented a deep learning method for the prediction of COVID-19 affected zones in Virudhunagar district in India. The results of the analysis revealed a significant increase in the diagnosis rate of Virudhunagar district with the use of deep learning. Deep learning has been used to improve COVID-19 infection ratio detection. This problem can be solved by using a deep learning algorithm. The overall results show that the deep learning model effectively predicted the COVID-19 affected zones from the data as compared with the C5.0 decision tree model. There are other algorithms, for example, the support vector machine, which has performed substantially better on learning performance. However, considering the decision tree model, the Deep learning model performed on average well (8.06% accuracy) in the test. This study helped to assign the risk scores of the different taluks headed for predicting the current COVID-19 which helped to substantiate and strengthen our perceptive of the COVID-19 disease.

Acknowledgements The authors would like to show gratitude to the management of Kalasalingam Academy of Research and Education for providing the fellowship to carry out this research work. We are also thankful to our alumni student Arun Pandian, who provided the real-time covid-19 dataset for Virudhunagar district.

References

1. El Wahid, A. A., Patel, P., Heidenreich, D., Hubert, F. T., & Weidmann, M. (2013). Reverse transcription recombinase polymerase amplification assay for the detection of Middle East respiratory syndrome coronavirus. *PLoSCurr*
2. Lessler, J., et al. (2009). Incubation periods of acute respiratory viral infections: A systematic review. *The Lancet Infectious Diseases, 9*(5), 291–300.
3. Anwar, S., Nasrullah, M., & Hosen, M. J. (2020). COVID-19 and Bangladesh: Challenges and how to address them. *Frontiers in Public Health, 8*(154), 1–8.
4. Sehgal, D. (2020). Analysis of vaccines to tackle Covid-19 with patent. *The Pharma Innovation Journal, 9*(7), 498–513.
5. Punn, N. S., Sonbhadra, S. K., & Agarwal, S. (2020). *COVID 19 epidemic analysis using machine learning and deep learning algorithms*. medRxiv.
6. Shinde, G. R., Kalamkar, A. B., Mahalle, P. N., Dey, N., Chaki, J., & Hassanien, A. E. (2020). Forecasting models for coronavirus disease (COVID-19): A survey of the state-of-the-art. *SN Computer Science, 1*(4), 1–15.
7. Sujath, R., Chatterjee, J. M., & Hassanien, A. E. (2020). A machine learning forecasting model for COVID-19 pandemic in India. *Stochastic Environmental Research and Risk Assessment, 34*(7), 959–972.
8. Al-Qaness, M. A. A., Ewees, A. A., Fan, H., & Aziz, M. A. E. (2020). Optimization method for forecasting confirmed cases of COVID-19 in China. *Applied Sciences, 9*(3), 1–9.
9. Elmousalami, H. H., & Hassanien, A. E. (2020). Day level forecasting for coronavirus disease (COVID-19) spread: Analysis, modeling and recommendations. *Quantitative Biology*. http://arxiv.org/abs/2003.07778
10. Yang, Z., Zeng, Z., Wang, K., Wong, S. S., Liang, W., Zanin, M., et al. (2020). Modified SEIR and AI prediction of the epidemics trend of COVID-19 in China under public health interventions. *Journal of Thoracic Disease, 12*(3), 165–174.
11. Yudistira, N. (2020). COVID-19 growth prediction using multivariate long short term memory. *Quantitative Biology, 14*(8), 1–8.

12. Tomar, A., & Gupta, N. (2020). Prediction for the spread of COVID-19 in India and effectiveness of preventive measures. *Science of the Total Environment*.
13. Prabira, K. S., & Santi, K. B. (2020). Detection of coronavirus disease (COVID-19) based on deep features, 1–9. https://doi.org/10.20944/preprints/202003.0300.v1
14. Li, Y., Guo, F., Cao, Y., Li, L., & Guo, Y. (2020). Insight into COVID-2019 for pediatricians. *Pediatric Pulmonology*. https://doi.org/10.1002/ppul.24734
15. Ardabili, S. F., Mosavi, A., Ghamisi, P., Ferdinand, F., Varkonyi-Koczy, A. R., Reuter, U., Rabczuk, T., & Atkinson, P. M. Covid-19 outbreak prediction with machine learning.
16. Xiong, P., Xu, K., & Xiao, G. (2020). How to deal with 2019 novel coronavirus (COVID-19): Public health practices from the centers for disease control and prevention in Zhang-gong district, Ganzhou city, China. *Infection Control & Hospital Epidemiology, 14*(8), 976–977. https://www.cambridge.org/core/journals/infection-control-and-hospital-epidemiology/issue/174788131C200159B9E88F0310CAAEE6
17. Pinter, G., Felde, I., Mosavi, A., Ghamisi, P., & Gloaguen, R. (2020). COVID-19 pandemic prediction for Hungary; a hybrid machine learning approach. *Mathematics, 8*(6), 890.
18. Salau, A. O., & Jain, S. (2021). Adaptive diagnostic machine learning technique for classification of cell decisions for AKT protein. *Informatics in Medicine Unlocked, 23*(1), 1–9. https://doi.org/10.1016/j.imu.2021.100511
19. Prakash, K. B., Imambi, S. S., Ismail, M., Kumar, T. P., & Pawan, Y. N. (2020). Analysis, prediction and evaluation of covid-19 datasets using machine learning algorithms. *International Journal, 8*(5).
20. Revathy, R., Balamurali, S., & Lawrance, R. (2019). Classifying agricultural crop pest data using Hadoop mapreduce based c5.0 algorithm. *Journal of Cyber Security and Mobility,* 393–408.
21. Chen, E., Lerman, K., & Ferrara, E. (2020). Tracking social media discourse about the covid-19 pandemic: Development of a public coronavirus twitter data set. *JMIR Public Health and Surveillance, 6*(2), e19273.
22. https://edition.cnn.com/2020/03/16/asia/china-pollutioncoronavirus-hnk-intl/index.html

Artificial Intelligence and an Edge-IoMT-Based System for Combating COVID-19 Pandemic

Joseph Bamidele Awotunde, Rasheed Gbenga Jimoh, Opeyemi Emmanuel Matiluko, Babatunde Gbadamosi, and Gbemisola Janet Ajamu

1 Introduction

The emergence of coronavirus (COVID-19) is currently a challenge that has physical, economic, social, and pedagogical boundaries, thus became global attention. The present global COVID-19 pandemic challenge has crossed the regional, extreme, scientific, cultural, social, and pedagogical boundaries [1, 2]. In the current epidemic circumstances, every nation around the world is grappling with the epidemic and is also searching for a genuine and lucrative approach to address the glitches that arise in diverse methods. It seems the epidemic that started in Wuhan, China, is unchecked. More than 35,897,739 people have been infected by the virus, with at least 1,048,781 deaths globally as of 10:33 am CEST, 08 October 2020.

The Huanan Seafood Market was linked to the outbreak. The virus belongs to the species of beta coronavirus and is associated with diseases that bring about [3]. The WHO was first notified on December 31, 2019, even though several cases of

J. B. Awotunde (✉) · R. G. Jimoh
Department of Computer Science, University of Ilorin, Ilorin, Nigeria
e-mail: awotunde.jb@unilorin.edu.ng

R. G. Jimoh
e-mail: jimoh_rasheed@unilorin.edu.ng

O. E. Matiluko
Center for System and Information Services, Landmark University, Omu Aran, Nigeria
e-mail: matiluko.emmanuel@lmu.edu.ng

B. Gbadamosi
Department of Computer Science, Landmark University, Omu-Aran, Nigeria
e-mail: gbadamosi.babatunde@lmu.edu.ng

G. J. Ajamu
Department of Agricultural Extension and Rural Development, Landmark University, Omu Aran, Nigeria
e-mail: ajamu.gbemisola@lmu.edu.ng

A. K. Tyagi et al. (eds.), *Intelligent Interactive Multimedia Systems for e-Healthcare Applications*, https://doi.org/10.1007/978-981-16-6542-4_11

unidentified etiology pneumonia were identified a lot former (Dec 8, 2019) [4, 5]. The epidemiological and clinical characteristics: a descriptive review. The Lancet, number 395(10,223), 507–513. This delay in announcing the epidemic and failure to immediately alert foreign authorities resulted in the unrestrained transmission of the virus. The pandemic is presently the focal point of worldwide concern.

In an attempt to prevent the circulation of the sickness, several countries were extending the lockdown and affecting millions of people. Initially, experts raised questions about the feasibility of this initiative and cautioned that certain countries were at risk of repeating a SARS-like epidemic [4, 6]. By this time, the pandemic appears to be under control in most countries, although there is still criticism of the utilization of what others have called "draconian" steps to stifle its circulation. The globe is presently trying to monitor the exceptional virus circulation that involves the greatest sum of indispositions plus deaths. As there is no such thing as definite medical care for coronaviruses and attempts to control the circulation have yet remained unsuccessful [7, 8], there's a crucial necessity for worldwide investigation of persons with intense COVID-19 contagion.

The combination of AI and IoT called (AiIoT) in medical sectors are advantageous and enabled suitable control of diseases by using interrelated wearable sensors and networks. IoT is an evolving area of investigation within infectious disease epidemiology. However, the augmented dangers of communicable ailment transmitted over worldwide integration and the pervasive obtainability of smart types of machinery, including interrelatedness of the world requires its utilization for monitoring, averting, predicting, and managing transmittable viruses.

AiIoT is an innovative way of combining healthcare gadgets and their applications to interact with the systems of human resources and data innovation. An inquiry on the possible outcomes of defying progressive diseases by adopting the AiIoT strategy when providing care to all groups of the patient without any partiality in poor and wealthy. The various cloud-based IoT administrations are the exchange of knowledge, report verification, investigation, patient monitoring, data social affair, cleanliness clinical consideration, and so on. It can change the working format of the medical services while rewarding the huge volume of patients with a prevailing degree of treatment and more fulfilment, especially during infectious disease diagnosis and monitoring. By functioning as an early warning system, IoT devices such as the geographic information system may be used as an important tool to curb the spread of these pandemics. Sensors like temperature and other signs might be used to detect people with any disease.

The emerging of new trends in technologies contributed to the commencement of the Internet of Medical Things (IoMT) an extension of the Internet of Things (IoT) that is acquiring worldwide concentration as well as becoming obtainable for monitoring, diagnosing, forecasting, and preventing arising from infectious diseases. IoMT in the healthcare system is advantageous and enabled suitable for controlling the COVID-19 outbreak by using interrelated wearable sensors and networks. IoMT is an evolving area of investigation within infectious disease epidemiology. However, the augmented dangers of communicable ailment transmitted over worldwide integration and the pervasive obtainability of smart types of machinery, including interrelatedness of the world requires its utilization for monitoring, averting, predicting, and managing transmittable viruses. This has helped in reducing the circulation rate in the hospital and helps to increase patient satisfaction.

A unified inclusion of an automated sickness management scheme could be key to managing this virus. Scientists in physical science and engineering are trying to resolve these glitches, formulate new ideas, clarify innovative research difficulties, construct user-centred clarifications, and establish themselves including the civilians overall. The healthcare system allowed by the IoMT is valuable for tracking COVID-19 sufferers properly, using an integrated system. This expertise assists to improve patient contentment and lowers hospital readmission rates. The IoMT is a distinct scheme of interconnected computing procedures, digital and automatic gadgets proficient in transmitting records across the system lacking people's interference at somewhat stage.

Many of those tools mentioned are labelled with their specific credential numbers or codes. IoMT is presently deep-rooted and tested expertise that incorporates numerous techniques, for instance, analytics, machine learning concept, and sensual possessions. Also, IoMT in traditional day-to-day operation is recognized as the usefulness of goods or devices serving people's real-life needs in several ways such as; home protection devices, smart illumination activities, and several others that are effortlessly manageable over our everyday use of smart reciters, smartphones, among others [9].

A multitude of innovative machinery in the mode of the IoT are acquiring intensifying worldwide consideration [10] and are increasingly available for the prediction, deterrence, and curbing of emerging transmittable sicknesses [11]. IoMT denotes an integrated network of smart gadgets, sensors, and persons from which information can be obtained in a fresh mode and distributed over cyberspace to be investigated for directions. Advanced IoMT-implemented Medical Care Management Schemes (Fitness Management Schemes) deliver actual monitoring by using wearable health tracking tools, cloud-centred inaccessible medical care research, and artificial intelligence (AI).

These control schemes incorporate the utilization of supervised, unsupervised, and machine learning in actual periods, social networks, public data, and medical data. As AI and machine learning integrate with the dispersed cloud, functional blockchain, device process mechanization, and AI language identification, medical care management schemes allow patients and doctors to create a robust remote monitoring system.

Therefore, this chapter proposes an architecture of an intelligent Edge-IoMT-Based monitoring system. The paper also elucidates the important role of Edge-IoMT-Based wearable body sensor networks during COVID-19 to minimize the need for caregivers and help people live an independent life, and besides providing people with quality care: The remaining part of this chapter is organized as follows: Sect. 2 discusses the opportunities for deploying the AI and IoMT technology during COVID-19 pandemic. Section 3 presents the supplication of edge computing during coronavirus outbreak, Sect. 4 reviews AI in fighting COVID-19 pandemic. Section 5 presents the proposed framework for monitoring COVID-19 patients, Sect. 6 discusses the practical implementation scenario of the proposed framework, and finally, Sect. 7 presents the conclusion and the possible future directions.

2 Opportunities for Deploying the Artificial Intelligence and IoMT Technologies During COVID-19 Pandemic

Digital wellness innovations provide huge incentives to reshape current health care programmes. Digital health innovations have offered improved quality of care at a more affordable cost, from the introduction of automated therapeutic annals to portable medical devices to other innovative technology. When part of health care programmes, politicians are continually researching, embracing, and implementing information and communication technology (ICT) [12], it forms the way people and patients view the structures and communicate with them. The road to digital medical care (eHealth) is a systemic evolution of the conventional medical care system that incorporates numerous aspects, together with universal entry to automated medical annals, online tracking systems, inmate services, wearable devices, portable medical applications, data analytics, and further transformative innovations [12, 13].

There is an urgent need to make good use of current technology due to the global outbreak of COVID-19 pandemic. IoMT is known to be one of the greatest innovative innovations with tremendous promise in combating coronavirus outbreak [14]. The IoMT consists of a sparse network where the IoMT systems feel the world and transmit valuable data across the Network.

The IoT-based system creates a huge amount of data named Big Data and thereby Influences the creation and growth of better-customized healthcare systems. Wearable medical devices can have active surveillance functionality that can gather a vast amount of medical data, resulting in Big Data, from which physicians can foresee the future condition of the patient [15]. This observational study and the extraction of information is a dynamic process that must ensure enhanced security methods [16]. The used of AI on generated Big Data from IoT-based system offer several opportunities for healthcare systems [17]. The application of AI in the process of generated Big Data can significantly improve global healthcare systems [18]. The IoT-based system has been used to reduce the global cost of infectious disease prevention. The IoT-based system can be used in real-time data capture to help patients during self-administration treatments. The integration of mobile apps is commons in IoMT-based sensors data capture for telemedicine and mHealth systems [19].

The data interpretation becomes easier with AI-based data analytics, and decrease the time needed for data performance analysis [20]. Besides, a new system has been created, "Personalized Preventative Health Coaches". It retains relationships and can be used to clarify and understand data on health and well-being [21]. For efficient health monitoring, the networked sensors enable people without direct access to medical facilities to be appropriately monitored [22]. The use of an AI-based system with wireless communication has helped physicians to make appropriate recommendations to patients. A thorough analysis of the IoMT framework in the medical areas has greatly helped in reducing the cost of diagnosing a patient in the healthcare system. Furthermore, the Internet of medical things helps in several healthcare systems like the generation of big data through the use of sensors and devices for vital physiological and biophysical parameters supervision, and big data analytics can be performing on them in other medical decision-making support methods. Hence, the combination of AI and IoT will greatly improve the healthcare system and significantly help in disease diagnosis, monitoring, predicting, and patient treatment [23–25].

The use of a broad variety of advanced technology brought about the IoT that transform conventional objects into intelligent objects, from implanted devices and networking technologies to Internet protocols. The potential impact of IoT in driving the economic development of IoT-based services are expected to offer many business opportunities. Furthermore, industries like transport, agriculture, urban infrastructure, defence, and retail, have an IoT market of approximately 15% overall [26, 27]. These estimates show the enormous and sharp progress of IoT products and produced data within a short period. In the years ahead, the estimated market share is expected to improve drastically [28, 29].

Figure 1 displayed potential applications of IoT-based during COVID-19

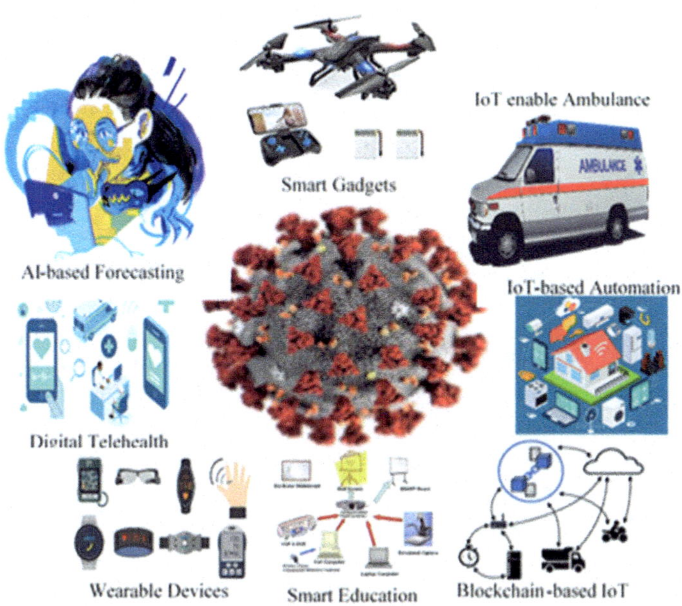

Fig. 1 Potential applications of IoT-based during COVID-19 Pandemic

pandemic. Ideally, engineers and technicians would avoid warehouses, isolated locations, or busy places travelling and visiting because they fear being infected with the virus. Nevertheless, their physical appearance on site is needed because they can't get away with manually operating the equipment available. By the use of special sensors mounted in machinery and enhanced knowledge, real-world overlays, and remote expert feedback, IoT may help solve their repair problems, conduct machine operation remotely, and AI may also anticipate when machines need repair (predictive maintenance) or when they might be faced with a challenge. In this way, physical visits will be significantly decreased, helping to safeguard workers' health and welfare, thus enhancing efficiencies at the level of service of the facilities. When supermarkets continue imposing limits on sales of goods per customer, future alternatives have also been produced by IoMT and AI.

A couple of years ago, a major US retail chain put IoT trackers in its trolleys to prevent daily theft. Perhaps it is time to start applying this to the store shelves of important homes, sanitizers, and everything else that is already over-selling, in an attempt to properly control supplies and prevent hoarding behaviour. Smart-watches and fitness trackers will be readily available in the not-too-distant future and people with chronic conditions will be able to record temperature, asthma, heartbeat without the use of intrusive instruments. For this fact, patients will be able to opt to transmit real-time and past data to public or private hospitals anytime they feel unwell so that medical health IT departments will interact with the wearables and mobile devices of patients. In this way, the treatment of coronavirus or other diseases may be prepared even more effectively and with minimal resources expended optimally. Smart connected medical devices, such as smart home ventilators, together with video and wearables, may support patients monitoring at home, give updates to those in distress, or even alert when paramedics are required to come and move them to hospital.

Ventilators are important in treating people that have become contaminated. The health services have not been prepared to deal with this magnitude of a pandemic, and a resulting shortage is now widespread in only the most developed hospitals. An IoT-3D printing may be a lifesaver in the face of coronavirus-induced supply shortages. With an IoT-3D printer that offers critical medical equipment, for example, replacement valves. This is what an Italian company called Isinnova does, taking a 3D printer to a Milan hospital and manufacturing incomplete valves to be shipped to a hospital in Brescia, Northern Italy. Touch screens have been the chosen user interface (UI) until recently: among them are tablets, computers, and even doors. Nonetheless, the fact that coronavirus is more quickly transmitted from a contaminated surface than by air has made direct contact sound risky.

Many UIs that don't need any physical contact are also usable. Voice has already triumphed over tactile user interfaces, especially through smart speakers and digital helpers. Despite people confining themselves inside the building, there will be increased interest in smart home apps, and the voice apps of smart speakers. Another functionality that gains ground in smartphones is beyond speech, biometrics, and their use for eye/face identification, such as the use of facial picture identification to open phones or make payments. The largest penetration is in China but the opportunity for the remaining part of the biosphere is enormous. Wearables, for instance, smart payment watches and other use cases (enabled by voice or close contact) can allow us to escape physical surface contact.

IoMT is the medical-care-precise variant of IoT which could be introduced to deliver remedy or cure to health care professionals, guarantee isolation compliance which tracks disease sources [30]. With the assistance of radars embedded in smart headsets, drones, robotics, and COVID-19 self-sampling experiments, as well as data collection may be performed. The data obtained by these techniques would be forwarded for processing to a central cloud repository. And such data can be used by medical personnel, government and other related personnel for policymaking, and for the projection of COVID-19 outbreak.

With these results, care professionals will be able to offer more tailor-made electronic wellness appointments for patients. Such electronic facilities will also allow patients to seek more effective treatment while reducing their access and further spread of the virus at the same time. Agency departments, together with resident public medical offices and the CDC, will be well prepared to distribute resources, assess quarantine needs, track outbreaks, and use this information to enforce emergency plans [30].

These technologies are now being implemented in major cities to reduce the pandemic. For example, for simultaneous tracking of COVID-19 inmates, the Shanghai Public Health Clinical Center utilizes physique fever monitors laterally utilizing facts transfer directly to the nurse post, thus minimizing possible sensitivity to healthcare workers [31]. Similarly, a device now used for medical interviews with sensors was installed in Boston to assess the breathing degree and physique fever of patients. In Singapore, a contact-tracing mobile programme utilizes Bluetooth wireless technologies to identify individuals who were similar to COVID-19 patients [32]. Apple and Google are working on touch monitoring and detection software that will be made available to many countries around the world that are intended to significantly step up the recognition that warns users who have been naively near to COVID-19 inmates. IoMT won't solitarily combat the present pandemic but could also be used to deter potential outbreaks.

3 Application of Edge Computing During Coronavirus Outbreak

In building and designing a reliable and convenient framework greater effort has been made in the area of the smart healthcare system for IoMT-based device systems [27]. In the biomedical industry, smart healthcare system gradually reshapes the conventional medical system with the rising of portable wearable devices and sensors [33, 34]. These devices and sensors are majorly used for collecting blood pressure, respiratory rate, motion function, blood glucose data, ECG, EEG, and body temperature among others for primary medical examinations. These capture data are primarily concerned with the preservation of health in providing early investigations to extricate the perception of other complications [35].

IoMT-based is used in the medical system to manage doctor's advice to patients, medical tools, patients' records, disease diagnosis, and patient treatment. The application of Machine Learning (ML) algorithms with the IoMT-based system makes the smart healthcare system highly effective in the area of disease diagnosis, prediction, health monitoring system, and before human utilization [36]. The IoMT-based in this direction allows telemedicine like telesurgery, telerehabilitation, and telehealth that remotely monitoring, treating, and diagnosing patients' in real-time. These used the IoMT-based model to transferred medical data to the database using IoMT-based cloud models. The models comprised of three major components namely, Body Sensor Network (BSN), the gateways, and the cloud server centre. The IoMT-based in recent years supports healthcare services in real-time to distant stakeholders. The capture data using IoMT-based devices are provided to physicians and relevant stakeholders to validate and provide useful information to patients' whenever it is needed.

The IoMT-based with edge computing lower latency services, energy-effective, cost-effective, and maximum satisfaction for healthcare contributors. Most IoMT-based environments depend on a cloud platform for massive smart health systems [37]. The model can be used to forward capture data produced from IoMT devices through the Internet to the cloud, and thereby used for diagnosis to provide useful reports using learning algorithms like ML or deep learning. But the IoMT-Cloud system is inappropriate, especially where lower latency is necessary. Hence, IoMT-based systems require a faster and low latency protection technique with delay-sensitive, smart, secure, stable smart healthcare management. Edge computing is the answer to this with a prolonged type of cloud computing where IoMT-based data can be computed closer to the edge of the network where data are produced [38].

The Edge computation reduced latency, data traffic, and data distance to the network since is running at a local processing level closed to the cloud database. Edge computing has become relevant and important since devices can recognize data instinctively, thus become useful in IoMT-based systems to reduce the latency to a lower level. Figure 2 depicted the edge computing architecture, the first part of a network uses the IoMT-based devices and sensors to collects data to be processed through a gateway using a Radio Access Network that uses edge devices to compute data aggregated by the network locally. Once the data processing has been done, the full computing operations and memory storage have been processed to the cloud.

The edge layer is like a junction point where enough networking, computing, and storage resources are available to manage local data collection, which can be readily obtainable and deliver fast results. Low-power system-on-chip (SoC) systems are used in most situations because they are meant to preserve the trade-off between processing performance and power consumption. Cloud servers, on the other hand, have the power to conduct advanced analytics and machine learning jobs to combine time series generated by a variety of heterogeneous or mixed kinds of items [39].

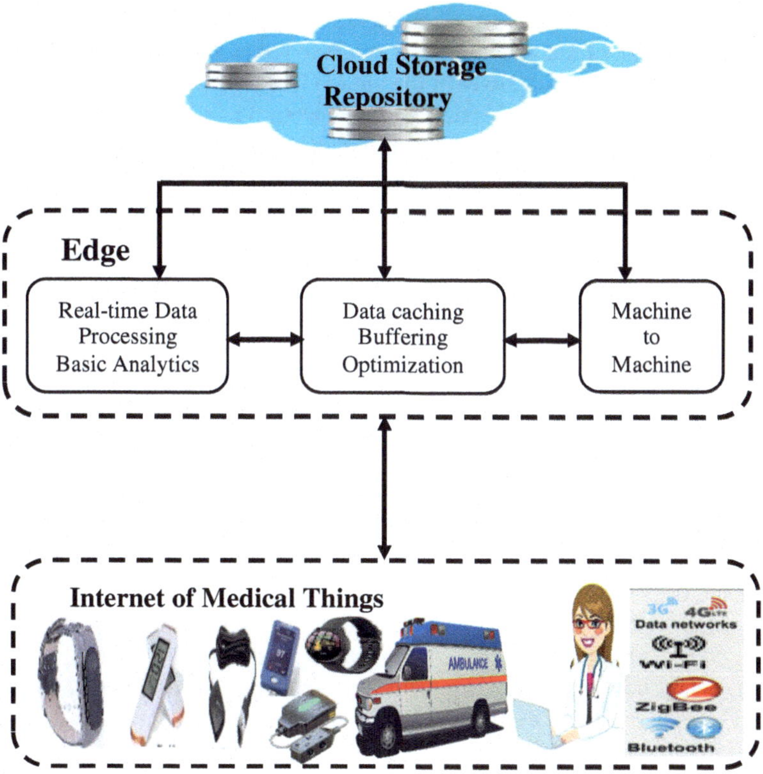

Fig. 2 The Architecture structure of edge computing in IoMT-based system

With the rapid development in wireless technology, IoT can generate a huge amount of medical data, smart devices, and customized enhance services. Such big medical data can be of countless types, like text, multimedia, and image, which the cloud server needs to store, analyze, and process [40]. The high latency, security problems, and network traffic that arises as a result of the handling of big cloud medical data. Fog computing was introduced to minimize the burden of the cloud been a new computing platform. The fog also helps in bringing the cloud service closer to the network edge, the layer acts as a flyover between the terminal device and the conventional cloud server. Hence, fog computing allows refined and secured healthcare services.

The edge of the network is an ideal place for analyzing real-time health information where data is created. The feature of edge computing placed it ahead of cloud computing like data pre-processing, local data analytics, data security and privacy, temporary storage, data trimming, distributed, decentralized storage. Both distributed edge and centralized cloud servers are needed in an IoMT-based application like health monitoring systems to efficiently perform big data analytics. The use of edge computing as an intermediary has created a better way of handling cloud databases on IoMT-based devices for real-time healthcare systems [40]. Edge computing takes resources to the edge of the network as an extension to cloud computing. This effectively brings the benefits and power of the cloud closer to the place where the data is produced, thereby assisting and speeding up "on-the-fly solutions" for applications in a smart healthcare system. This decentralized model's main objective is to bring devices and software to the edge of the network where the data is generated. Edge computing's main aim is to reduce the amount of data that is transmitted to cloud data centres for processing and analysis. It also improves security, a key issue in the IoMT industry [41, 42].

4 Artificial Intelligence in Fighting COVID-19 Pandemic

Advent of Coronavirus generated a large amount of medical datasets that call for the adoption of machine learning (ML) techniques and applications as it enables computers to imitate and adapt human-like behaviour. ML techniques can interact with different applications to perform actions, and produce something the system can learn and use as experience for the next action(s). The overview of analytics data method which enables computers to learn and do what comes naturally to human's mind was carried out. It includes machine learning's nomenclature and applications' describing what, how and why. The technology roadmap of machine learning was discussed to understand and verify. The primary objective of the study was to give insight into why machine learning is the future [43, 44].

Artificial intelligence (AI) will create smart framework to automatically track and forecast the spreading of this outbreak [25, 28, 45]. A genetic algorithm may also be built to remove the visual characteristics of this infection. It has the potential to provide patients with daily alerts and also to offer better options for COVID-19 epidemic follow-up. AI can easily determine this virus' level of transmission by recognizing the fragments and 'hot spots' and can effectively track the individuals' contacts and even monitor them. It can foresee this spread of the disease future path, and possibly reoccurrence. These technologies can also monitor and predict the existence of the epidemic from the data, social media and broadcasting channels present, about the threats of the outbreak and its probable spreading. It can also forecast the number of useful cases and deaths in any area. AI will help recognize the areas, citizens and communities most affected and take effective measures [23, 29].

An empirical investigation was done using AI/ML with the implementation of Plotly and Matplotlib visualization tools that may be used with IoT to support contact tracing in future were initiated, and results show the locations that are affected. This data-driving innovation can assist engineers and scientists for clinicians, and healthcare experts around the world for deployment of vaccines, contact tracing and curb the spread of the coronavirus that is ravaging the whole world. The degrees of COVID-19 active cases vary in various counties of the world, Canada, Russia, the United States, Brazil were among the countries of the world that have a higher number of COVID-19 active cases while Madagascar, Angola and most of the African countries has low active cases.

The extent of COVID-19 confirmed cases also vary in various counties of the world, Brazil, Canada, China, Russia, United States were among the countries with higher number of confirmed cases while Angola, Libya, Madagascar, Zambia and most of the African countries have low confirmed cases. The extent of COVID19 death cases also varies in various counties of the world like other cases Brazil, Canada, China, Russia, United States were among the countries of the world that have higher death cases. Many African countries on the other hand have very low death cases. This may be due to the climatic and other environmental conditions in African.

The extent of COVID-19 recovered cases also varies in various counties of the world as usual. Bolivia, Canada were among the countries with high recovery cases, very low recovery cases of COVID-19 in Algeria, Australia, Brazil, Kazakhstan and Russia. The higher level of recovery cases in Bolivia, Canada and few other countries may not be unconnected with the use and implemented contact tracing for that might have reduced the spread. Most European countries implemented this at the early stage of the pandemic as a measure of curbing the spread. The forecasting results of active, confirmed, death and recovered cases for the next seven days were done using Artificial Intelligence/machine learning model built with Facebook prophet.

The evaluation of the model built for prediction and forecasting shows high degree of accuracy, having used three evaluation metrics to measure its performance. The model performance for forecasting model was evaluated using three performance metrics, the R-score, mean square error and absolute mean error.

These evaluation metrics help to measure performance of univariance time-series forecasting models in this AI/ML medical dataset study. The Active, Death, Confirmed and Recovered cases forecasting models were evaluated. The evaluation results of forecasting model shown that R-Score of 0.9999, 0.9999, 0.9999, and 0.9998, Mean square error of 32,950,433.47, 43,988,753.26, 724,820.40 and 43,611,232.23 for Active, Death, Confirmed and Recovered cases respectively. Also, absolute mean error of 4229.98, 4776.94, 603.04 and 3814.23.

So far, researchers use machine learning models to predict and forecast deaths, confirm, survival/ recovered of COVID -19 cases especially in separate studies, there is no critical investigation of COVID-19 medical dataset across various countries of the world, that has forecasted four different cases (active, confirmed, death and recovered cases) of Coronavirus at the same time with the same dataset using state-of-the-art techniques lying in AI/ML tools and visualizing the degrees of infection of the pandemic across various countries of the world. To address the concerns raised by the spread of COVID-19, this chapter proposed a comprehensive research framework responsible for the investigation of COVID-19 medical data across various countries of the world.

Combating Coronavirus can be contributed to, immensely but its contributions have not been impactful due to the lack of robust COVID-19 medical data which is also hindered by the requirement of data privacy, healthcare sector and human-AI interaction. Massive diagnostic data gathering of infectious people and their contacts will be essential AI-based solutions to curtail economic loss and save lives. The proliferation of data on COVID-19 has cost World Health Organization (WHO) a huge investment to collect data for predicting, forecasting and monitoring the Coronavirus disease in other to ensure the curtailment of the disease [46, 47].

Artificial Intelligence is a revolutionary technology that can be used to tackle disease outbreak COVID-19. This innovation helps to better scan, monitor, and forecast current and potential patients. The key implementation of AI is to identify and diagnose the infection early on. An AI can be used to produce medicines and vaccines, and to reduce the strain of medical personnel. The techniques of AI may be outlined in two groups based on two separate styles of learning: supervised and unsupervised machine learning. Supervised learning is the process of introducing a feature from the training samples, including SVM, Decision Tree, Random Forest, Naïve Bayes (NB), Artificial Neural Network (ANN), Bootstrap Aggregating, AdaBoost, that could easily manage the regression and classification problem in health information [48, 49].

All these approaches may be beneficial in assessing diagnostic accuracy and in recommending effective care for patients with COVID-19. In particular, the predictive results from these approaches may be used to alert authorities and the populace in anticipation and recommend suitable strategies for prevention and management. Unattended learning techniques such as Principal Component Analysis (PCA) may be used to minimize data proportions, making it possible for scientists to recognize some primary COVID-19 disease outbreak causes [50]. Some unsupervised principles of learning, like K-means, might classify COVID-19 victims and identify suspicious patients which might direct scientists to concentrate on these medical situations. Furthermore, topic models like the Latent Dirichlet Allocation (LDA) may be used to remove the issues from the medical book record. Recently, deep learning models were widely used in prediction and diagnosis, filtering social networks, and computational biology and are considered effective techniques for analyzing infectious diseases.

AI can scrutinize the abnormal symptoms as well as other 'obvious signs' swiftly and alerts patients and medical officials [51, 52]. It provides great quicker policy-making, which is cost-effective. It tends to help, through valuable techniques, establish new treatment and monitoring skills for the COVID 19 cases. Using diagnostic imaging innovations such as Computed Tomography (CT), Magnetic Resonance Imaging (MRI) scanning of human organs, AI helps diagnose highly contagious cases.

AI will provide relevant information with the aid of real-time analysis, which is useful in preventing this infection. It could be used to forecast possible sites of an outbreak throughout this epidemic, the proliferation of the epidemic, the need for spaces, and health care providers. AI is useful for the potential detection of viruses and illnesses, with the aid of prior coached data over data that are present at various times. It describes the features, sources, and factors why infection has dispersed. This will be a promising technique in the future for fighting other outbreaks and infectious diseases. It can provide precautionary action and tackle various illnesses. In the future, AI can play a crucial role in making healthcare more informative and reactive. AI will create a smart framework to automatically track and forecast the spreading of this outbreak [53–55]. A genetic algorithm may also be built to remove the visual characteristics of this infection. It has the potential to provide patients with daily alerts and also to offer better options for COVID-19 epidemic follow-up.

AI can easily determine this virus' level of transmission by recognizing the fragments and 'hot spots' and can effectively track the individuals' contacts and even monitor them. It can foresee this spread of the disease's future path, and possibly reoccurrence. These technologies can also monitor and predict the existence of the epidemic from the data, social media, and broadcasting channels present, about the threats of the outbreak and its probable spreading. It can also forecast the number of use cases and deaths in any area. AI will help recognize the areas, citizens, and communities most affected and take effective measures.

Analysis of available data on COVID-19 allows the use of AI for drug testing. It's suitable for the production and creation of therapeutics. This innovation is used to expedite drug screening in real-time, where normal screening takes a lot of time and thus enables to greatly achieve a better result, which a person would not be able to accomplish [28, 53]. Identifying useful drugs for treating COVID-19 patients can help. This has become a strong instrument for designing diagnostic tests and improving vaccinations [56–58]. AI helps to produce vaccines and therapies much quicker than normal and is also effective in clinical trials during vaccine production.

Healthcare workers have such a heavy workload because of a rapid and unprecedented rise in the number of patients during the COVID-19 outbreak. Here AI is being used to minimize health professionals' duties [59–64]. It assists with initial screening and effective medication using digital methodologies and decision-making skills, provides the best exercise for students and health professionals on this new virus [65–67]. AI can greatly impact clinical outcomes and address more future problems that reduce the physicians' burden.

5 Proposed Architecture for the Monitoring of COVID-19 Patient

The IoMT-based wearable sensor network monitoring system uses smartphones and wearable sensors to track aged people in real-time, hence improved medical productivity during COVID-19 by offering a more efficient and effective healthcare network that provides home-based supervision. The key purpose of the system is to track the clinical data obtained from the wearable system of the aged, then a data record generated in the data centre, and eventually to provide access to these data by registered health care providers and physicians anywhere at any period. The process is composed of three key layers that function together to accomplish system objectives. For instance, in older people layers, each layer has its specifications and strategies, the main components are that the devices, as well as the pathways, should be able to link to the cloud services to store patient collected data. The system's principal layers are shown in Fig. 3.

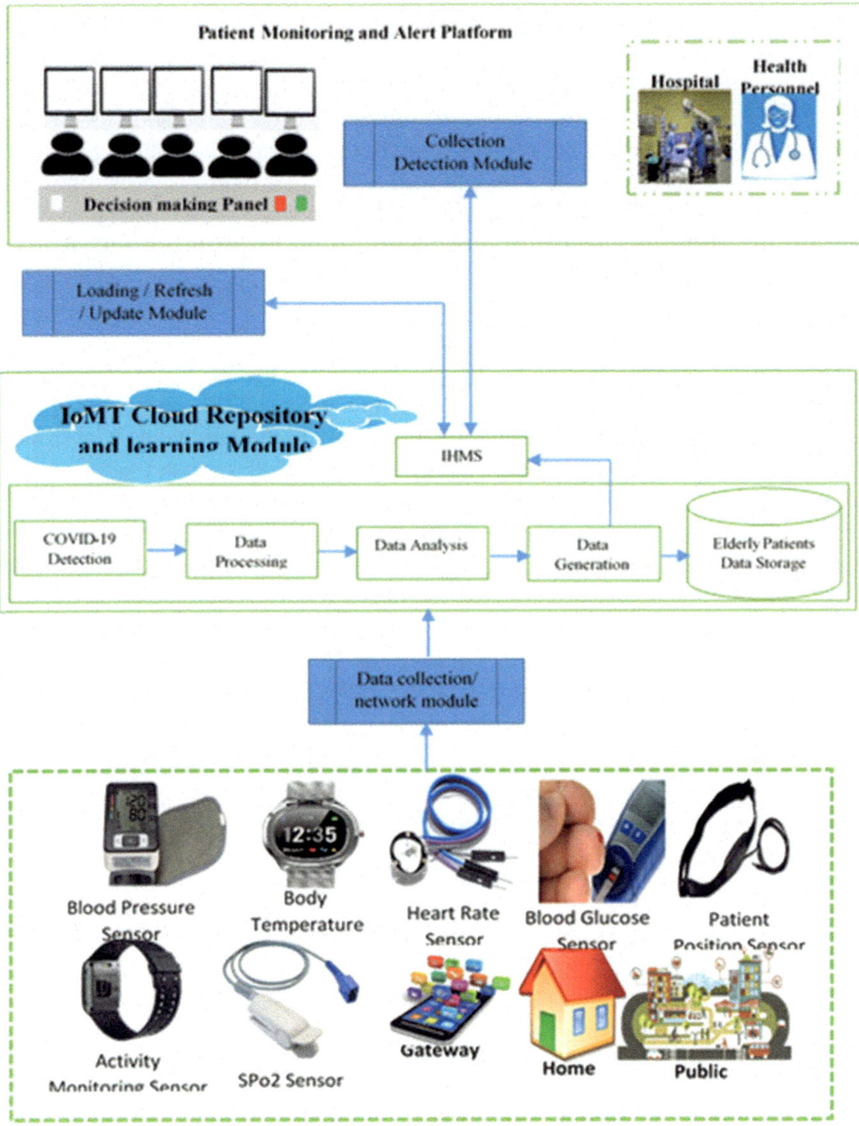

Fig. 3 The proposed architecture of IoMT-based wearable sensor

Patients' Layer (Wearable Devices): To gather clinical data, a wearable monitor and smartphone sensors are attached to the patient's body. These sensors calculate vital signs, including inundation of blood oxygen, temperature, pulse rate, blood glucose, and SPo2, a variety of healthcare sensors are available today [68–72]. It is extremely important to track these symptoms in the patient's body, because any suspicious data may potentially result in infection [69, 70].

For example, a decrease in the human body's level of oxygen triggers sleeps apnea, leading to death. Unusual blood pressure also causes kidney disease or diabetes; all these are symptoms of the COVID-19 outbreak thereby make them important in an elderly patient for monitoring. The sensitive data is transmitted through a Bluetooth connection to the patient's mobile app, and eventually to a database server. Also, sensors can work to calculate and send data daily without patient intervention to automate it (IoMT), thereby improving interface design efficiency and making it more convenient.

Cloud-IoMT-Based (Data Layer): The cloud includes the location where information is deposited and processed on the network. Cloud allows patient data to be processed from their mobile over the network and then it is eligible for doctor assessments. Therefore, for any condition identification in medical information, all documents collection and handing out will be stored in the cloud, therefore, the irregular modifications in patient information will be categorized dependent on patient condition and illness. All documents resulting will be either submitted to the patient and/or doctor's website or emergency room, or both will depend on the patient's condition. Therefore, the IoMT web promotes cooperation and transmission of data through its platform that allows healthcare experts to store customer records, analysis, and diagnostics so that other specialists can automatically read the information around common interests. It shows the patient records in faster medications and real-time updates [73].

Monitoring and Alert Platform (Hospital Layer): This framework is the medium for the doctor to track the information and sensory data of customers. The physicians can review data from the cloud produced by the programme and can take action. Information replication in this application in real-time by deleting all information from the IoMT server as soon as it arrives to use to ensure physicians are up-to-date with the patient's condition, as well as helping paramedics take an immediate decision in the event of an emergency until the situation gets worse and avoiding hospital admission.

The other elements of a supported sensor network are mostly used in the management of network pattern settings and connections between device stages and their objects. Besides, domain-specific management inside the computer system is accessible in the software application to access and configure similar activities of the device, such as active/inactive timestamps and sensing frequency. Domain-specific management, therefore, works with both the public network to deploy sensor network configuration and updates and the component to inform/update the services operating on the network about the new changes. Likewise, according to the services given, the data analysis aspect exists within the cloud server to handle data processing activities, such as statistical analysis.

Gateway: This component is responsible for communicating with patient devices used to identify symptoms of patients and conduct primary data analysis. The result of this section is a description of the circumstances of patients sent to healthcare. Also, the Framework can respond to signs of irregularity when it is identified, e.g. submitting a request for assistance (e.g. demand for an assistant care provider) or an urgent request (e.g. call for an ambulance) when an urgent condition is detected.

6 The Practical Implementation Scenario of the Proposed Framework

The conceptual architecture consists of four main components of advanced technology: Cloud servers, IoMT gateway, network apps, and IoMT systems, and sensors. Since IoMT devices and sensors produce an immense volume of data (Big Data), which is thereafter forwarded to a TCP (Transmission Control Protocol) port where an analytics platform is previously in succession and heeding to this channel. The tool mediator is set up with the actual data streams created by IoMT as the origin and the Apache as the sink so that after listening from the TCP port the data is stored on Apache tools. The proposed analytics solutions are simplified (i.e. the big data analytics platform uses all of the Apache environment's virtual machines) to store the data. The IoMT-based instruments and monitors are single or multiple practical IoMT instruments such as blood pressure monitors, glucose sensors, temperature sensors, oxygen sensors, luminosity sensors, smoke/hazardous gas detectors, and others. Cloud storage is typically used to store the huge amount of data produced by IoMT devices and sensors before submitting it to the computing software used by big data analytics.

The network tools are used to connect via any wireless network accessible among other components. The IoMT sensor data collection, optimization, and simulation can be conducted in the Big Data Analytics software and even how the building environment is managed based on the effects of the real-time data analysis. The data is processed in real-time from any database Apache application and will be saved in the cloud database for future use depending on the findings of the analytics.

6.1 The Following are Practical Applications of the Proposed Framework

For tracking purposes, smartphone applications are empowered with IoMT-based devices providing real-time information using wireless network gateways, Wi-Fi networks, RFID, etc. They have been used in different ways extensively useful to intensification the chance of monitoring and detecting infected people [5, 30]. The implementation of smartphone applications with IoMT-based platforms during COVID-19 an outbreak might have the benefits of having a complete cloud database with COVID-19 outbreak data and information that government, physicians, and healthcare experts can be used to monitor and allow the infected person receiving treatment from home. The online hospital and real-time health information are possible for people to upload their health-related information to the cloud using an IoMT-based cloud database and get health advice from physicians' online within physically present at the clinic. Treatment is being administered within this platform, and without expanding the contamination, the patient will be cured at home. The system is cost-effective when compared with the existing methods with direct contact and appointment with physicians, and the report can be used by the government to make better decisions and actions in future pandemics. They will be able to manage the outbreak effectively [30].

The application of wearable smart glasses in IoMT-based devices has also proved useful in detecting the COVID-19 outbreak among people. This can also be replaced with thermometer guns with their characteristic of less human interaction. The smart glass empowers with a thermal camera and with the functionality of optical have been used to monitor people in a crowd [74]. The face recognition technology within the sensor captures the user's body temperature, and tracking an infected person becomes more comfortable. The data from smart glasses become more reliable with the help of Google Location History, which can be used to track the infected patient contact within a given time. The report of the captured data can be handy from the IoMT-cloud database or sent to the physicians' smartphone for further actions [74]. For example, a Chinese company Rokid smart glasses with infrared devices to fight the COVID-19 outbreak, which can monitor up to 200 people [74]. The combination of Vuzix intelligent glasses with Onsight Cube camera thermal is another excellent example of these devices; in detecting high temperature the device is very helpful and provides a real-time report for medical centres.

Different IoMT smart thermometers that can be used to record constant measurements of body temperatures have been developed. They are created in various types such as radiometer, touch and patch, very accurate devices, and cost-effective [75]. The tools are beneficial in early diagnosis, treatment, and monitoring of COVID-19 patients and any suspicious cases that can arise from the outbreak. Also, infrared thermometers can spread the COVID-19 outbreak when used for taking body temperature because of the nearness of the infected person and physician; thus smart thermometers will be of help in such cases (Mohammed et al. [76]).

Different wearable thermometers can be used during this period such as IFiever, ISense, Ran's Night, Tempdrop among others, which report the body temperature in real-time on smartphones and can be used as sensors on IoMT-based devices. These touchable devices can be a stick or worn on the skin under clothing [75]. For example, In the USA, Kinsa's thermometers have been used to predict the most suspicious areas based on the recorded reports using temperature measurement to detect the highest of being infected with the COVID-19 virus [77–79]. This thereby helps the system to diagnose new COVID-19 patients without stress and increase people's daily lives.

Another acceptable sensor is the smart helmet with a thermal camera results when compared with the infrared thermometer gun due to its lower human interactions [80]. The image and location of the user's face are taken when an optical camera detects the high temperature on the smart helmet and reports it to the IoMT-cloud database. Experts can differentiate the infected person, and take necessary action immediately. The use of the devices allows physicians and other related officers to have access in the crowd to personal information, dark spot visioning temperature, and facial recognition of the user.

The smart helmet has the storage capacity to keep all of the captured data within the helmet, and thus serve as a backup for the IoMT-cloud database [80]. Moreover, the smart helmet integrated Google Location, and the history of the infected person can be used to find the places after discovery [81]. This wearable device has been used successfully in countries like Italy, the United Arab Emirates (UAE), and China to monitor crowds within two meters and has shown promising results [82]. For instance, a Chinese company produced a smart helmet called KC N901 used for body temperature discovery with an accuracy of 96% and has been used by the countries as mentioned earlier [73, 82–85].

Based on the specifications of popular therapeutic organizations and the physiognomies of entirely all forms of disease community, by offering primary diagnostic services for targeted remote health identification, experts can get the technical diagnostic facility at all periods and appropriately access their well-being information. At the same time, it is possible to monitor the development of all types of growing acute, chronic sickness inmates. Bettering care, antecedent detection, antecedent intervention, and early recovery will advance the value of the life of people with severe illness and decrease the risk of sickness. A delayed diagnosis will significantly reduce federal health benefits, revolving to prevent crucial diseases [84].

Sustainable healthcare Based on the IoMT-based sensor [85]. Since IoMT-based incorporates several physiological sensors into the body of patients, it could collect a range of critical physical markers and has the benefits of being relaxed, appropriate for ageing, progenies, and persons with physical and psychological sickness [73, 86]. Hence, consuming these innovative wearable devices will create a modern medical infrastructure that incorporates less-power radio receiver networking, cloud computing, big data, and deep learning technologies to comprehend customized healthcare services based on simple physiological knowledge tracking [73, 87]. The core therapeutic services are primarily focused on a handful of huge sanitoria.

IoMT-based expertise offers a way to exchange different sections of current medical services and is one of the critical steps for ensuring parity of health [84, 85]. Cloud and IoMT-based systems satisfy the demand of consumers in a timely way, consider the patient's current state of health, enhance contact between physicians and sick persons, and reduce the waiting period for therapeutic care, which will boost client loyalty and at the same time maximize hospital performance. Right telemedicine may achieve a standardized norm. Apart from smart healthcare, this theoretical system could be applied to other uses. Smart agriculture, intelligent vehicles, smart cities, and aircraft may be used to track and regulate sensors and equipment rates to ensure convenience, health, and protection.

7 Conclusion and Future Research Directions

The integration of computer and biomedical technologies in medical systems has supported healthcare events, for instance, real-time disease analysis, remote monitoring of patients, and real-time drug prescriptions, among others. The methods have helped greatly to store both patients' personal information and their symptoms on the cloud, which can help during the COVID-19 pandemic. This aids the quality of services provided by the physicians thereby improve patients' satisfaction. IoMT and wearable sensors and devices can aid early diagnosis of COVID-19 pandemics and create an efficient type of measurement in response to the outbreak. These devices have a remarkable impact on the prompt detection of the COVID-19 outbreak. For instance, cloud and IoMT-wearable sensors have the power to show any part of them that is not functioning well, by capturing every single health data from the user thereby creates big data. As a result of these devices, users can notice any change in their health condition frequently and book an appointment with a physician before it is generated to a real disease of any symptoms appear. The COVID-19 pandemic might be easier to fight with the implementation of cloud and IoMT with smart wearables in the healthcare system. Also, monitoring COVID-19 patients remotely would be more convenient and reduce the number of a patient admitted into hospital or isolation centres. The proposed framework is a platform that incorporates various wearable sensors and includes generic onboard computational resources for detecting individual incidents, warnings, and interacting with numerous health information systems providers. Our programme is designed to provide enhanced supervision for patients during COVID-19, collection of data in certain specific cases, and remote assessment for patients. In the time of the ongoing COVID-19 disease outbreak, IoMT is offering so many innovative cloud-based services and infrastructure to more effectively serve aged patients. During such a crucial period of lockout, the remote healthcare network has much sense. The Edge-IoMT-based collects biomedical data from patients through smart technologies and transmits it to the IoMT server to analyze and process the data. Thus any identification of abnormality in patient information will be reported through the hospital portal to the patient's physicians. The Edge-IoMT-based system has a treatable framework that can easily scale and extend, thereby offering efficient, cost-effective applications for remote monitoring of patients. Furthermore, the performance of the system can make a positive contribution accurately to the improvement of healthcare services by using the impeccable CI-WBSN system that can monitor the symptoms of older patients wirelessly and promptly. The Edge-IoMT helps to control and manage elderly people, patients who are in remote areas for their medical needs. We agree that conventional healthcare is certain to see a major conceptual change in the nearest future, as the technological revolution will put sophisticated software and its related services at the patients' fingertips and offer greater connection to reliable healthcare services for both patients and doctors in different areas. For future research purposes, the security challenges of the IoMT-based system can still be enhanced using encryption algorithms with edge computing to secure medical information on the cloud, and the research questions and operational problems need to be addressed. In this study, various challenges concerning information safety and confidentiality. There is a need to concentrate on the challenges related to AiIoT in prediction, diagnosis, examinations, and monitoring of disease. In this context, an intelligent security model should be thoroughly studied to minimize the risks identified.

References

1. Singh, R. P., Javaid, M., Haleem, A., & Suman, R. (2020). Internet of things (IoT) applications to fight against COVID-19 pandemic. *Diabetes & Metabolic Syndrome: Clinical Research & Reviews.*
2. Folorunso, S. O., Awotunde, J. B., Adeboye, N. O., & Matiluko, O. E. (2022). Data classification model for COVID-19 pandemic. In *Studies in systems, decision and control* (Vol. 378, pp. 93–118).
3. Fung, S. Y., Yuen, K. S., Ye, Z. W., Chan, C. P., & Jin, D. Y. (2020). A tug-of-war between severe acute respiratory syndrome coronavirus 2 and host antiviral defence: Lessons from other pathogenic viruses. *Emerging Microbes & Infections, 9*(1), 558–570.
4. Ogundokun, R. O., Lukman, A. F., Kibria, G. B., Awotunde, J. B., & Aladeitan, B. B. (2020). Predictive modeling of COVID-19 confirmed cases in Nigeria. *Infectious Disease Modelling, 5*, 543–548.
5. Awotunde, J. B., Jimoh, R. G., AbdulRaheem, M., Oladipo, I. D., Folorunso, S. O., & Ajamu, G. J. (2022). IoT-Based wearable body sensor network for COVID-19 pandemic. In *Studies in systems, decision and control* (Vol. 378, pp. 253–275).
6. Allam, Z., & Jones, D. S. (2020). Pandemic stricken cities on lockdown. Where are our planning and design professionals [now, then, and into the future]? *Land Use Policy*, 104805.
7. Pullano, G., Pinotti, F., Valdano, E., Boëlle, P. Y., Poletto, C., & Colizza, V. (2020). Novel coronavirus (2019-nCoV) early-stage importation risk to Europe, January 2020. *Eurosurveillance, 25*(4), 2000057.
8. Zhao, S., Lin, Q., Ran, J., Musa, S. S., Yang, G., Wang, W., Lou, Y., Gao, D., Yang, L., He, D., & Wang, M. H. (2020). Preliminary estimation of the basic reproduction number of novel coronavirus (2019-nCoV) in China, from 2019 to 2020: A data-driven analysis in the early phase of the outbreak. *International Journal of Infectious Diseases, 92*, 214–217.
9. Bai, L., Yang, D., Wang, X., Tong, L., Zhu, X., Zhong, N., Bai, C., Powell, C. A., Chen, R., Zhou, J., & Song, Y. (2020). Chinese experts' consensus on the internet of things-aided diagnosis and treatment of coronavirus disease 2019 (COVID-19). *Clinical eHealth, 3*, 7–15.
10. Wan, J., Al-awlaqi, M. A., Li, M., O'Grady, M., Gu, X., Wang, J., & Cao, N. (2018). Wearable IoT enabled real-time health monitoring system. *EURASIP Journal on Wireless Communications and Networking, 2018*(1), 298.
11. Christaki, E. (2015). New technologies in predicting, preventing, and controlling emerging infectious diseases. *Virulence, 6*(6), 558–565.
12. Sust, P. P., Solans, O., Fajardo, J. C., Peralta, M. M., Rodenas, P., Gabaldà, J., Eroles, L. G., Comella, A., Muñoz, C. V., Ribes, J. S., & Monfa, R. R. (2020). Turning the crisis into an opportunity: Digital health strategies deployed during the COVID-19 outbreak. *JMIR Public Health and Surveillance, 6*(2), e19106.
13. Meskó, B., Drobni, Z., Bényei, É., Gergely, B., & Győrffy, Z. (2017). Digital health is a cultural transformation of traditional healthcare. *Mhealth, 3.*
14. Awotunde, J. B., Ogundokun, R. O., & Misra, S. (2021). Cloud and IoMT-based big data analytics system during COVID-19 pandemic. In *Internet of things* (pp. 181–201).
15. Marques, G., & Pitarma, R. (2018, November). Smartwatch-based application for an enhanced healthy lifestyle in indoor environments. In *International conference on computational intelligence in information system* (pp. 168–177). Springer, Cham.
16. Manogaran, G., Varatharajan, R., Lopez, D., Kumar, P. M., Sundarasekar, R., & Thota, C. (2018). A new architecture of internet of things and big data ecosystem for secured smart healthcare monitoring and alerting system. *Future Generation Computer Systems, 82*, 375–387.
17. Özdemir, V., & Hekim, N. (2018). Birth of industry: Making sense of big data with artificial intelligence, "the internet of things" and next-generation technology policy. *Omics: A Journal of Integrative Biology, 22*(1), 65–76.
18. Allam, Z., & Dhunny, Z. A. (2019). On big data, artificial intelligence and smart cities. *Cities, 89*, 80–91.

19. Marques, M. S. (2016). G., Pitarma, R. (2016) Smartphone application for enhanced indoor health environments. *Journal of Information Systems Engineering & Management, 1*, 4.
20. Dimitrov, D. V. (2016). Medical internet of things and big data in healthcare. *Healthcare Informatics Research, 22*(3), 156–163.
21. Marques, G., Ferreira, C. R., & Pitarma, R. (2019). Indoor air quality assessment using a CO_2 monitoring system based on internet of things. *Journal of Medical Systems, 43*(3), 1–10.
22. Kaur, P., Kumar, R., & Kumar, M. (2019). A healthcare monitoring system using random forest and internet of things (IoT). *Multimedia Tools and Applications, 78*(14), 19905–19916.
23. Ayo, F. E., Awotunde, J. B., Ogundokun, R. O., Folorunso, S. O., & Adekunle, A. O. (2020). A decision support system for multi-target disease diagnosis: A bioinformatics approach. *Heliyon, 6*(3), e03657.
24. Oladele, T. O., Ogundokun, R. O., Awotunde, J. B., Adebiyi, M. O., & Adeniyi, J. K. (2020, July). Diagmal: A malaria coactive neuro-fuzzy expert system. *Lecture notes in computer science (including subseries lecture notes in artificial intelligence and lecture notes in bioinformatics)* (Vol. 12254, pp. 428–441). LNCS.
25. Ayo, F. E., Ogundokun, R. O., Awotunde, J. B., Adebiyi, M. O., & Adeniyi, A. E. (2020, July). Severe acne skin disease: A fuzzy-based method for diagnosis. *Lecture notes in computer science (including subseries lecture notes in artificial intelligence and lecture notes in bioinformatics)* (Vol. 12254, pp. 320–334). LNCS.
26. Darkins, A., Ryan, P., Kobb, R., Foster, L., Edmonson, E., Wakefield, B., & Lancaster, A. E. (2008). Care Coordination/home telehealth: The systematic implementation of health informatics, home telehealth, and disease management to support the care of veteran patients with chronic conditions. *Telemedicine and e-Health, 14*(10), 1118–1126.
27. Pham, M., Mengistu, Y., Do, H., & Sheng, W. (2018). Delivering home healthcare through a cloud-based smart home environment (CoSHE). *Future Generation Computer Systems, 81*, 129–140.
28. Awotunde, J. B., Matiluko, O. E., & Fatai, O. W. (2014). Medical diagnosis system using fuzzy logic. *African Journal of Computing & ICT, 7*(2), 99–106.
29. Solanki, A., & Nayyar, A. (2019). Green internet of things (G-IoT): ICT technologies, principles, applications, projects, and challenges. In *Handbook of research on big data and the IoT* (pp. 379–405). IGI Global.
30. Yang, T., Gentile, M., Shen, C. F., & Cheng, C. M. (2020). *Combining point-of-care diagnostics and the internet of medical things (IoMT) to combat the COVID-19 pandemic.*
31. Koh, D. (2020). *SPHCC employs IoT tech and wearable sensors to monitor COVID-19 patients.* Mobi Health News. https://www.mobihealthnews.com/news/Asia-pacific/sphcc-employs-IoT-tech-and-wearable-sensors-monitor-covid-19-
32. Baharudin, H., & Wong, L. Coronavirus: Singapore develops a smartphone app for efficient contact tracing. https://www.straitstimes.com/singapore/coronavirus-singapore-develops-smartphone-app-for-efficient-contact-tracing
33. Lu, L., Zhang, J., Xie, Y., Gao, F., Xu, S., Wu, X., & Ye, Z. (2020). Wearable health devices in health care: Narrative systematic review. *JMIR mHealth and uHealth, 8*(11), e18907.
34. Wen, F., He, T., Liu, H., Chen, H. Y., Zhang, T., & Lee, C. (2020). Advances in chemical sensing technology for enabling the next-generation self-sustainable integrated wearable system in the IoT era. *Nano Energy*, 105155.
35. Athavale, Y., & Krishnan, S. (2020). A telehealth system framework for assessing knee-joint conditions using vibroarthrographic signals. *Biomedical Signal Processing and Control, 55*, 101580.
36. Pustokhina, I. V., Pustokhin, D. A., Gupta, D., Khanna, A., Shankar, K., & Nguyen, G. N. (2020). An effective training scheme for deep neural network in edge computing enabled Internet of medical things (IoMT) systems. *IEEE Access, 8*, 107112–107123.
37. Janet, B., & Raj, P. (2019). Smart city applications: the smart leverage of the internet of things (IoT) paradigm. In *Novel practices and trends in grid and cloud computing* (pp. 274–305). IGI Global.

38. Raj, P., & Pushpa, J. (2018). Expounding the edge/fog computing infrastructures for data science. In *Handbook of research on cloud and fog computing infrastructures for data science* (pp. 1–32). IGI Global.
39. Rehman, H. U., Khan, A., & Habib, U. (2020). Fog computing for bioinformatics applications. *Fog Computing: Theory and Practice*, 529–546.
40. Devarajan, M., Subramaniyaswamy, V., Vijayakumar, V., & Ravi, L. (2019). Fog-assisted personalized healthcare-support system for remote patients with diabetes. *Journal of Ambient Intelligence and Humanized Computing, 10*(10), 3747–3760.
41. Pan, J., & McElhannon, J. (2017). Future edge cloud and edge computing for internet of things applications. *IEEE Internet of Things Journal, 5*(1), 439–449.
42. Xu, X., Liu, Q., Luo, Y., Peng, K., Zhang, X., Meng, S., & Qi, L. (2019). A computation offloading method over big data for IoT-enabled cloud-edge computing. *Future Generation Computer Systems, 95*, 522–533.
43. Alzubi, J., Nayyar, A., & Kumar, A. (2018, November). Machine learning from theory to algorithms: An overview. In *Journal of physics: Conference series* (Vol. 1142, No. 1, p. 012012). IOP Publishing.
44. Zivkovic, M., Bacanin, N., Venkatachalam, K., Nayyar, A., Djordjevic, A., Strumberger, I., & Al-Turjman, F. (2021). COVID-19 cases prediction by using hybrid machine learning and beetle antennae search approach. *Sustainable Cities and Society, 66*, 102669.
45. Lu, F. S., Hou, S., Baltrusaitis, K., Shah, M., Leskovec, J., Hawkins, J., Brownstein, J., Conidi, G., Gunn, J., Gray, J., & Santillana, M. (2018). Accurate influenza monitoring and forecasting using novel internet data streams: A case study in the Boston metropolis. *JMIR Public Health and Surveillance, 4*(1), e4.
46. Naudé, W. (2020). Artificial intelligence vs COVID-19: Limitations, constraints and pitfalls. *AI & Society, 35*(3), 761–765.
47. Ajagbe, S. A., & Adesina, A. O. *Design and development of an access control based electronic medical record* (Emr). CPJ, 2020008, 26108.
48. Kononenko, I. (2001). Machine learning for medical diagnosis: History, state of the art and perspective. *Artificial Intelligence in Medicine, 23*(1), 89–109.
49. Foster, K. R., Koprowski, R., & Skufca, J. D. (2014). Machine learning, medical diagnosis, and biomedical engineering research-commentary. *Biomedical Engineering Online, 13*(1), 94.
50. Wang, Y., Fan, Y., Bhatt, P., & Davatzikos, C. (2010). High-dimensional pattern regression using machine learning: From medical images to continuous clinical variables. *NeuroImage, 50*(4), 1519–1535.
51. Ai, T., Yang, Z., Hou, H., Zhan, C., Chen, C., Lv, W., Tao, Q., Sun, Z., & Xia, L. (2020). Correlation of chest CT and RT-PCR testing in coronavirus disease 2019 (COVID-19) in China: A report of 1014 cases. *Radiology*, 200642.
52. Luo, H., Tang, Q. L., Shang, Y. X., Liang, S. B., Yang, M., Robinson, N., & Liu, J. P. (2020). Can Chinese medicine be used for prevention of corona virus disease 2019 (COVID-19)? A review of historical classics, research evidence and current prevention programs. *Chinese Journal of Integrative Medicine*, 1–8.
53. Haleem, A., Javaid, M., & Vaishya, R. (2020). Effects of COVID 19 pandemic in daily life. *Current Medicine Research and Practice.*
54. Biswas, K., & Sen, P. (2020). *Space-time dependence of corona virus (COVID-19) outbreak.* arXiv preprint arXiv:2003.03149
55. Stebbing, J., Phelan, A., Griffin, I., Tucker, C., Oechsle, O., Smith, D., & Richardson, P. (2020). COVID-19: Combining antiviral and anti-inflammatory treatments. *The Lancet Infectious Diseases, 20*(4), 400–402.
56. Sohrabi, C., Alsafi, Z., O'Neill, N., Khan, M., Kerwan, A., Al-Jabir, A., Iosifidis, C., & Agha, R. (2020). World health organization declares global emergency: A review of the 2019 novel coronavirus (COVID-19). *International Journal of Surgery.*
57. Chen, S., Yang, J., Yang, W., Wang, C., & Bärnighausen, T. (2020). COVID-19 control in China during mass population movements at New Year. *The Lancet, 395*(10226), 764–766.

58. Bobdey, S., & Ray, S. (2020). Going viral–Covid-19 impact assessment: A perspective beyond clinical practice. *Journal of Marine Medical Society, 22*(1), 9.
59. Gozes, O., Frid-Adar, M., Greenspan, H., Browning, P. D., Zhang, H., Ji, W., Bernheim, A., & Siegel, E. (2020). *Rapid AI development cycle for the coronavirus (covid-19) pandemic: Initial results for automated detection & patient monitoring using deep learning CT image analysis.* arXiv preprint arXiv:2003.05037
60. Pirouz, B., Shaffiee Haghshenas, S., Shaffiee Haghshenas, S., & Piro, P. (2020). Investigating a serious challenge in the sustainable development process: Analysis of confirmed cases of COVID-19 (new type of coronavirus) through a binary classification using artificial intelligence and regression analysis. *Sustainability, 12*(6), 2427.
61. Whitelaw, S., Mamas, M. A., Topol, E., & Van Spall, H. G. (2020). Applications of digital technology in COVID-19 pandemic planning and response. *The Lancet Digital Health.*
62. Wan, K. H., Huang, S. S., Young, A. L., & Lam, D. S. C. (2020). Precautionary measures needed for ophthalmologists during pandemic of the coronavirus disease 2019 (COVID-19). *Acta Ophthalmologica, 98*(3), 221–222.
63. Li, L., Qin, L., Xu, Z., Yin, Y., Wang, X., Kong, B., Bai, J., Lu, Y., Fang, Z., Song, Q., & Cao, K. (2020). Artificial intelligence distinguishes COVID-19 from community acquired pneumonia on chest CT. *Radiology.*
64. Smeulders, A. W., & Van Ginneken, A. M. (1989). An analysis of pathology knowledge and decision making for the development of artificial intelligence-based consulting systems. *Analytical and Quantitative Cytology and Histology, 11*(3), 154–165.
65. Gupta, R., & Misra, A. (2020). Contentious issues and evolving concepts in the clinical presentation and management of patients with COVID-19 infection with reference to use of therapeutic and other drugs used in co-morbid diseases (Hypertension, diabetes etc). *Diabetes & Metabolic Syndrome: Clinical Research & Reviews.*
66. Hussain, A., & do Vale Moreira, N. C. (2020). Clinical considerations for patients with diabetes in times of COVID-19 pandemic. *Diabetes & Metabolic Syndrome, 14*(4), 451
67. Gupta, R., Ghosh, A., Singh, A. K., & Misra, A. (2020). Clinical considerations for patients with diabetes in times of COVID-19 epidemic. *Diabetes & metabolic syndrome, 14*(3), 211.
68. Nienhold, D., Dornberger, R., & Korkut, S. (2016, October). Sensor-based tracking and big data processing of patient activities in ambient assisted living. In *2016 IEEE international conference on healthcare informatics (ICHI)* (pp. 473–482). IEEE.
69. Patel, S., Park, H., Bonato, P., Chan, L., & Rodgers, M. (2012). A review of wearable sensors and systems with application in rehabilitation. *Journal of Neuroengineering and Rehabilitation, 9*(1), 1–17.
70. Shnayder, V., Chen, B. R., Lorincz, K., Fulford-Jones, T. R., & Welsh, M. (2005). *Sensor networks for medical care.*
71. Chauhan, J., & Bojewar, S. (2016, August). Sensor networks based healthcare monitoring system. In *2016 International conference on inventive computation technologies (ICICT)* (Vol. 2, pp. 1–6). IEEE.
72. Pantelopoulos, A., & Bourbakis, N. G. (2009). A survey on wearable sensor-based systems for health monitoring and prognosis. *IEEE Transactions on Systems, Man, and Cybernetics, Part C (Applications and Reviews), 40*(1), 1–12.
73. Awotunde, J. B., Jimoh, R. G., Oladipo, I. D., Abdulraheem, M., Jimoh, T. B., & Ajamu, G. J. (2021). Big data and data analytics for an enhanced COVID-19 epidemic management. In *Studies in systems, decision and control* (Vol. 358, pp. 11–29).
74. Mohammed, M. N., Hazairin, N. A., Syamsudin, H., Al-Zubaidi, S., Sairah, A. K., Mustapha, S., & Yusuf, E. (2020). 2019 Novel coronavirus disease (Covid-19): Detection and diagnosis system using IoT based smart glasses. *International Journal of Advanced Science and Technology, 29*(7 Special Issue).
75. Tamura, T., Huang, M., & Togawa, T. (2018). Current developments in wearable thermometers. *Advanced Biomedical Engineering, 7*, 88–99.
76. Mohammed, M. N., Hazairin, N. A., Al-Zubaidi, S., AK, S., Mustapha, S., & Yusuf, E. (2020). Toward a novel design for coronavirus detection and diagnosis system using IoT based drone technology. *International Journal of Psychosocial Rehabilitation, 24*(7), 2287–2295.

77. Chamberlain, S. D., Singh, I., Ariza, C. A., Daitch, A. L., Philips, P. B., & Dalziel, B. D. (2020). *Real-time detection of COVID-19 epicenters within the United States using a network of smart thermometers*. medRxiv.
78. Dubov, A., & Shoptaw, S. (2020). The value and ethics of using technology to contain the COVID-19 epidemic. *The American Journal of Bioethics*, 1–5.
79. McNeil, D. G. (2020). Can smart thermometers track the spread of the coronavirus? *The New York Times*.
80. Mohammed, M. N., Syamsudin, H., Al-Zubaidi, S., AKS, R. R., & Yusuf, E. (2020). Novel COVID-19 detection and diagnosis system using IOT based smart helmet. *International Journal of Psychosocial Rehabilitation, 24*(7).
81. Ruktanonchai, N. W., Ruktanonchai, C. W., Floyd, J. R., & Tatem, A. J. (2018). Using Google location history data to quantify fine-scale human mobility. *International Journal of Health Geographics, 17*(1), 28.
82. Ghosh, S. (2020). Police in China, Dubai, and Italy are using these surveillance helmets to scan people for COVID-19 fever as they walk past, and it may be our future regular. *Business Insider*.
83. Adeniyi, E. A., Ogundokun, R. O., & Awotunde, J. B. (2021). IoMT-based wearable body sensors network healthcare monitoring system. In *IoT in healthcare and ambient assisted living* (pp. 103–121). Springer, Singapore.
84. Awotunde, J. B., Folorunso, S. O., Bhoi, A. K., Adebayo, P. O., & Ijaz, M. F. (2021). Disease diagnosis system for IoT-based wearable body sensors with machine learning algorithm. In *Intelligent systems reference library* (Vol. 209, pp. 201–222).
85. Awotunde, J. B., Folorunso, S. O., Jimoh, R. G., Adeniyi, E. A., Abiodun, K. M., & Ajamu, G. J. (2021). Application of artificial intelligence for COVID-19 epidemic: An exploratory study, opportunities, challenges, and future prospects. In *Studies in systems, decision and control* (Vol. 358, pp. 47–61).
86. Awotunde, J. B., Bhoi, A. K., & Barsocchi, P. (2021). Hybrid cloud/fog environment for healthcare: An exploratory study, opportunities, challenges, and future prospects. In *Intelligent systems reference library* (Vol. 209, pp. 1–20).
87. Bright, J., & Liao, R. (2020). Chinese startup Rokid pitches COVID-19 detection glasses in the US.

Artificial Intelligence Based Diagnostic Model for the Detection of Malaria Parasites from Microscopic Blood Images

Golla Madhu and A. Govardhan

1 Introduction

Malaria is a severe global health issue that causes morbidity and mortality of vector-borne disease that is caused by a Plasmodium parasite of the genus Plasmodium, as declared by the World Health Organization (WHO). In 2020, the WHO analysis report has found around 229 million malaria cases in the world's population [1]. In India, 2.861 million malaria cases were reported in 2020, till October [2]. India has shared the highest decrease in malaria cases region-wide, from about 20 million to 6 million. It has been observed a reduction rate of 83.34% in morbidity and 92% mortality of malaria between the year 2000–2019 [2].

In general, microscopic assessments are the most reliably and frequently used technique for malaria diagnosis in thin blood smears. However, thick blood smears assist with recognizing the presence of parasites while thin blood smears help with distinguishing the types of the parasites [3, 4]. Consequently, these procedures heavily depend on human expertise and are very tedious, require a clinical expert that has limited reliability [5]. Unfortunately, such expert resources are very much limited in rural areas where malaria has an observed majority [4]. However, there is an immediate need for prevention and cure for saving lives by making early detection and diagnosis. A pathologist examines parasites under the microscope, to examine the image color and morphological features toward the diagnosis of malaria [6]. The estimation precision of the diagnosis process usually depends on the medical experts

G. Madhu (✉)
Department of Information Technology, VNR Vignana Jyothi Institute of Engineering and Technology, Hyderabad, Telangana 500090, India
e-mail: madhu_g@vnrvjiet.in

A. Govardhan
Department of Computer Science and Engineering, JNTUH College of Engineering, J.N.T. University, Hyderabad, Telangana 500085, India
e-mail: govardhan_cse@jntuh.ac.in

A. K. Tyagi et al. (eds.), *Intelligent Interactive Multimedia Systems for e-Healthcare Applications*, https://doi.org/10.1007/978-981-16-6542-4_12

who will decide to more for the further process [6]. This process might be implicated in humanistic errors in the provision of subjective, which leads to uncertainty and reduces diagnosis accuracy [6].

The procedure of utilizing machine learning (ML) approaches to medical image analysis, has enormous contributions for achieving significant feature representation for higher diagnostic precision [6–8]. In order, to increase such a diagnostic process by minimizing inconsistency, and for developing a machine learning-based computer-aided diagnosis model for malaria-infected cell detection which gives attention for a better decision toward early and accurate diagnosis [6]. In the past decade, most of the clinical diagnosis methods are the Polymerase Chain Reaction method, the Quantitative Buffy Coat method, the Rapid Diagnosis Test method, and other procedures [9, 10]. Further, these methods had the constraint of human resistance and time taking process. From the previous studies, researchers have been attempting several image processing methods pursue by machine learning techniques to diagnosis malaria. The biggest challenging issues are feature crafting and optimal feature set selection from microscopic images.

To overcome these limitations the making of a modern automated diagnosis system is required to figure out useful insights from the microscopic images. The microscopic images are processed and diagnosed, but each of the blood cells is represented by a different feature serving as size, shape, and textures. To diagnose the parasite cell and to segregate the different life cycles of malaria, its performance a dynamic role in the diagnosis process. However, the feature extraction and the classification hit a vital role to detect, differentiate, and diagnosis of the parasite stages, which makes sense to take the decision-making process. This research develops a computer-assisted diagnosis model for malaria detection and selection of important features set to classify parasites from thin microscopic blood images, which give better performance than the other approaches.

The remaining chapter is organized as follows: Section 2 highlights the related works pertaining to machine learning techniques for malaria detection and classification. The major contribution of the proposed diagnosis process and its comprehensive workflow model is described in Sect. 3 and each subsection describes the denoising, segmentation, and its algorithms, and feature extraction. Section 4 presents the feature selection process using a random forest algorithm that includes both textural and morphological features of malaria parasites from microscopic blood images. Section 5 presents a brief discussion of the malaria parasite classification using machine learning methods. Section 6 outline the experimental outcomes and the performance assessment of the proposed versus other up-to-date methodologies. Section 7 presents the conclusions and future research highlights which are mainly to assist the pathologist in the malaria diagnosis process.

2 Related Works

In literature, several researchers have proposed and have implemented various techniques for malaria diagnosis, but the microscopic procedure is a golden method in the diagnosis of malaria [11]. Thiran et al. [12] proposed a morphologically feature extraction for the analysis of image shape, size, and texture features of the cancerous tissues. Manjunath and Ma [13] proposed Gabor wavelet-based feature extraction for texture analysis in image data. This method shows a higher pattern retrieval accuracy on large image data. Recht [14] patent works presented a low-level morphological feature extraction approach for the classification of premalignant or malignant cells. Nasser et al. [15] suggested an automated procedure for feature extraction in microscopic images. Using this procedure six features were extracted such as moment, inverse difference moment, entropy, correlation, dissimilarity, and contrast, it achieves an overall accuracy of 88.2%. Marghani et al. [16] presented texture feature extraction using a morphological feature approach on the segmented cancer tissues of microscopic images. Results have shown significant improvement in the separation of normal and malignant cancer. Tek et al. [17] presented an automatic diagnosis model for detection and recognition of malaria in thin blood smears. For detection used a customized k-NN classifier and identification considered and evaluated the three-class classification methods. Al-Kadi [18] presented a morphological gradient approach that depends on optimum texture measure combination used for the region of interest and meningioma texture feature extraction used for texture feature analysis and the model achieved an overall accuracy of 92.50%. However, combining more than two texture measures decreases the model accuracy which leads to higher complexity. Das et al. [19] presented a texture and morphological-based feature extraction using geometrical and Haralick texture measures in malaria images. This method is statistically important for feature extraction that is adapted through a multivariate regression prototype. Das et al. [6] computed 80 textural and 16 morphological features in light microscopic images of malaria-infected erythrocytes. Besides, 94 features are statistically significant with six classes of infected and non-infected malaria. Hanung et al. [20] presented a histogram-based feature extraction method for malaria parasite cell features. The limitation of the histogram method is the dependence on the representation of the color of the item and ignoring its contour and textures. Vinayak et al. [21] presented similarities of texture features and its classification of malaria parasite life cycles. This approach extracts textural features and statistical features of malaria parasites from microscopic images. This approach has been achieved has higher accuracy in the diagnosis of malaria detection. Yochay et al. [22] given a feature extraction method based on size, intensity location, and morphology. This approach examines the unique morphological features for the detection of malaria diagnosis. Loddo et al. [23] reviewed various feature extraction approaches such as mathematical morphology for size distribution, characterization, and granulometry used for the extraction of parasite cells. Devi et al. [24] proposed a method for error prediction, chrominance channel histogram, LBPGLCM, and RG color channel. This method is used for the feature extraction of Plasmodium species of malaria-infected erythrocytes classification. This includes various feature extraction such as geometric features, which include, area, perimeter, eccentricity, convex hull, and convex area, and other texture features. Jan et al. [25] presented an analysis on automatic malaria diagnosis for microscopic images and presented state-of-the-art methods and their limitations. Torres et al. [26] demonstrated a prototype diagnostic model for malaria diagnosis by using machine learning methods and it was assessed for Giemsa-stained blood films in Peru. Poostchi et al. [8] developed an automated diagnostic model for malaria detection from Giemsa-stained thin blood images using image processing and machine learning methods. Multiscale LoG filter and C-EPAC utilized for malaria detection and segment malaria parasites. Linear SVM and ANN have used the classification of human and mouse slides. Abbas et al. [27] presented an inductive approach for malaria parasite recognition in thin blood smears. The Gaussian mixture model is used for malaria parasite segmentation and classifies diseased and non-diseased RBCs. Mohanty et al. [28] proposed an automatic model for malaria identification from blood smear images using self-organizing maps which attained an accuracy of 87.5%. Mwanga et al. [29] developed a supervised machine learning approach for the recognition of malaria parasites in dried human blood places from mid-infrared spectroscopy. Logistic Regression (LR) is used for this model and it attained overall predicting accuracies of 92%. Iradukunda et al. [30] presented feedforward neural network with single hidden layer (Extreme Learning Machine) model that is used to classify and predict malaria or non-malaria. This model was compared with other machine learning methods and achieved an accuracy of 99% in 28 s. Abbas et al. [31] proposed malaria parasite quantification and life cycle phase classification in thin blood smears. For life cycle stage classification employed k-NN, Naïve Bayesian algorithm, and SVM based on histograms and local binary pattern features. Taneja et al. [32] discussed two Bayesian networks types for malaria diagnosis employing clinical signs and symptoms. The first model is the manual model, and the second model is an augmented naïve Bayesian model, the first model performed an accuracy of 63.6% and the other model achieved an accuracy of 62.7%. Gitta and Kilian [33] presented current strategies on the diagnosis of malaria in endemic areas and discussed the history of *Plasmodium falciparum* detection and limitation of various diagnostic methods has been applied and assessed toward malaria detection. In our previous works [34], we proposed a computer vision and machine learning-based methodology for malaria detection from microscopic blood smears. Specifically, we addressed the improved k-SVD strategy for image denoising, fuzzy type-II functions are utilized for segmentation. Subsequently, Extra Trees were utilized for the classification of malaria stages. Smith and Kirby [35] presented a review on AI-based image analysis on clinical microbiology and which is reviewed future trends in the same field. Additionally, illustrated progress in smear and plate interpretation and the potential of AI diagnostic tools in clinical microbiology laboratories. Fatima and Farid [36] presented a computer-assisted diagnosis for automated malaria parasite detection and classification in microscopic images. Bilateral filters are used to eliminate the noise and improve the image quality in microscopic images, and image processing procedures are employed to detect malaria parasites. Devi et al. [37] presented a review on various malaria predictions as well as screening methods and analyzed the significance of disease prediction with different techniques. The forecast model includes big data analysis-based datasets like environmental data, clinical data, and others. Nag et al. [38] presented an application of the machine intelligence approach for the identification of malaria in thin blood smears. Which incorporates supervised, unsupervised, and rule-based algorithms for the segmentation of parasites and classification of malaria. Yoon et al. [39] built up an automated system for malaria parasite detection using digital image analysis. This framework contains microscopy, chip, fluorescent dye, and image analysis program. Consequently, assessed with linearity, accuracy, and threshold of detection that was compared with traditional microscopic examinations, and flow cytometry. Lee et al. [40] proposed a machine learning model for malaria detection using patient information from parasite case reports. Moreover, the minority oversampling technique was utilized for balancing problems. Parveen et al. [41] presented a Bayesian network approach for malaria detection that is constructed on different attributes of the patient's symptoms and environmental data. this model achieved an accuracy of 81%. Sushma et al. [42] presented a comparative study on malaria recognition using microscopic blood images. The Otsu, global threshold methods, and artificial neural networks, and support vector machine classifiers have shown efficient performance in the diagnosis of malaria.

In this research review, it is noticed that several machine learning techniques have been utilized texture or color of the feature for classification and use geometric features for recognition of parasite cells in thin blood smears for the diagnosis of malaria and deep learning techniques are required more computational space and time. Previous works propose that an AI-based automated diagnostic system could significantly improve the malaria diagnosis process.

3 Proposed Methodology

This methodology presents the progression of the proposed works which relies on parasite detection and classification of unhealthy and healthy malaria from microscopic blood images. The conventional and comprehensive workflow diagrams for malaria detection and classification are shown in Fig. 1. the proposed methodology for the detection and classification of malaria parasites from microscopic blood images can be partitioned into five phases (see Fig. 1): (i) Image denoising using k-SVD method, (ii) Blood image cell segmentation, (iii) Feature extraction (Local and global features), (iv) Feature selections and classification through Random forest algorithm, (v) Diagnosis of Malaria.

The initial step is typically the obtaining of microscopic blood images which are relied upon the hardware and materials being to be used. These blood images are gathered (shown in Fig. 2) from Vivekananda Hospitals, Begumpet, Hyderabad, Telangana 500016, India, and are set up under the management of pathologists and Dr. Sree Mukesh. Non-infected malaria blood images were downloaded from the NIH, U.S.A [see 43].

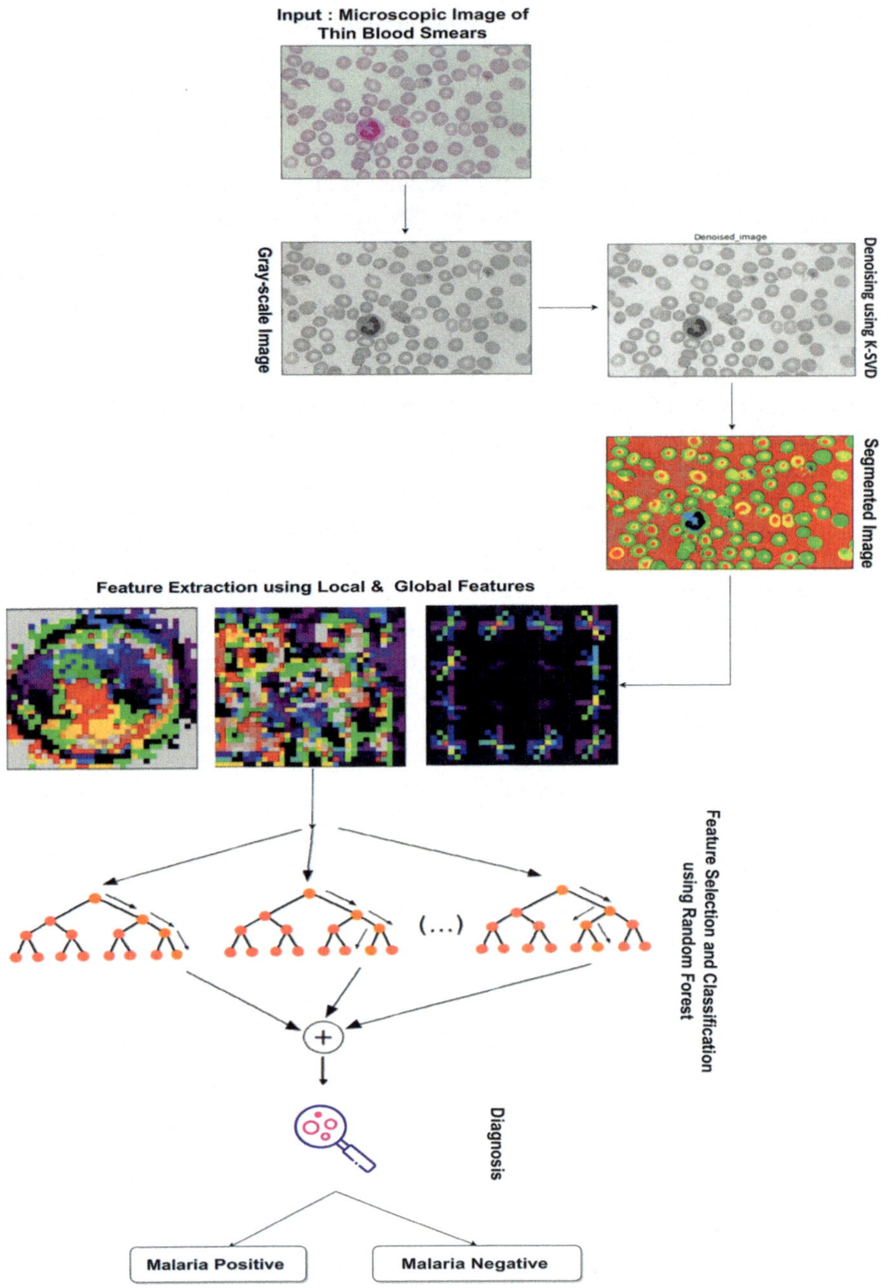

Fig. 1 The block diagram for the proposed malaria detection system

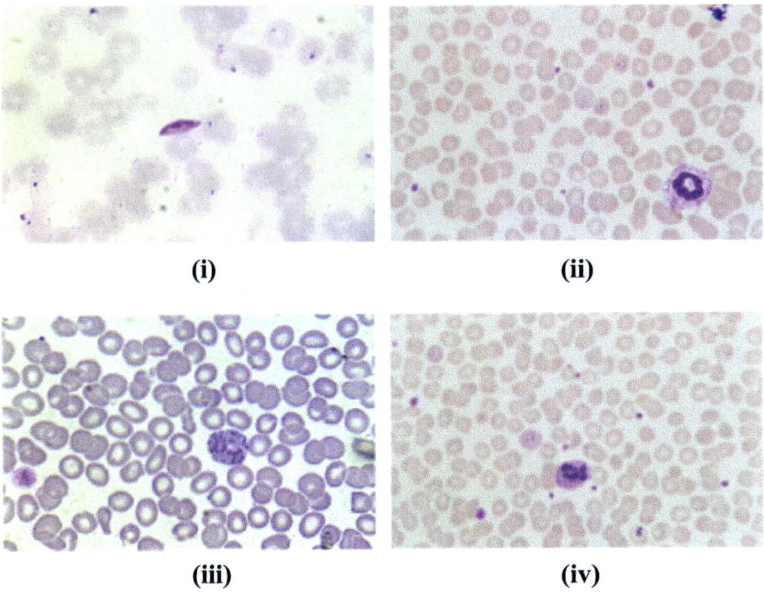

Fig. 2 Plasmodium (i) Gametocyte image, (ii) Ring form Image, (iii) Schizont image, (iv) Trophozoite image

3.1 Image Denoising Using k-SVD

The denoising approach is developed by authors Madhu and Sudipta

Rudra [44] by using the method of *k*-means clustering and singular value decomposition (*k*-SVD) with pursuit approaches for overcoming dictionary learning. However, this approach achieves the best performance on microscopic images with higher accuracy. This innovative method utilizes denoising phenomena of the *k*-SVD procedure. This study utilizes knowledge of the enhanced dictionary learning approach of the image patches by the heapsort mechanism, which is tailed via dictionary learning update process [See 44]. The developed algorithms are computed on varied malaria test images and denoised results are shown in Fig. 3(i) to (iii). This procedure shows more legitimate execution than any traditional denoising strategies which is acceptable execution on the quality enhancement of the clinical pictures, yet it has minimal computational speed with huge computational multifaceted nature.

3.2 Blood Image Segmentation

The segmentation method is developed by author Madhu [45], which presents a unique method for the segmentation of cells and the detection of parasites from microscopic images, and its outcomes were presented in Fig. 4, and description is

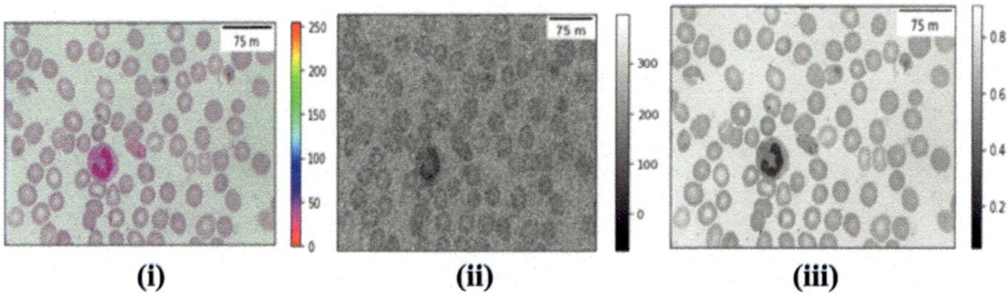

Fig. 3 (i) Plasmodium ovale trophozoite image, (ii) Noised image, (iii) Denoised image

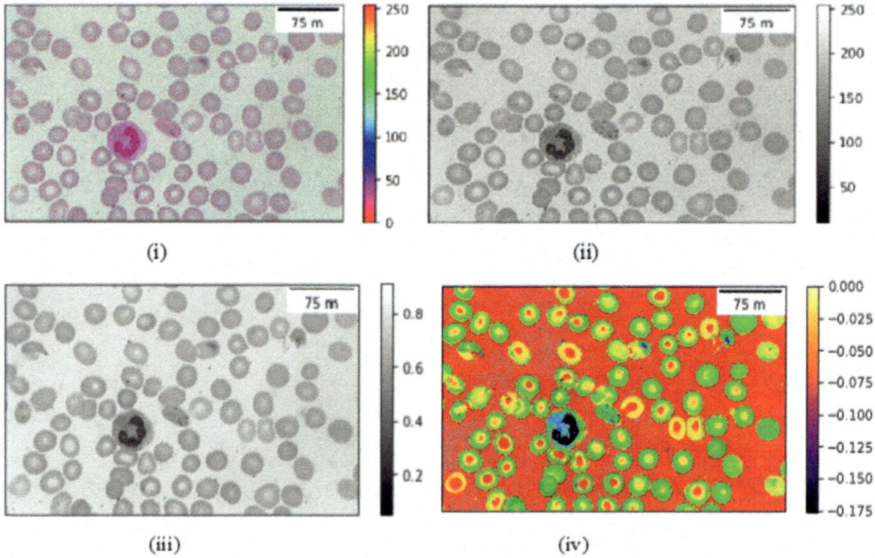

Fig. 4 (i) Plasmodium ovale trophozoite image, (ii) Grayscale image (iii) Denoised image (iv) Segmented image

presented in Algorithm-I [45].

Algorithm-I: A New Algorithm for Malaria Parasites Segmentation

Input: Microscopic image of Thin blood smears A = (m, n).

Output: Segmented image.

Step 1: Thin blood smears collected from microscopy with various labs that consist of *Plasmodium falciparum*, vivax of malaria.

Step 2: Transformed the Step-1 images into grayscale images.

Step 3: Calculated a non-local mean with denoising method on grayscale images which reduces the various noise stages in the image.

Step 4: Applied to normalization process to achieved grayscale images by utilizing the function $g'(a, b) = \frac{(g(a,b) - g\_\min(a,b))}{(g\_\max(a,b) - g\_\min(a,b))}$

Step 5: Calculate the membership values using the formula: $\mu_{\tilde{A}}(x_{i,j}) = \exp\left(-\frac{1}{2}\left(\frac{\vec{x}_n - \vec{m}_j}{\sigma_j}\right)^2\right)$ on step 4.

Step 6: Compute the membership function, $M = \frac{(\mu_L(x_{i,j}) - \mu_U(x_{i,j}))}{(1+2*\delta)+\mu_L(x_{i,j})*\mu_U(x_{i,j})}$ for $\delta \geq 0$ by utilizing the Einstein t-conorm function.

Step 7: Finally, inverse Gaussian gradient function and Otsu functions are applied to these membership functions which is obtained from step 6, then the cell images are segments effectively.

Step 8: Repetition the above advances (2) to (7) for isolated microscopic blood smears.

Step 9: Stop

At last, it applies the inverse Gaussian gradient measure to generate the segmented erythrocytes from microscopic images. This technique achieved a 0.99% DICE coefficient measure, SSIM similarity is 0.99%. It is observed that the proposed segmentation technique achieves robust performance for parasite segmentation in microscopic images. The proposed model is verified on different malarial test images and the results are shown in Fig. 3(i) to (iv).

3.3 *Feature Extraction*

The feature extraction procedures are presented by the same author in [see 46] which characterizes some meaningful patterns relative to an image. This study adapted Shannon entropy [47], SpeedUp Robust Features (SURF) [48, 49] as local features, Hu moments [50, 51], Haralick textural features [52, 53], and Histogram features [54] as global features. The goal of this research is to study the important features of parasite cells in microscopic images that lead to accurate detection.

In this study, Shannon Entropy was utilized as one quantify for feature extraction that is utilized to calculate the randomness of grayscale images. SURF descriptors are used to measure the local regions of malaria blood smears. Here, the POI (point of interest) is computed of the whole blood image, thus these image regions are very close up to those activity points that are to be measured for analysis. Hu moments are committed of seven types of moments of the image which are constant to image makeover (see in 46). These Hu moments are often producing high-level related features which address significant features in our study and evaluates the parasite shape. Haralick feature set was utilized to measure the texture feature of the microscopic blood images in the diagnosis of malaria. Hence, histograms relay to the strength values of the pixels in an image which is an eight-bit grayscale image that comprises 256 unique boxes within the range 0–255.

4 Feature Selection Through Random Forest

This section includes both textural features and morphological features for the categorization of parasites in microscopic blood images. These features are taken for further analysis with the Random forest feature selection algorithm implemented in a package of Python [55].

4.1 Feature Selection

In this study, Random forest decision trees are used for feature selection in the workflow model because of their optimal strategies of ranks that increase the purity of each node in the tree. Also, the mean reduction in impurity causes in all decision trees, the maximum reduction in impurity arises at the root of the decision tree. The node with a minimum drop in impurity occurs at the bottom of the decision trees, after the pruning of the tree that generates a highly influenced feature subset. The datasets are used in this research are malaria microscopic blood images that contain four hundred microscopic blood images, which are obtained from various clinical labs in Hyderabad city regions, India. Among the entire four hundred malaria images, three hundred are the images of malaria infected and a hundred are the images of non-malaria infected that are utilized for the experimentations.

Table 1 shows the size of the malaria dataset and Table 2 shows the results of various blood cell features that are taken from the malaria images and the top 30 features are generated through Random forest feature selection method with help of Python library [55] shown in Table 2 and top-30 blood cell features are computed from SURF features that include feature-4, 33,34,46,49 50,62,66, from Haralick Textural Features such as feature-87,88, and Histogram Features like feature-95,140,270 and others, which are generated through the Random Forest algorithm showed in Fig. 5.

The SURF descriptors are quantifying the local regions of microscopic blood cell images which are useful to determine the infected image regions of malaria parasites. Haralick Fs describe the texture of the microscopic image for identifying the spatial relationships in the images and other Histogram Fs quantify the substantial variation in their illumination of the image.

Table 1 Characterization of the given malaria dataset and its selected features

S. No.	Datasets	Input sizes	Feature selections
1	Train set	[360, 603]	[360,185]
2	Test set	[40, 603]	[40,185]

Table 2 Top-30 features generated by the random forest algorithm

S. No.	Features	Rank (Gini-index)	S. No.	Features	Rank (Gini-index)
1	F 4	0.02098	*16*	F-584	0.01013
2	F-583	0.02037	*17*	F-383	0.01006
3	F-591	0.01965	*18*	F-231	0.00993
4	F-50	0.01649	*19*	F-405	0.00973
5	F-587	0.01589	*20*	F-589	0.00949
6	F-88	0.01225	*21*	F-340	0.00946
7	F-585	0.0121	*22*	F-592	0.00943
8	F-596	0.01201	*23*	F-33	0.00886
9	F-46	0.01194	*24*	F-62	0.0087
10	F-66	0.01163	*25*	F-594	0.00866
11	F-595	0.01148	*26*	F-87	0.00849
12	F-34	0.01105	*27*	F-270	0.00846
13	F-95	0.01077	*28*	F-396	0.00829
14	F-593	0.01069	*29*	F-49	0.00825
15	F-349	0.01032	*30*	F-140	0.00823

Note Here F = features

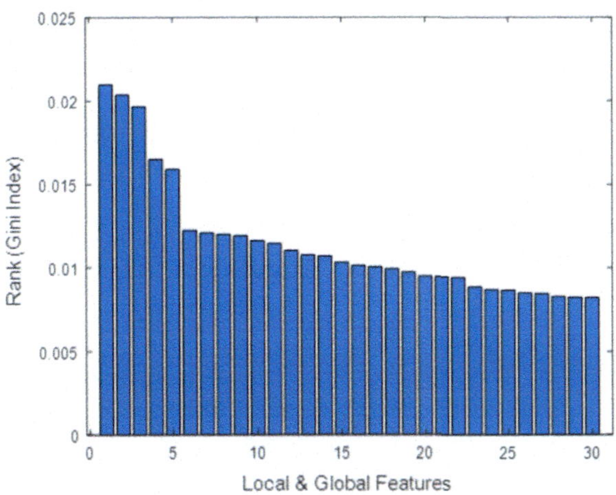

Fig. 5 Local and global top-30 Fs generated through random forest algorithm

5 Malaria Parasites Classification Through Machine Learning Techniques

This section gives a brief review of a machine learning algorithm that is called Random forest and has been used for malaria classification on digital pathological images and, it fascinates the initial need for clinicians for their decision-making under-diagnosis process.

5.1 *Random Forest*

Breiman et al. 1984 [56] presented about Random Forests is an ensemble of Classification And Regression Trees (CART). This builds decision trees at the training module and predicts the class as output time, it reduces the overfitting issues in decision trees. These forests are trained on the given data of the equivalent size as the training set, this is known as bootstraps, which are formed from the random sampling on the training data set to itself [57]. Previously, a forest is created with a set of bootstraps that are not already enclosed from the given dataset (also called out of the bag (OOB)) that is utilized as the testing dataset. The error rate is computed based on OOB estimation which is the prediction error rate of random forests. To estimate the error rate gives empirical evidence that shows the OOB estimation accuracy by utilizing a test dataset of the equal number as the training dataset [58].

In this study, the random forest (RF) classifier is trained on microscopic images using the bootstrap aggregation method, where each new tree is suitable from a bootstrap test of the train set $f_i = (x_i, y_i)$ and the out-of-bag (OOB) error is computed (See Fig. 6) which measures at the count of each new tree during the training period. Here, the OOB error is the average error of each f_i that is calculated by predictions from the trees which don't contain f_i in their individual bootstrap test. The results plot shown in Fig. 6 that Fs an expert to estimate a suitable value of *n_estimators* at

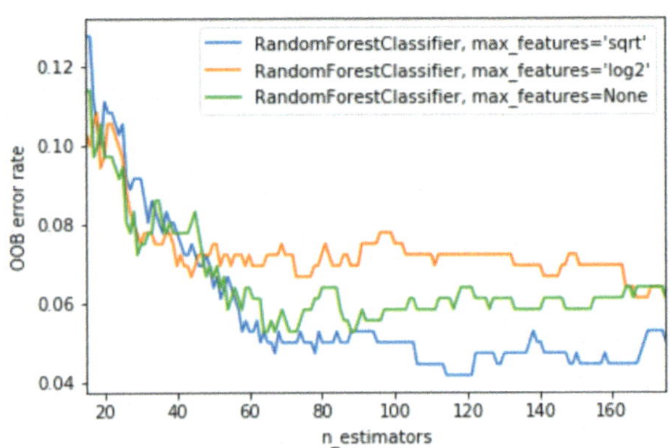

Fig. 6 OOB error rate calculation during the training period of each new decision ree

which the error stabilizes during the training period of each new decision tree and it is useful to estimate F vector importance in image data.

6 Experimental Results and Discussions

In this section, the model assessed malaria datasets which are collected from Vivekananda Hospitals, Begumpet, and Hyderabad, India, and is prepared under the supervision of pathologists. Non-infected malaria blood images are downloaded from the U.S. Public Library [43]. This study uses a *k*-fold validation test strategy [59] to avoid the problems of overfitting on malaria datasets. Table 2 shows F-185 an important F out of 603 are statistically significant, which are estimated by the Random forest F selection algorithm using a package in Python [60]. Table 3 shows the confusion matrix table that is often employed to describe the implementation of the classification tasks, the terms true malaria positive, true malaria negative, false malaria positive, and false malaria negative.

In Table 3 across the top is the predicted class names and the downside are actual class names, and every cell contains the number of expectations made by the classifier which fall into that cell. This study used four metrics, called accuracy, precision, recall, and F1-score for measuring the performance of the system. Here, accuracy is used as the proportion of true malaria retrieved, both positive and negative. Precision measures the number of correct malaria instances retrieved divided by all malaria retrieved instances, given in formula (2). Recall measures the number of correct malaria instances retrieved divided by all correct malaria instances, given formula (3), and F1-score measures the weighted average of both precisions and recall de-pending on the weight parameter $\beta = 1$, see formula (4).

$$\text{Accuracy} = \frac{\text{TMP} + \text{TMN}}{\text{TMP} + \text{TMN} + \text{FMP} + \text{FMN}} \tag{1}$$

$$\text{Precision} = \frac{\text{TMP}}{\text{TMP} + \text{FMP}} \tag{2}$$

Table 3 Confusion matrix (2 × 2 contingency table)

Actual class	Predicted class		
		Malaria negative	Malaria positive
	Malaria negative	True malaria negative (TMN)	False malaria positive (FMP)
	Malaria positive	False malaria negative (FMN)	True malaria positive (TMP)

Table 4 Performance evaluation of random forest classifier and other methods on malaria and non-infected malaria

S. No.	Methods	Accuracy	Precision	Recall	$F1$-score
1	Proposed approach	98.02	0.987	0.984	0.974
2	Logistic regression	87.50	0.885	0.882	0.872
3	Linear discriminant analysis	97.50	0.981	0.973	0.973
4	CART	87.40	0.893	0.881	0.884
5	Decision tree (C4.5)	97.50	0.986	0.972	0.975
6	*k*-NN	82.50	0.846	0.822	0.836
7	Naïve_Bayes	80.00	0.803	0.800	0.795

$$\text{Recall} = \frac{\text{TMP}}{\text{TMP} + \text{FMN}} \tag{3}$$

$$F1 - \text{Score} = 2 \times \frac{\text{Precision} \times \text{Recall}}{\text{Precision} + \text{Recall}} \tag{4}$$

Table 4 shows classification efficiency of the random forest algorithm. Also, the obtained optimal F set for achieving the highest classifier accuracy of 98.02%. Similarly, the k-fold stratified cross-validation method ($k = 10$) generates a confusion matrix and these experiments are performed in the Python language. From the confusion matrix, it is observed that the number of infected and infected parasite prediction made by the Random forest classifier. This can be utilized to assess the performance of a classification sample. Here, accuracy, sensitivity, specificity, and $F1$-score metrics are used for the quantitative analysis of parasite cell classification. Table 4 shows the outcomes of the random forest classifier with various parameters.

From these outcomes, the proposed approach shows significant performance and accomplished an accuracy of 98.02%. The performance of other classifiers like LDA achieved a classifier accuracy of 97.5%, and the CART classifier achieved an accuracy of 87.5%, on the training set. Thus, the C4.5 classifier produced similar consequences of LDA Analysis which achieved an accuracy of 97.5%. The k-NN classifier performs an accuracy of 82.5%, respectively.

However, Naïve Bayesian classifier gives a precision of 80%, with an accuracy of 80.01%, and f1-scores a total of 79% respectively. The Random forest classifier accuracies presented in Table 3 show an outperformed result with other classifier approaches. Certainly, a comparative study cited in Table 4 shows that this method is accurate and effective in comparison with other existing malaria diagnostic methods. In Fig. 7, Receiver Operating Characteristic (ROC) is utilized to select a threshold for different classifiers which boosts the true positive (TP) rate while minimizing the false positives (FP) rate. However, different types of issues have diverse optimal classifier thresholds. The ROC curve depicted the ability to assess the performance of the classifier over its entire operating range. ROC curve sketches of the trade-off between the TP rate and FP rate that tested on the suggested model are shown

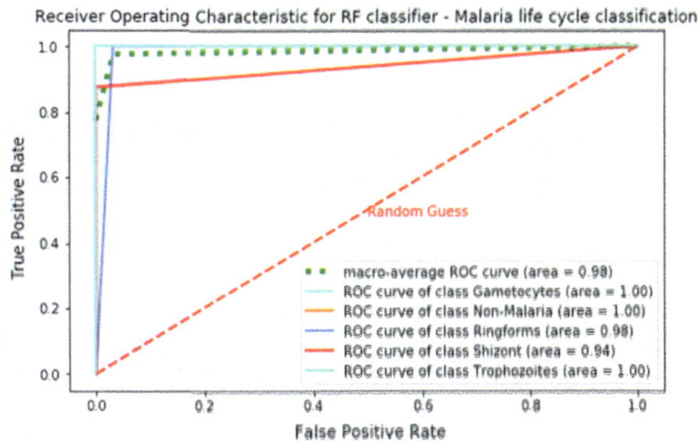

Fig. 7 ROC curve and malaria life cycle classes

in Fig. 7, which is important to identify the possible malaria cases. The TP rate is characterized as the quantity of true positive values split by a total amount of levels in all malaria images. The FP rate is characterized as the quantity of false positive rates divided by the number of malaria blood images.

Table 5 shows the comparative study results where the proposed model generalizes better than the other methods. From Table 5, it has been seen that many of the experiments have been describing for only *P. falciparum*, *Plasmodium vivax* infection stage classification using microscopic images. The proposed machine learning technique using Random forest classifier attained an accuracy of 98.02%. Finally, we concluded that the proposed model generates significant results that may be useful in the diagnosis of malaria and it is also useful to other precise diagnoses.

Table 5 Relative consequences of this method with state-of-the-art models

S. No.	Authors	Types of malaria	Sensitivity (%)	Specificity (%)
1	Tek et al. (2006) [17]	*Plasmodium falciparum*	76.50	97.50
2	Ross et al. (2006) [7]	*P. falciparum*	98.34	85.57
3	Sio et al. (2007) [61]	*P. falciparum*	92.50	85.20
4	Diaz et al. (2009) [62]	*P. falciparum*	94.50	99.60
5	Das et al. (2013) [19]	*P. falciparum, Plasmodium vivax*	97.27	88.82
6	Devi et al. (2018) [24]	*P. falciparum, P. vivax*	95.90	98.91
7	*Proposed approach*	*P. falciparum, P. vivax*	98.02	97.58

7 Conclusions

This research presents the artificial intelligence based diagnostic model for malaria parasite detection. This diagnostic model can significantly characterize both *P. falciparum, P. vivax* for superior diagnosis. In addition, it validates that, feature extraction of microscopic images with infected regions of malaria parasite and feature selection algorithm which are capable of discerning between relevant or irrelevant feature values of an image. This investigation unifies both local and global features which include textural features and morphological features to segregate malaria and non-malaria parasites from microscopic images. The feature dataset consists of 603 features which are designed by the local and global features. The feature vector is reduced with wavering classifier accuracy while the feature's reined ability measure by the random forest selection technique. Additionally, the attainment of the Random forest classifier has been assessed by the feature selection data. From these experiments, it is acceptable that this recommended method outperforms all other detection methods with significant results in terms of malaria detection with good accuracy and its life cycle classification. Therefore, this diagnostic model can perform accurate parasite recognition in the diagnosis of malaria for a better understanding of test samples. In addition, this tool can be used in telemedicine to provide quick and accurate diagnoses in remote areas where pathologists are not regularly easy to use. In the future scope of the work, the proposed model can be utilized for identifying the various stages of the malaria life cycles. Additionally, it would be interesting to explore AI strategies, for example, deep learning methods for stagewise malaria classification.

Acknowledgment The authors acknowledge DRDO/DRL-TEZPUR, for providing financial support to carry out this works (Ref: No. DRLT-P1-1205/Task-64). We would like to acknowledge Dr. Sree Mukesh, Vivekananda Hospitals, Begumpet, Hyderabad, Telangana 500016, India, for providing malaria datasets during this research, and we would like to thank the National Institutes of Health (NIH), the USA for providing online malaria datasets for open access.

Funding Statement This research was supported by the DRDO/DRL-TEZPUR, India under Grant Letter No. DRLT-P1-1205/Task-64.

References

1. World Health Organization. *World malaria report 2020*, ISBN: 978-92-4-001579-1.
2. WHO World Malaria Report 2020: India continues to make impressive gains in reduction of malaria burden, press information bureau. [Online]. Retrieved March 10, 2020, from https://pib.gov.in/PressReleasePage.aspx?PRID=1677601#:~:text=The%20total%20number%20of%20malaria,2019%20(2%2C86%2C091
3. Madhu, G., Govardhan, A., Srinivas, B. S., Sahoo, K. S., Jhanjhi, N. Z., Vardhan, K. S., & Rhit, B. (2021). Imperative dynamic routing between capsules network for malaria classification. *Computers, Materials & Continua, 68*(1).

4. Pan, W. D., Dong, Y., & Wu, D. (2018). Classification of malaria-infected cells using deep convolutional neural networks. *Machine learning: Advanced Techniques and Emerging Applications, 159.*
5. Mitiku, K., Mengistu, G., & Gelaw, B. (2003). The reliability of blood film examination for malaria at the peripheral health unit. *Ethiopian Journal of Health Development, 17*, 197–204.
6. Das, D. K., Ghosh, M., Pal, M., Maiti, A. K., & Chakraborty, C. (2013). Machine learning approach for automated screening of malaria parasite using light microscopic images. *Micron, 45*, 97–106.
7. Ross, N. E., Pritchard, C. J., Rubin, D. M., & Duse, A. G. (2006). Automated image processing method for the diagnosis and classification of malaria on thin blood smears. *Medical and Biological Engineering and Computing, 44*(5), 427–436.
8. Poostchi, M., Silamut, K., Maude, R. J., Jaeger, S., & Thoma, G. (2018). Image analysis and machine learning for detecting malaria. *Translational Research, 194*, 36–55.
9. World Health Organization (2010) *Basic malaria microscopy, Part I learners guide* (2nd ed.) World Health Organization, Geneve, Switzerland.
10. Jain, P., Chakma, B., Patra, S., & Goswami, P. (2014). Potential biomarkers and their applications for rapid and reliable detection of malaria. *BioMed Research International.*
11. Tangpukdee, N., Duangdee, C., Wilairatana, P., & Krudsood, S. (2009). Malaria diagnosis: A brief review. *The Korean Journal of Parasitology, 47*(2), 93.
12. Thiran, J. P., & Macq, B. (1996). Morphological feature extraction for the classification of digital images of cancerous tissues. *IEEE Transactions on Biomedical Engineering, 43*(10), 1011–1020.
13. Manjunath, B. S., & Ma, W. Y. (1996). Texture features for browsing and retrieval of image data. *IEEE Transactions on Pattern Analysis and Machine Intelligence, 18*(8), 837–842.
14. Recht, J. M. (1997). Intensity texture-based classification system and method. U.S. Patent 5,625,705 issued April 29, 1997.
15. Esgiar, A. N., Naguib, R. N., Sharif, B. S., Bennett, M. K., & Murray, A. (1998). Microscopic image analysis for quantitative measurement and feature identification of normal and cancerous colonic mucosa. *IEEE Transactions on Information Technology in Biomedicine, 2*(3), 197–203.
16. Marghani, K. A., Dlay, S. S., Sharif, B. S., & Sims, A. J. (2003, May). Morphological and texture features for cancer tissues microscopic images. In *Medical imaging 2003: image processing* (Vol. 5032, pp. 1757–1764). International Society for Optics and Photonics.
17. Tek, F. B., Dempster, A. G., & Kale, I. (2010). Parasite detection and identification for automated thin blood film malaria diagnosis. *Computer Vision and Image Understanding, 114*(1), 21–32.
18. Al-Kadi, O. S. (2010). Texture measures combination for improved meningioma classification of histopathological images. *Pattern Recognition, 43*(6), 2043–2053.
19. Das, D., Ghosh, M., Chakraborty, C., Maiti, A. K., & Pal, M. (2011). Probabilistic prediction of malaria using morphological and textural information. In *2011 International conference on image information processing* (pp. 1–6). IEEE.
20. Nugroho, H. A., Akbar, S. A., & Murhandarwati, E. E. H. (2015). Feature extraction and classification for detection malaria parasites in thin blood smear. In *2015 2nd International conference on information technology, computer, and electrical engineering (ICITACEE)* (pp. 197–201). IEEE.
21. Bairagi, V. K., & Charpe, K. C. (2016). Comparison of texture features used for classification of life stages of malaria parasite. *International Journal of Biomedical Imaging.*
22. Eshel, Y., Houri-Yafin, A., Benkuzari, H., Lezmy, N., Soni, M., Charles, M., & Salpeter, S. J. (2017). Evaluation of the parasight platform for malaria diagnosis. *Journal of Clinical Microbiology, 55*(3), 768–775.
23. Loddo, A., Di Ruberto, C., & Kocher, M. (2018). Recent advances of malaria parasites detection systems based on mathematical morphology. *Sensors, 18*(2), 513.
24. Devi, S. S., Roy, A., Singha, J., Sheikh, S. A., & Laskar, R. H. (2018). Malaria infected erythrocyte classification based on a hybrid classifier using microscopic images of thin blood smear. *Multimedia Tools and Applications, 77*(1), 631–660.

25. Jan, Z., Khan, A., Sajjad, M., Muhammad, K., Rho, S., & Mehmood, I. (2018). A review on automated diagnosis of malaria parasite in microscopic blood smears images. *Multimedia Tools and Applications, 77*(8), 9801–9826.
26. Torres, K., Bachman, C. M., Delahunt, C. B., Baldeon, J. A., Alava, F., Vilela, D. G., Proux, S., Mehanian, C., McGuire, S. K., Thompson, C. M., & Bell, D. (2018). Automated microscopy for routine malaria diagnosis: A field comparison on Giemsa-stained blood films in Peru. *Malaria Journal, 17*(1), 1–11.
27. Abbas, N., Saba, T., Mohamad, D., Rehman, A., Almazyad, A. S., & Al-Ghamdi, J. S. (2018). Machine aided malaria parasitemia detection in Giemsa-stained thin blood smears. *Neural Computing and Applications, 29*(3), 803–818.
28. Mohanty, I., Pattanaik, P. A., & Swarnkar, T. (2018, May). Automatic detection of malaria parasites using unsupervised techniques. In *International conference on ISMAC in computational vision and bio-engineering* (pp. 41–49). Springer, Cham.
29. Mwanga, E. P., Minja, E. G., Mrimi, E., Jiménez, M. G., Swai, J. K., Abbasi, S., & Okumu, F. O. (2019). Detection of malaria parasites in dried human blood spots using mid-infrared spectroscopy and logistic regression analysis. *Malaria Journal, 18*(1), 1–13.
30. Iradukunda, O., Che, H., Uwineza, J., Bayingana, J. Y., Bin-Imam, M. S., & Niyonzima, I. (2019). Malaria disease prediction based on machine learning. In *2019 IEEE international conference on signal, information and data processing (ICSIDP)* (pp. 1–7). IEEE.
31. Abbas, N., Saba, T., Rehman, A., Mehmood, Z., Kolivand, H., Uddin, M., & Anjum, A. (2019). Plasmodium life cycle stage classification-based quantification of malaria parasitaemia in thin blood smears. *Microscopy Research and Technique, 82*(3), 283–295.
32. Taneja, S. B. (2020) *Bayesian networks for diagnosing childhood malaria in Malawi.* Ph.D. dissertation, University of Pittsburgh.
33. Gitta, B., & Kilian, N. (2020). Diagnosis of malaria parasites plasmodium spp. in endemic areas: Current strategies for an ancient disease. *BioEssays, 42*(1), 1900138.
34. Madhu, G. (2020). Computer vision and machine learning approach for malaria diagnosis in thin blood smears from microscopic blood images. In *Machine learning for intelligent decision science* (pp. 191–209). Springer.
35. Smith, K. P., & Kirby, J. E. (2020). Image analysis and artificial intelligence in infectious disease diagnostics. *Clinical Microbiology and Infection, 26*(10), 1318–1323.
36. Fatima, T., Farid, M. S. (2020, March). Automatic detection of Plasmodium parasites from microscopic blood images. *Journal of Parasitic Diseases, 44*(1), 69–78. https://doi.org/10.1007/s12639-019-01163-x
37. Devi, S. S., Solanki, V. K., & Laskar, R. H. (2020). Recent advances on big data analysis for malaria prediction and various diagnosis methodologies. *Handbook of data science approaches for biomedical engineering* (pp.153–184).
38. Nag, S., Basu, N., & Bandyopadhyay, S. K. (2020). Application of machine intelligence in digital pathology: Identification of falciparum malaria in thin blood smear image. In *Advancement of machine intelligence in interactive medical image analysis* (pp. 65–97). Springer.
39. Yoon, J., Jang, W. S., Nam, J., Mihn, D.-C., & Lim, C. S. (2020). An automated microscopic malaria parasite detection system using digital image analysis. *Diagnostics, 11*(3), 527.
40. Lee, Y. W., Choi, J. W., & Shin, E.-H. (2021). Machine learning model for predicting malaria using clinical information. *Computers in Biology and Medicine, 129*, 104–151.
41. Parveen, R., Song, W., Qiu, B., Bhatti, M. N., Hassan, T., Liu, Z. (2021). *Probabilistic model-based malaria disease recognition system, complexity* (Vol. 2021, Article ID 6633806, 11 pages, 2021). https://doi.org/10.1155/2021/6633806
42. Sushma, D., Rao, N. T., & Bhattacharyya, D. (2021). A comparative study on automated detection of malaria by using blood smear images. In *Machine intelligence and soft computing* (pp. 1–18). Springer.
43. Malaria Datasets—LHNCBC. U.S. National Library of Medicine. Retrieved December 22, 2020, from https://lhncbc.nlm.nih.gov/publication/pub9932

44. Golla, M., and Rudra, S. (2019). A novel approach of *k*-SVD-based algorithm for image denoising. In *Histopathological image analysis in medical decision making* (pp. 154–180). IGI Global.
45. Madhu, G. (2018). Gaussian membership function and type II fuzzy sets based approach for edge enhancement of malaria parasites in microscopic blood images. In *International conference on ISMAC in computational vision and bio-engineering* (pp. 651–664). Springer, Cham.
46. Pharwaha, A. P. S., & Singh, B. (2009, October). Shannon and non-shannon measures of entropy for statistical texture feature extraction in digitized mammograms. In *Proceedings of the world congress on engineering and computer science* (Vol. 2, pp. 20–22).
47. Bay, H., Tuytelaars, T., & Van Gool, L. (2006, May). Surf: Speeded up robust features. In *European conference on computer vision* (pp. 404–417). Springer, Berlin, Heidelberg.
48. Bay, H., Ess, A., Tuytelaars, T., & Van Gool, L. (2008). Speeded-up robust features (SURF). *Computer Vision and Image Understanding, 110*(3), 346–359.
49. Hu, M. K. (1962). Visual pattern recognition by moment invariants. *IRE Transactions on Information Theory, 8*(2), 179–187.
50. Structural Analysis and Shape Descriptors—Open CV 2.4.13.7 documentation. http://docs.opencv.org/modules/imgproc/doc/structural_analysis_and_shape_descriptors.html?highlight=cvmatchshapes#humoments
51. Haralick, R. M., Shanmugam, K., & Dinstein, I. H. (1973). Textural features for image classification. *IEEE Transactions on Systems, Man, and Cybernetics, 6*, 610–621.
52. Haralick, R. M. (1979). Statistical and structural approaches to texture. *Proceedings of the IEEE, 67*(5), 786–804.
53. Summer School Session 2: Histogram equalisation, filters and image enhancement. (2018, July 07). https://iitmcvg.github.io/summer_school/Session2/
54. Breiman, L., Friedman, J., Stone, C. J., & Olshen, R. A. (1984). *Classification and regression trees*. CRC Press.
55. Sarica, A., Cerasa, A., & Quattrone, A. (2017). Random forest algorithm for the classification of neuroimaging data in Alzheimer's disease: A systematic review. *Frontiers in Aging Neuroscience, 9*, 329.
56. Breiman, L. (1996). Bagging predictors. *Machine Learning, 24*(2), 123–140.
57. Pedregosa, F., Varoquaux, G., Gramfort, A., Michel, V., Thirion, B., Grisel, O., & Duchesnay, E. (2011). Scikit-learn: Machine learning in Python. *The Journal of machine Learning Research, 12*, 2825–2830.
58. Patrick, M. T., Raja, K., Miller, K., Sotzen, J., Gudjonsson, J. E., Elder, J. T., & Tsoi, L. C. (2019). Drug repurposing prediction for immune-mediated cutaneous diseases using a word-embedding–based machine learning approach. *Journal of Investigative Dermatology, 139*(3), 683–691.
59. Sio, S. W., Sun, W., Kumar, S., Bin, W. Z., Tan, S. S., Ong, S. H., & Tan, K. S. (2007). MalariaCount: An image analysis-based program for the accurate determination of parasitemia. *Journal of Microbiological Methods, 68*(1), 11–18.
60. Madhu, G. (2020). Computer vision and machine learning approach for malaria diagnosis in thin blood smears from microscopic blood images. In *Machine learning for intelligent decision science* (pp. 191–209). Springer, Singapore.
61. https://chrisalbon.com/machine_learning/trees_and_forests/F_selection_using_random_forest/
62. Díaz, G., González, F. A., & Romero, E. (2009). A semi-automatic method for quantification and classification of erythrocytes infected with malaria parasites in microscopic images. *Journal of Biomedical Informatics, 42*(2), 296–307.

Issues and Challenges Towards Intelligent System in Healthcare

Imposing Security and Privacy in the Healthcare Industry Using Blockchain Technology

J. Bheemeswara Sastry and Barnali Gupta Banik

1 Basic Concepts of Blockchain

Blockchain Technology is a crucial accessory Technology of Bitcoin [1] that has been operating continuously for numerous being not including federal functionality and organization. This piece of writing is a general case of how to use Blockchain in digital currencies using Bitcoin. Although Blockchain technology is advancing rapidly, there is no strict global definition of Blockchain in the industry. The Blockchain description mainly compares to the following definition. Wikipedia manages the data over time and identifies distribution databases where the data likely to corrupt. Each block has an occasionally organized cycle in the data structure representing this time and encrypts the previous set.

The Satoshi Nakamoto White Paper is a rich, reliable, and collectively protected database of Blockchain distribution documents [2]. Blockchain believes that reliable machines can rely on Internet protocols such as the HTTP protocol without third party supervision. Interconnect technology considers as the primary procedure for the next generation Internet called "Value Internet." Now the default protocol level is similar to HTTP. Blockchain, according to economists, is a trust system that transforms trust and builds long-term relations.

J. Bheemeswara Sastry (✉)
Research Scholar, Department of Computer Science & Engineering, Koneru Lakshmaiah Education Foundation, Deemed to be University, Hyderabad, Telangana 500075, India
e-mail: shastri.06@klh.edu.in

B. G. Banik
Associate Professor, Department of Computer Science & Engineering, Koneru Lakshmaiah Education Foundation, Deemed to be University, Hyderabad, Telangana 500075, India
e-mail: barnali.guptabanik@ieee.org

A. K. Tyagi et al. (eds.), *Intelligent Interactive Multimedia Systems for e-Healthcare Applications*, https://doi.org/10.1007/978-981-16-6542-4_13

1.1 Structure of Blockchain

Blockchain is a new method of creating, storing, and distributing data using innovative technologies from a technological end of sight. In short, Blockchain is a distributed database based on a network architecture that connects blocks over time using cryptography to prevent fraud and deception. Blockchain is a new decentralized infrastructure and system model that allows viewing and storing data using Blockchain data structures in a broader perspective and the process of generation and updating of the data using this method similar to distributed nodes. Using encryption, we can make sure data transport and right of admission security. Program and manage applications using smart contracts with automated script code. Blockchain is an intermediate meadow that wants to discuss with starting many angles. To understand, first look at the process of creating blocks and Blockchains. Table 1 gives the summary of different Blockchain structures [1–4].

Manacles link the block. A module is a database tool designed to describe transaction information during a transaction example database log [3]. Create a plug-in for each block. In the Bitcoin system, blocks are created in about 10 min using block body and block header. Blockchain themes play a significant and vital position in the Blockchain network. Block headers operate to evidence the meta-information about existing modules and to describe their structure, relevance, and application. It also includes the version figure, the confusion of the preceding Blockchain headers, the

Table 1 Summary of objectives, contributions, and improvements of different Blockchain structures

Author's	Objectives	Contributions	Improvements	Remarks
Hasanova et al. [1]	To create a currency alternative (Bitcoin)	Miners to maintain a decentralized basin is a challenge	To predict the mines attack, we use game theory	Bitcoins viability teeters precipitously
De la Rosa et al. [2]	Proved to be compatible with many Bitcoin applications	Open Innovation describes it as a "transboundary" process	Development of openness and cooperation around the world	Data Stored on the Blockchain consider as Incorruptible
Smith et al. [3]	Bitcoin Blockchain database has potential to spread large data	Data management projects based on learning outcome	Bitcoin Blockchain timestamps improve the security	Inherently complex and expensive technology
Antonopoulos et al. [4]	Discusses the need to review currency programs	Blockchain used for E-Governance	Bitcoin and Crypto currencies gained acceptance in several fields	Focus on currency rather than key Blockchain core Technologies

Merkle root, the timestamp, the chunk complexity, and the random value. Blockchain description numbers apply to conclude block rating rules.

The block's difficulty is that the Blockchain headers' previous hash has to be less than or equivalent to its worth. Merkle origin hashes for every Blockchain function to ensure the transaction integrity, and each valid Bitcoin transaction must be signed by employing a unique key digitally to get a confusion worth. In the Merkle tree, every deal's hash worth is stored maliciously on the surface of a set of hash values as many hash functions gradually take up the hash value, so the hash function attribute cannot copy easily. Merkle trees belong to block buildings. Unix Time [4] refers to the time when the miner started mining. An important timeline exceeds 11 volumes. Also, other modules do not receive a time label after 2 h. The mess algorithm can convert a communication of a certain extent into a character of a certain length. The hash function has two functions associated with Blockchain. First, functions like hash $(a) = b$ do not change, but you can define a predefined hash system even if p is the hashing result. Second, the value of the transaction record changes slightly, completely changing the results obtained.

1.2 Module Creation in Blockchain Technology

Blocks are not equal to nodes. Because Blockchain has network terminals, the number of blocks in Blockchain is large, so the number of blocks in Blockchain is small and does not augment the following attainment of a certain number [5]. Table 2 procedure of creating the module is as follows.

Finally, it integrates all the modules to create a Blockchain that converts information quickly and efficiently [6]. The structure of the information block is shown in Fig. 1.

Table 2 Procedures of creating the module

S. No.	The procedure of creating the module
1	Block body records transaction details to local memory
2	To get information about each block transaction, create a Merkle tree in the first, block and select the original Merkle tree object from the block header
3	Enter the chunk subtitle data before the SHA-256 algorithm and get the input the previous worth with the hash value above the present chunk
4	Hoard the present time in the Timestamp meadow
5	This field controls the entire network transition's total value during the average output of the previous value. The system will become more efficient and complex. Reducing system power will reduce the problem, so additional modules will take longer to complete

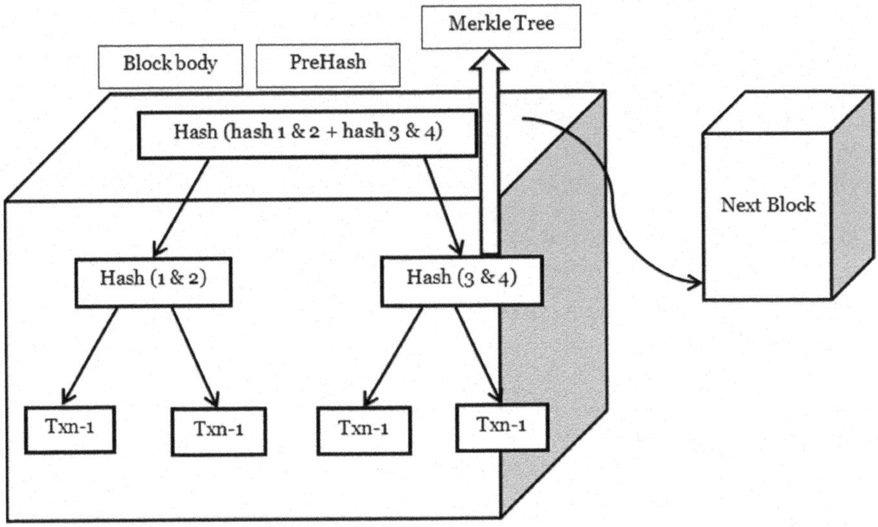

Fig. 1 Structure of information block

2 Research Background of Blockchain

Blockchain knowledge is a fast-growing wonder. Blockchain is silent in its childhood, but it is previously in its next stage. The individuality of Blockchain is that extra and extra practitioners and researchers are focusing on this knowledge. The evolution of Blockchain describes as in Fig. 2. Then, the general characteristics and the three types of Blockchain are describing in detail. Two Blockchain-based sites and applications use for a real-time process are Ethereum and HyperLedger.

2.1 Developing Trend

Swan (2015) describes Blockchain's comprehensive development, mainly dividing into three carpets as streams [7] that have the same classification. The primary brook is Blockchain 1.0, which mainly includes Bitcoin and extra cryptocurrencies in the assets market. The next watercourse is Blockchain 2.0, which primarily integrates critical technologies such as distributed ledger contracts, smart contracts, and updated protocol. The next age bracket Blockchain is an extending Blockchain. It changes the lives of people and relationships. The systems with variety of functions can communicate without restrictions.

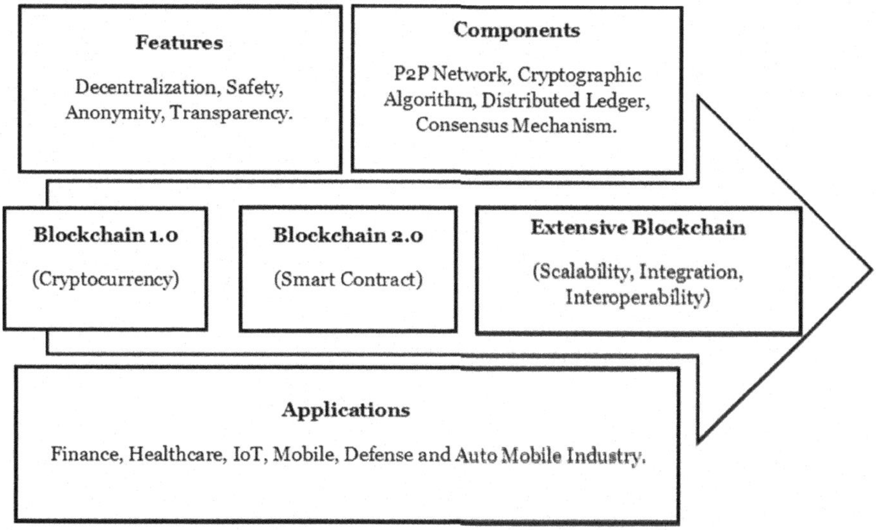

Fig. 2 The evolution of Blockchain potential development

2.2 Blockchain 1.0 and 2.0

Bitcoin and other cryptocurrencies based on Blockchain 1.0 are essential technology that solves a problem that attracts people's attention regarding integrity, security, and reliability [8]. Blockchain technology ensures the integrity, breach, and safety of business data from side to side digitally installed business networks, Blockchains with Pre-Hash blocks, and subsidiaries. Satoshi Nakamoto introduces and explains Bitcoin and Blockchain's notion, which slowly confirms and implements its significance in the money market, and subsequent skin tone attracted much attention. Table 3

Table 3 Features of Blockchain technology

Features	Description
Decentralization	Centrally regulated Blockchain knowledge does not rely on third-party technology
Openness	Blockchain Technology is release basis, and information is unfastening to the public. Anyone can search Blockchain information and create affiliate programs through the open interface
Freedom	With authentication and protocol, all nodes can be automatically verified and send data without system interruption
Safety	It is a multifaceted subject that affects both internal and external factors. In principle, if anyone manages 51% of data, nodes can overwrite or modify the Blockchain scheme's data. No one uses it
Anonymity	The law does not require disclosure or verification of the identity and associated information of each terminal

describes the features of Blockchain technology.

Figure 2 Evolution of Blockchain. For instance, in July 2013, MasterCoin (Omni) expanded its Bitcoin operations from side to side the meta-protocol. In December 2013, the NCX (prospect Currency) become the first total PoS Blockchain. Bitshares (bitstock) appeared in 2013, and NXT created a "digital asset." In addition to the Lisk, recommends by The DAO in May 2016. These cryptocurrencies are based on Blockchain knowledge. Elegant transactions increase the confidence of IoT customers and become a key technology in Blockchain 2.0. At present, it has two significant features. One of them is the digitalization of possessions, which can be digitized if needed or in Blockchain. Innovative transactions through additional programming languages such as golang, Java, and JavaScript can use the Frameworks Ethereum and HyperLedger, which provides simple Blockchain logic. More sophisticated Blockchain systems implement through intelligent functions. Digital assets and smart contracts are becoming more popular as they come in digital form. Blockchain technology used in digital assets and intelligent contracts monitors content effectiveness and shows its shortcomings and reliability.

2.3 Blockchain 3.0

The first two tabs were alike, but the description of the following age band Blockchain is not clear. Swan [7] Only potential projects are considered future capital, implementation, and consolidation projects. Due to the rapid development, it is not simple to define the next age group Blockchain accurately. In the prospect, Blockchain will be wise to collaborate with budding technology like Internet of Technology, Artificial Intelligence, and Cloud Computing to give lofty excellence social military. Blockchain becomes a venture organization and a diverse database of the entire Internet. Blockchain 3.0 describes various programmable themes. The proliferation and integration of Blockchain technology simultaneously take human ideology and social structure to a new level. This stage is the third stage of Blockchain growth. Blockchain knowledge has the potential to be used at all levels of human life and society.

2.4 Common Aspects of Blockchain

Blockchain has a decentralized arrangement lacking middle management, and it is not dependent on third parties or hardware [9]. Blockchain does not have a centralized or hierarchical management system but a macro auto-adapted system that prevents competition between micro-interactions and subnet networks. All Blockchain nodes have the same authority and responsibilities, and each node has a complete transaction log. Therefore, damage or defeat of one or more nodes or nodes does not influence the Blockchain scheme. Blockchain uses an asymmetric data update method.

Newly created data or most of the Blockchain nodes check in the shared book before storing the letter. Therefore, it is difficult to modify or create 235 journals in management analysis: PoW (Proof of Work), PoS (Proof of Stake), DPoS (Delegate Proof of Stake), or PBFT (Practical Byzantine Fault Tolerance). The dissimilarity between the first three agreement organizations is who gets the fundamental civil rights. In particular, evidence that all computer nodes struggle for computer system power. PoW is currently the most widely used integrated system in Blockchain.

The likelihood of obtaining a block with PoW depends on the job done by the miner. PoS accounts provide a significant portion of the direct nodes under attack. Replace the PoS with an energy-saving device. Depot stakeholders select agents to verify account credentials. DPoS is the backbone of Bitcoin, and PBFT is an unnecessary way to deal with Byzantine errors. HyperLedger is a Blockchain platform implemented by PBFT. How to increase the size is one thing to create an integrated system. Various modified protocols are developing for Blockchain applications with different requirements.

The Blockchain system creates a reliable public data reading system based on privacy agreement and protocol that allows all nodes to send and receive data automatically and securely without computer intervention. Blockchain encrypts computer data and makes names anonymous at various levels. The SHA-256 series is one of the most popular confusion functions used in Blockchain and Crypto Currency. Do not post or verify device identification or related information unless required by law. The data should verify according to the previous timestamp of the Blockchain character. The complete Blockchain system is unlocked and clear, and the technical features allow anyone to get and examine facts and nodes to search Blockchain numbers. It creates affiliate programs through the open interface.

2.5 *Modes of Blockchain*

Blockchain technology is transforming into three modes: public Blockchain, Federal (hybrid) Blockchain, and Private Blockchain. The public network is an entirely decentralized Blockchain, and a common cryptocurrency that represents a public network is Bitcoin. The Federal Blockchain is partially decentralized or multi-center into several topics like synchronization procedures, which control by predefined nodes. For instance, it needs to check at least five of the ten synchronization nodes preselect for Blockchain monetary market and health plans. The confidential Blockchain is a federal official that applies to the internal data organization and audit of exact companies that received written permission to read health and supremacy's cookies, an impending area for secret Blockchain adoption. Table 4 summarizes the Blockchain technology background and current studies [7–10].

Table 4 Summary of current research in Blockchain technology

Author's	Current research	Features
Swan [7]	Extended Blockchain	Different functions communicate without any restrictions
Tschorsch and Scheuermann [8]	NXC—Future currency	Transactions increase the confidence of IoT users
Croman et al. [9]	PoW, PoS, DPoS, and PBFT	SHA256 hash functions used for authentications
He et al. [10]	Pubic, Private, and Hybrid Blockchain	Applied to management and Auditing of internal data

3 Cyber Security Threats and Incidents on Blockchain

As companies in the digital and other sectors increasingly using Blockchain technology simultaneously, Cyber Security issues are becoming more modern. The organizational level's most crucial question is how to use Cyber Security in the organization and how much should be invested in Cyber Security to ensure network security and data [11]. Most recently, 61% of small businesses were able to back up this plan in 2017 using Cyber tax data.

Cyber Security attacks are so common today that they occur "with or without," but "when will it." Many theories describe personal safety goals and actual behavior in the context of information technology, including public safety theory, security motivation theory, the theory of Planned behavior, rational model, and naturalization.

However, these models and theories focus on external or scientific factors rather than internal factors such as decision-making styles that describe the Blockchain environment's essential functions. Even today, the attitudes of people, businesses, and individuals in personal and professional life are not able to prepare for these Cyber attacks. According to a survey conducted by Cyber Security companies, 96% of businesses believe that Cyber Security systems do not exist now or in the prospect. Businesses need to be more prepared to protect themselves from Cyber crime.

Many banks and other monetary institutions are currently testing and implementing a Blockchain safety system that reduces risk, Cyber threats, and fraud. Nasdaq recently announces plans to create a Blockchain-based digital book that enhances capital management skills shows that Nasdaq is concerned about Cyber Security for itself and its users. A complete shutdown of the Cyber Security network will not affect these modern systems. However, the security issues associated with Blockchain 3.0 technology are still significant because if the Cyber attack is successful, all the information storing in the digital ledger retrieving at once. Cyber criminals can make money through corporate networks, and companies like giant Black stratus, a Cyber Security industry, destroy the top five Cyber Security threats facing people today.

Threats include Malware, Phishing, Ransomware, File less attacks, and Human mistakes. Let us look at the first five Cyber Security attacks. The first is malicious programs that affect most Cyber fraud communities. These types of viruses can infect computer systems. 90% of malicious programs are sent by email, and when employees open them, they usually hide something else. The standard price of a company malware attack is $2.4 million, another major threat to the second phishing system. Advanced phishing software collects additional sensitive data from companies for reliable advertising and communication. The average value of data lost or stolen by businesses due to information break or phishing is $150 per evidence.

4 Categorization of Blockchain Threats and Vulnerabilities

The goal of Cyber Security is Blockchain technology. Some of them are unique in Blockchain function are generic. There are five types of vulnerabilities in Blockchain Cyber Security.

4.1 Client's Vulnerabilities

Because Blockchain addresses cannot use directly, they care about how individuals interact with Blockchain and do not need to identify a partner during the transaction process. There are digital signature vulnerabilities in corruption. Figure 3 shows various attacks of client vulnerability [12, 13].

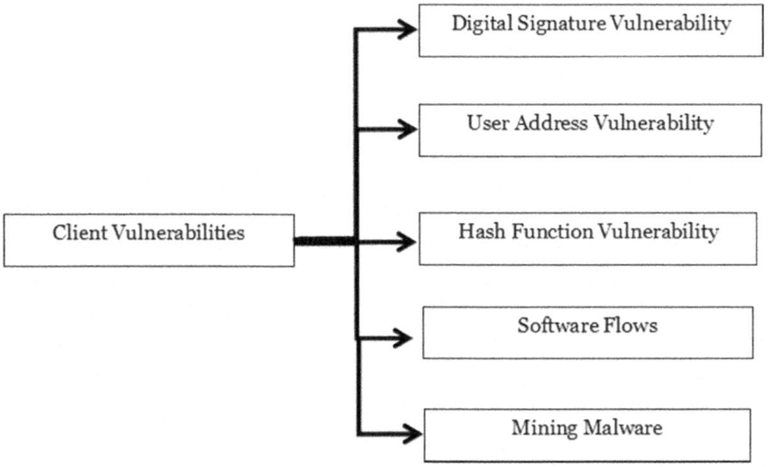

Fig. 3 Various attacks of client vulnerability

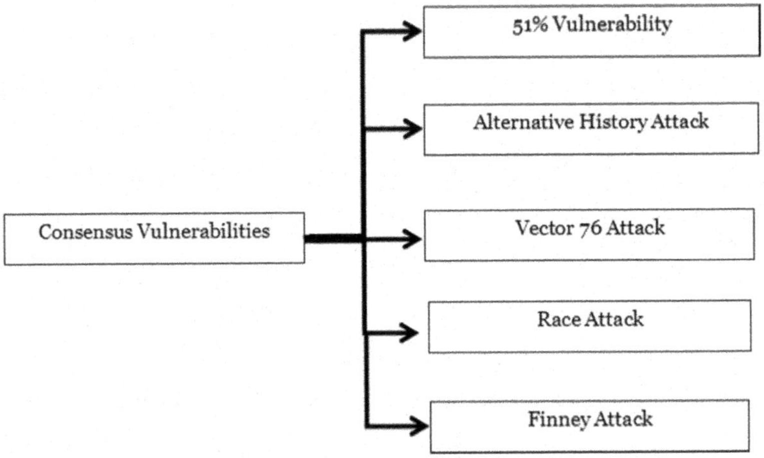

Fig. 4 Various attacks of consensus mechanism's vulnerability

4.2 Consensus Mechanism's Vulnerability

Since Blockchain is a decentralized database that depends on a peer-to-peer (P2P) network, each node in the Blockchain network must have a shared ledger's current status and a copy of the incorrect data for the new volume. For a Blockchain network to work correctly, nodes must meet specific Blockchain content requirements and compress data into a block done through a distribution synchronization procedure that ensures a continuous sequence of generated data.

The distribution synchronization procedure ensures that the quorum Blockchain system node matches the communal book's size, thus adding a new volume to the book. Figure 4 shows different attacks of Consensus Mechanism's Vulnerability.

4.3 Mining Pool Vulnerability

The mining pool facility's foundation is a centralized scheme in which miners gather a pool and solve the pit blocks a puzzle to increase the mines and quarries' intensity. Once the mining process is complete, the miners will earn a steady income based on personal contributions. For this purpose, various mining facilities are building, and mining strategies can test.

Though, centralized cryptocurrency mining pools pose evils. For example, the five Bitcoin mining pool controls 70% of the total hash energy, while the other two Ethereum pools control 50% of the total hash energy is a severe problem because it requires Blockchain localization. The mine's prominent role is to increase the pool-based mine's damage and expose the Blockchain network structure from DDoS attacks. Figure 5 shows different attacks of Mining Pool Vulnerability.

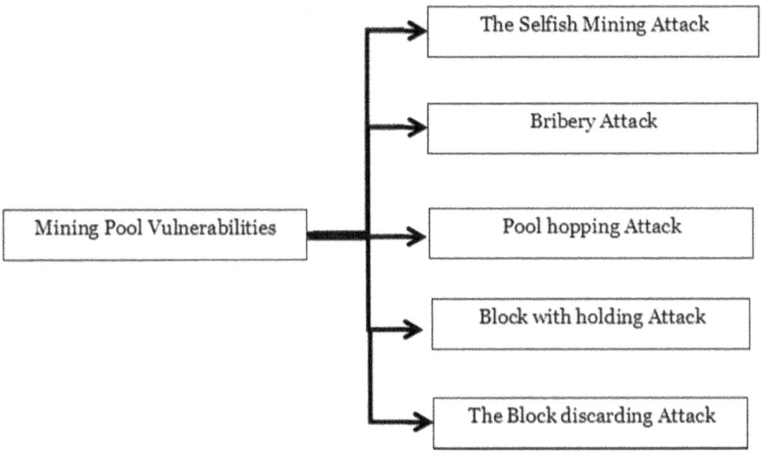

Fig. 5 Various attacks of mining pool vulnerability

As a solution, SMARTPOOL [14], a new procedure plan for decentralized removal. The author proposed two essential contributions. Figure 5 shows various attacks in mining pool vulnerability. First, it uses the pool extraction protocol used in the Ethereum network through intelligent functions. Second, their protocol is valuable and measurable for participants. SMARTPOOL maintains two main lists under the Agreement: Claim List, Claim List, and Certified Claim List verClaimList.

When a miner complains about an Ethereum block, it adds to the list of complaints. At this point, the miners can encrypt the requested list. Each claim has several partners defined by the miner and the machine operator who determine the following operator process's requirements. SMARTPOOL claim Verification. Once verification is complete, that will be redirected to the verClaimList list to confirm the complaints, and the Ethereum process will automatically review the complaint. Every claim allows miners to present a batch of shares example, one million shares. The submitted claim must contain sufficient metadata for verification.

In the first phase of the reserve, if the miner finds the correct chunk in Crypto Currency's aim, the block viewed from the smart pool address can be delivered directly to the beneficiary. Therefore, closing SMARTPOOL provides one or more block adds to miners on the target network. In the previous step, the system checks the Cryptographic agreement. There are many benefits to this group. In other words, the protocol does not require a central operator to control participants. It is a fully decentralized, minimally functional team protocol that rewards participants with communication costs, communication speed, area codes, and other costs. This protocol is justified because participants are rewarding for their contributions.

4.4 Network Vulnerability

As with most system security research, there are Blockchain security issues here. However, there may be other issues related to compatibility, security, access, and management. The introduction of diversified financial advertising has provided a business-based management service for digital attacks and advertising victims. Among the various attacks, a DDoS attack is a functional attack that steals computer data that interferes with management. In the Blockchain-based phase, DDoS attacks differ from traditional attacks in that they are complete P2P updates, and decentralized applications that are attempting to disrupt a system with certain transactions are often more complementary and complex than designing decentralized applications. The steps may be Blockchain-based.

In this way, the decentralized Blockchain configuration provides flexibility and greater availability, but DDoS attacks remain a threat to security outcomes. Money transactions play an essential role in the digital money environment, but overall, DDoS attacks occur as often as possible within this framework. Feder et al. spoke that few cash trades had been closed down since DDoS assaults. It is considered the leading broker of Bitcoin and the largest trader of Bitcoin. He, along with EVasekand Moore, conducted extensive surveillance investigations into the diode attacks against Bitcoin's biological system and published 58 attacks against Bitcoin transactions and management. In particular, 40 Bitcoin managements include more than 250 DDoS attack types, of which executives identify 7%.

Anyone who generates information about transactions, mining, race managers, wallets, and budget management does not have limited rights to attack other DDoS attack managers. According to various sources, 19.1% of small DDoS attacks and 56.8% of large DDoS attacks are enormous pools different from the official operating system. The legitimate Paradigm of resources allows players to add resources, turn them into reporting activities, and increase their chances of winning races. The construction alliance has launched more DDoS attacks to focus on mining groups and make greater use of the mining pool. Figure 6 shows various attacks of network vulnerabilities.

4.5 Smart Contract Vulnerability

During this attack, the attacker creates a fake contract and acts as the victim's entire contract. In general, other scientific articles discuss security violations and cause serious harm. Buterin, with the help of the public Blockchain, has compiled a list of critical drawbacks of intelligent contracts and identified common issues and risks associated with college courses in innovative contract programming. There are general studies on specific vulnerabilities such as vulnerability issues and privacy

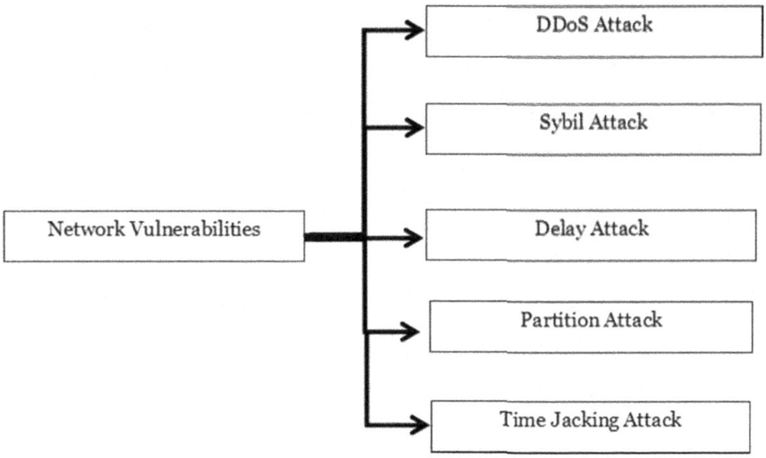

Fig. 6 Various attacks of network vulnerability

issues and the above. It integrates development challenges such as keeping critical functions confidential, using encryption algorithms correctly, and preventing inaccessible data entry.

The survey of non-smart contracts identified the criteria that Ethereum must meet to divide paper contracts. They conclude that it is not recommending to replace legally valid contracts with brilliant contract schemes due to significant privacy violations. Personal information stored in this document may compromise at the time of disclosure, and Blockchain will not protect the personal information. Not having confidentiality about transactions and not having the information flow are two main solitude concerns. Vulnerable smart contracts use to detect fraud and errors, i.e., damage to vulnerable devices. To create a list of unsafe intelligent contracts, we used existing academic articles, online resources, and social discussions to evaluate intelligent contract attacks and errors.

Synthetic smart contracts are pronouncing with the word "Sample" in their name. It also highlights because they will remove innovative contractors who may withdraw contract funds and solicit suicide, the code is no longer in use, and also, we are having reliability issues rather than errors or instability will not be displayed. Not all intelligent contracts scan all devices because all security fixes various damages. Figure 7 shows various attacks in smart contract vulnerability. However, for a general analysis of how vulnerable each device is, they determine all susceptible intelligent contracts. It also provides information on future improvements to security devices. Data psychoanalysis consists of four evaluations: performance, correctness, consistency, and overall evaluation [15]. The other three estimates contain an exact data psychoanalysis procedure and assessment technique in addition to the complete estimate.

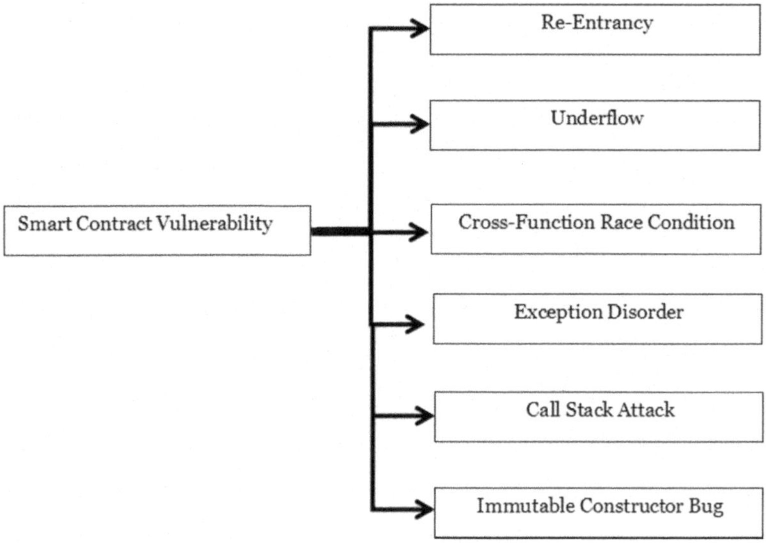

Fig. 7 Various attacks of smart contract vulnerability

5 Blockchain-Based Security

Blockchain is the single newest accepted technology in the IT industry and is still evolving. They did not hold hands, and the populace is still familiar with the technology and is trying to use it in places other than cryptocurrency. Blockchain technology first appeared in 2008 in Satoshi Nakamoto's White Paper. Satoshi Nakamoto is considered the nickname of the association, and some consider he is a natural person. Nevertheless, no sequence of records about this person or the organization. Blockchain recommends as the leading technology of cryptocurrency, also known as Bitcoin.

Blockchain introduces these colleagues to Blockchain research, an electronic money system that solves many of the problems that existed in the previous version of such a system. Blockchain is a list of posts that continue when new blocks add at the end of the post. Neighboring blocks are connected and protected with cryptography. Blockchain is nothing but the transfer of data across blocks. Former data add to the Blockchain, and all subsequent data sets must be changed. It is a desire in situations where changes are not allowed.

Blockchain technology has attracted much attention now as it has created many other things besides cryptocurrency. The Linux Foundation, IBM, Corda, Ethereum, and other business partners can integrate operating system technology into their platforms through intelligent trading. Since the removal of ransomware and Bitcoin payments, Blockchain and cryptocurrency have attracted much attention, mainly focused on Bitcoin, which has forced IT and other sectors to invest in Blockchain to explore its potential in various sectors. Cryptocurrency is a peer-to-peer operation without intermediaries between users. Network users use cryptography to verify transactions on the Bitcoin network, and these records stores publicly as a distributed Blockchain [16].

5.1 P2P Network

The M2M Application field specifies the required configuration service and application distribution using the P2P network. The program contains one or more essential services. Accordingly, the signal is activated through various M2M message protocols like CoAP, HTTP, SIP, and MQTT for communication and application use, depending on the subscription or notification policy. The described Service Management Framework (SMF) is an integral part of M2M based service and application distribution and allows each pair to create and customize M2M applications.

The feedback provided does not address the various safety issue in the P2P-based M2M environment and does not include security risk management strategies. Increasing attacks on M2M networks requires the development of technologies to prevent attack and scheme crashes. This paper aims to identify safety vulnerabilities in P2P and M2M networks and address various security issues in P2P based M2M applications. This test framework improves M2M armed forces security and applications and addresses M2M services and applications' dispersed natural world. The structure safety ensures by specific measures of reliability and trustworthiness will be considered based on various assessments. Besides, the Blockchain knowledge into a given safety structure enhances safety among peers.

5.2 P2P-Based M2M Applications and Security Issues

Figure 8 shows the arrangement of the P2P peers in the M2M society and the structure of the three armed forces for each program. Based on the process described in the M2M diagram, the subsequent universal classifications can be made based on general safety: (a) M2M network—M2M program, M2M service, M2M message protocol, (b) P2P network—P2P message, P2P overlay, (c) IP network. Many publications address IP networks and network security, describing various vulnerabilities and safety solutions. Though, the IP network layer on this system cannot be protected. Many security issues in M2M communication fall into three categories: physical attacks, side-channel attacks, software updates and malware, and M2M device damage or theft, rational attacks include personal fraud, denial of service, and relay attacks. Data attacks include attacks on privacy, data transfer, misinformation, and selective sharing or forgery. The current sensor security status and the temporary network of M2M communications provide an intelligent home application model. Owning a smart home poses a severe risk. The author argues that M2M commu-

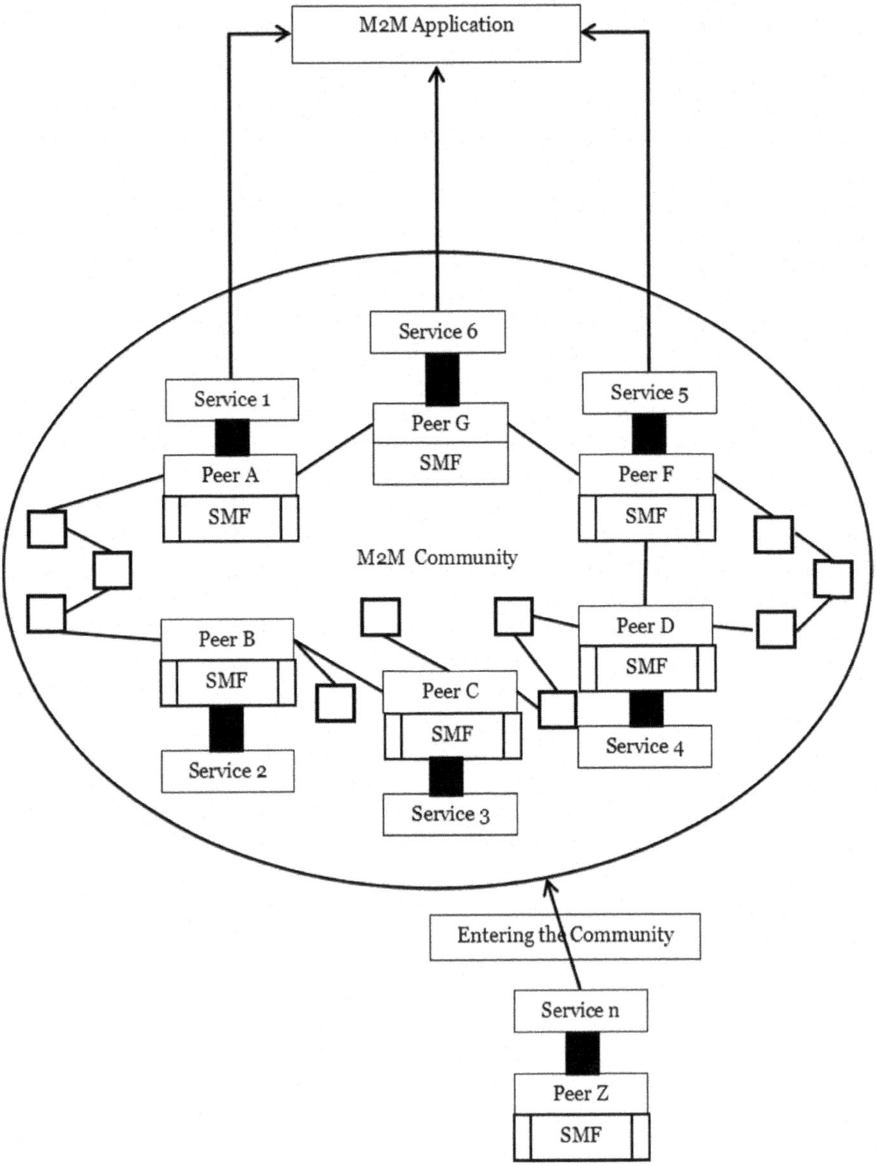

Fig. 8 P2P connected peers in M2M community

nications should provide all network communications security issues and provide multiple refuge features, counting node cooperation detection, location symbols, two-way verification, and dual scheme [17].

6 Blockchain-Based Security

6.1 Motivation

Vehicular Network has become very popular, and it has grown a lot in recent times. The employ of an Interplanetary file system (IPFS) and marginal transport nodes provides data transmission systems and a safe message over secure channels. Vehicular network solves security and privacy issues using Blockchain technology that offers open, distributed, distribution book system features. Though, Blockchain is a superior resource consumption skill that requires high maintenance. We offer a secure Blockchain-based data distribution system for Vehicular networks due to all these issues.

6.2 Problem Statement

With the advent of Blockchain technology, the expansion of a protected repair delivery system for IoT has become realistic. In IoT, several electronic devices connect to form a network. Due to the rapid development of IoT plans, a large amount of data is generating. A decentralized data control system is needed to manage this large amount of data efficiently and securely. Authors with IoT Blockchain provide secure Blockchain-based service delivery systems. Service codes protect accessible computer networks that can be connected to trusted servers using Blockchain technology. The resource management tools of computer evaluation using simulation results. However, neither the charging system nor the Cryptographic system provides a secure connection.

The authors advocate a collaborative, transparent central processing unit network for intelligent traffic with centralized and dispersed structures for a well-organized and compelling message. Boundary servers are worn in a dispersed mode to supply the necessary military and to attain localization. Though, the well-organized use of French servers, completion of caching technique, and data collection between IoT discussion are not complete yet now. As the population grows, so will the number of smart cars.

The Vehicular Network authors argued that the Blockchain-based Vehicular Network distribution network would enable efficient and effective use of large-scale vehicles. In addition to that, a file system provided by the trust administration requires ensuring reliable communication and data storage between vehicles. In V2V communications, the vehicle identification number is commonly using the communication purposes. However, this may lead to a privacy leak. An incentive system is needed to improve consumer attitudes. However, the vehicle development system is still not able to implement.

6.3 Contributions

The main contributions of our projected scheme are:

1. The Blockchain between shared nodes controlling resources based on sharing Vehicular Network data based.
2. A distribution file scheme, or IPFS, is used to amass data generated by intelligent devices.
3. All transactions are automated and verified by intelligent contract.
4. Proof of Work (PoW) and Proof of Authority (PoA) to decrease inactivity and add to scheme performance.
5. Edge offers a cryptocurrency-based incentive system on vehicle edges. If the operating service provides at the end of the vehicle, it gives some incentive.
6. Encryption system used for secure data sharing: Symmetric key encryption/decryption used [18].

6.4 Asymmetric Encryption

From a universal point of view, this comes intending for low population boundaries examples are natural boundaries such as mountains. Figure 9 shows an explanation of the present technique of not having any human intervention aerial vehicle observation atmosphere. This approach applies to the aerial vehicle distribution network's operation providing employment services, and base on the supposition that each being journey a restricted area observes numerous UAVs. All UAVs are regulating following Blockchain policy and information transmit to UAVs.

The Blockchain contains a list of minutes called modules. The link flanked by these minutes is encrypted, and each volume contains the previous level of hash contents. The record cannot change in this way without changing all subsequent volumes. Each module needs change, then the hash of the next module must be changed, and then the size of this update must be changed to the next module, and so on. All modules on different nodes store the data, and it is impossible to change the volume unless the majority does not change. This method, in turn, is stored securely and permanently on the peer-to-peer (P2P) network. Most nodes hijack, so it is challenging to carry out attacks. The present comes up to is enthused by this policy, and each UAV has a list of individual airline identifiers under the direct supervision of UAV claims. This information transmits to a UAV network, so most UAVs store this in order securely and enduring. If the compromising UAVs attempt to replace this Blockchain by providing incorrect information (e.g., adding a fake guest ID), other UAVs will be rejected under Blockchain P2P policy is compromising and rarely considering with common Blockchain assumptions. The compromising UAV is said to be another circumstance invented by a person. In this way, the P2P Blockchain network cannot deny this information. In this way, this misinformation deposit on the Blockchain supplied to the UAV. Furthermore, we have incorporated the principle

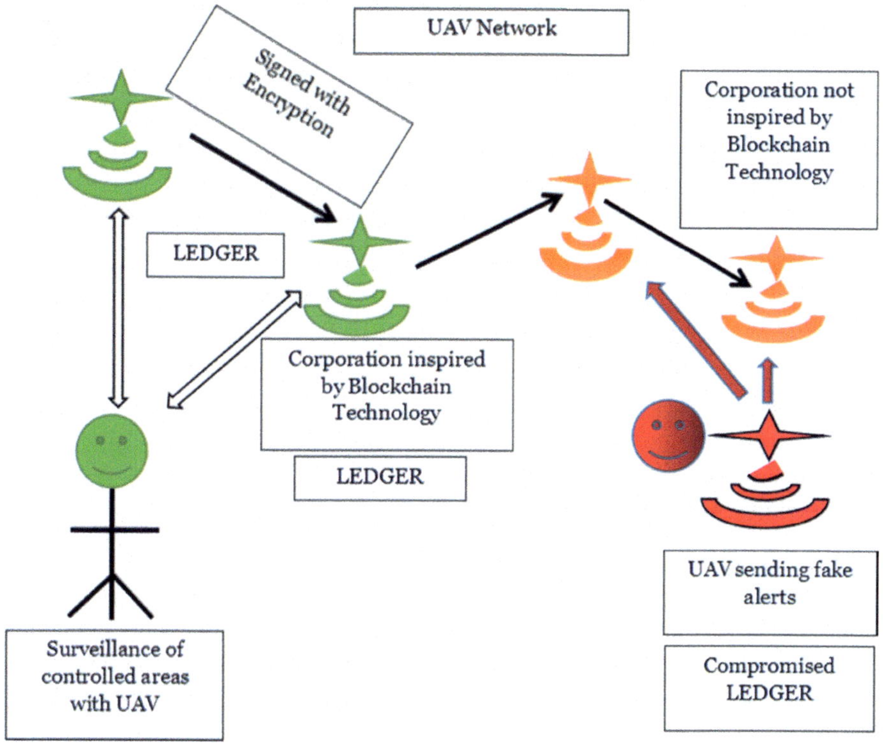

Fig. 9 Overview of the detection of compromised UAV's in surveillance

of trust to detect these events, i.e., to identify recurring events (i.e., across borders) that can only be repeated by a live observer, each event usually being monitored by many UAVs. The compromising UAV is another opportunity to prevent a person's discovery, although it is usually found by other UAVs [19].

6.5 Smart Contract

An intelligent agreement is an executable system that operates on a Blockchain to simplify, compile, and implement contract terms. The principal purpose of a smart contract is to comply with the contract conditions following specific terms mechanically. Therefore, smart contracts guarantee lower contract fees than fixed systems, necessitating a reliable third party to execute and enforce the contract's proviso.

The design for the elegant deal came from Sophie in 1994. However, this concept did not see the glow of day until the advent of Blockchain knowledge. Smart Deal is a complete digital asset distribution system for all parties with predefined terms.

For example, a Y coin receives a call, Alice Pop will send an X coin to the coins. Various definitions of elegant agreement contain been discuss in the text.

The system divides all meaning into two parts, the elegant agreement Code and the Smart Legal agreement. Smart treaty code "Blockchain Save, Verify, Activation Code." This application's contract effectiveness depends entirely on the programming language, and the module's network features used to express it. An innovative legal contract is a code for terminating or changing a legal contract. The focus of this study will be on the first definition of a smart contract code.

An intelligent deal includes account balance, personal savings, and executable code. Agreement status includes savings and contract balance. When the contract completes, the government maintains and renews the Blockchain. Figure 10 shows a sound, intelligent contract system. A unique 20-byte address adds to each transaction. After using the contract.

Blockchain is impossible to change the contract code. To fulfill the contract, the customer can send the transaction to the contract address. Each insurance terminal (so-called miners) in this transaction network agrees on its results. The status of the contract renews accordingly. Based on the transaction received, the contractor can read and write to his memory, save the remaining amount, send and receive messages from the user and another contract, or create a new contract. There are two types of smart contracts, permanent and unresolved smart contracts. A smart contract is a smart indenture that does not require any information from outside. An unspecified smart contract base on external party information [20]. Table 5 summarizes the Blockchain-based security [16–20].

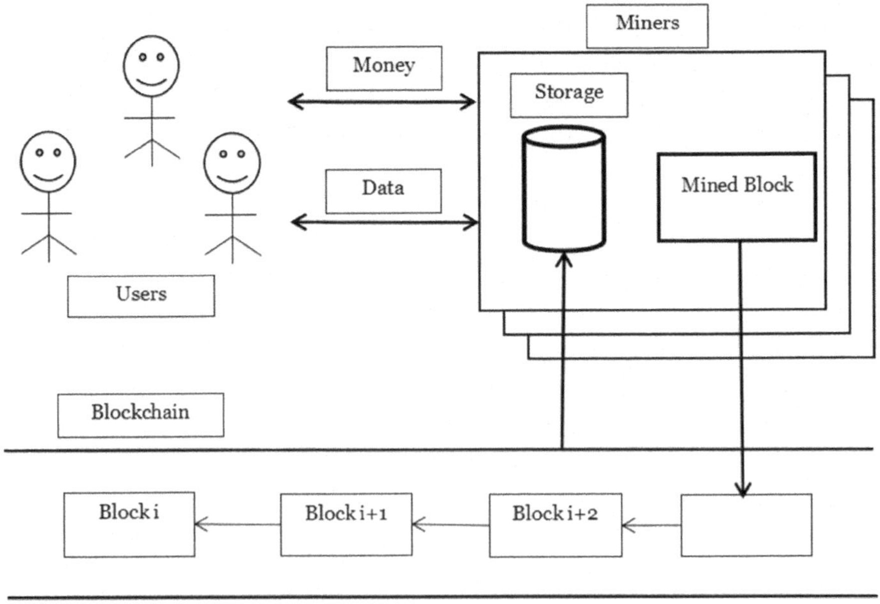

Fig. 10 Smart contract system

Table 5 Summary of Blockchain-based security

Author's	Objectives	Contributions	Improvements	Remarks
Krishnan et al. [16]	Data Collection and transmission over the Internet	Offers the safety framework which allows doing power grid	Insecurity systems, immune systems use in various fields	Nonsecure data collection and transmission causes catastrophic actions
Shala et al. [17]	Blockchain offers a safety the atmosphere for the utilization of M2M applications	To confirm the reliability of colleagues a new trust management system was introduced	Blockchain improves system security and data storage in Blockchain strategies	A P2P network needs to set up to share details among trusted agencies
Javed et al. [18]	To authenticate Channel State Information (CSI)	In a secure environment V2V communication is enabled	Blockchain improves the spectra efficiency	Lack of security, privacy, and lack trust
García-Magariño et al. [19]	UAV's supports surveillance in network infrastructure	Uses a secure asymmetric encryption	Blockchain improves the Security of distributed datasets	Detects threats in critical areas and the surveillance of military bases
Alharby et al. [20]	Recognizes map areas and associated smart contracts	Conducts a systematic mapping to study research related to smart contracts	As more contracts execute per second, the act of Blockchain systems would be improved	Transaction ordering dependency

7 Essential Technologies of Blockchain Security, Privacy, and Trust

7.1 Encryption Technology Related to Security

All Blockchain technologies provide encryption. After the encryption method fails, Blockchain data security is compromised, and there are no invisible changes to the Blockchain. The encryption algorithm is to alienate into asymmetric encryption algorithms, and asymmetric encryption algorithms use in Blockchain. Encryption is the leading Blockchain safety knowledge.

Asymmetric encryption involves the use of two different keys for encryption and encryption. Both of these keys are community and confidential. Bitcoin dealings are primarily performing by the sender, who encrypts the transaction using a public key recipient and sends it to the address. The addressee will encrypt the in sequence using his/her private key. The sender encrypts the digital signature with his key and sends it to the address. The sender encrypts the sender's community key, which confirms that the sender sent them in order.

7.2 Hash Function, Merkle Tree Related to Privacy

The hash algorithm considerably reduces the amount of data when penetrating the actual data because it has certain characters (hash function) to organize the data together. For instance, if the data is associated with a data key, this in a sequence should be store in the f (key) state of the hash meaning. So, if anyone wants to make sure that it is one of the two big data given in the Blockchain can reduce the data and compare the hash worth of the particular span.

The hash algorithm cannot change after the hash function, and the key to the actual value of the data cannot obtain with the hash value f (key). When transferring Blockchain data, send the data hash value simultaneously to avoid data corruption, and the data receiver must generate the data hash value, compare the previous hash value with the revised hash value and find out if the data is corrupt.

The problematic advantage of the confusion purpose is the agreement algorithm's foundation (PoW) for displaying the load on the Blockchain. PoW has a resource algorithm to check how much work is on Blockchains, which is the primary way to multiply Blockchains. The block's data is related to the selected values, and the hash worth is intending using computation control, and every first n bits of the confusion charge is zero. Illustrate the PoW algorithm with a flow example.

If anyone is entering a recognized "proof of work" line, the SHA-256 hash function of the workload request must be done thoroughly with the total value of the truth in the "proof of work" line is implementing on a "proof of work once" (the Bitcoin system load evidence purpose is SHA256). If the effect is a hexadecimal hash worth initial with "0000", a check will be sent. According to this algorithm, if anyone wants to increase the first 6-bit hash's value starting at nonce = 1, calculating 65,536 hash to find the value of the first 0—bit hash must perform 620,969 hash functions on "0".

There is no additional well-organized way to find a hash that meets the supplies. Consequently, a hash worth that meets the exact supplies obtained due to this process consider as a load. Merkle Tree (MT) is a Grind binary tree with leaf tips, intermediate tips, and root tips. The Bitcoin Blockchain system uses the Merkle binary tree to quickly summarize Blockchain data integrity to store the data packets in a Blockchain and continuously create new ones. Only one Merkle path saves in the block title. Each hash node has two consecutive blocks or their hash values, as shown in Fig. 11. Second, it supports Merkle's Simple Payment Verification Protocol (SPV) strategy, which tracks transaction data, including entire Blockchain network nodes. So, it is necessary to use a database, for example, a Merkle tree on a block network.

The Merkle tree is a tree arrangement in the data arrangement. It can be a double-tree or a multi-fruit tree in the broadest sense, but the Merkle tree in Bitcoin is a whole doubletree. It performs a hash function on all modules of the business module, and the hash function remains in pairs until the value of the received hash reaches the complete binary tree. Figure 11 shows that Trade A, Trade B, Trade C, and Trade D consider as data leaf nodes below and their associated hash value. H_A, H_B, H_C, and H_D are the leaf node at the top level, the hash value achieved by the hash data block (i.e., Trade A, Trade B, Trade C, and Trade D). By understanding this, the hash

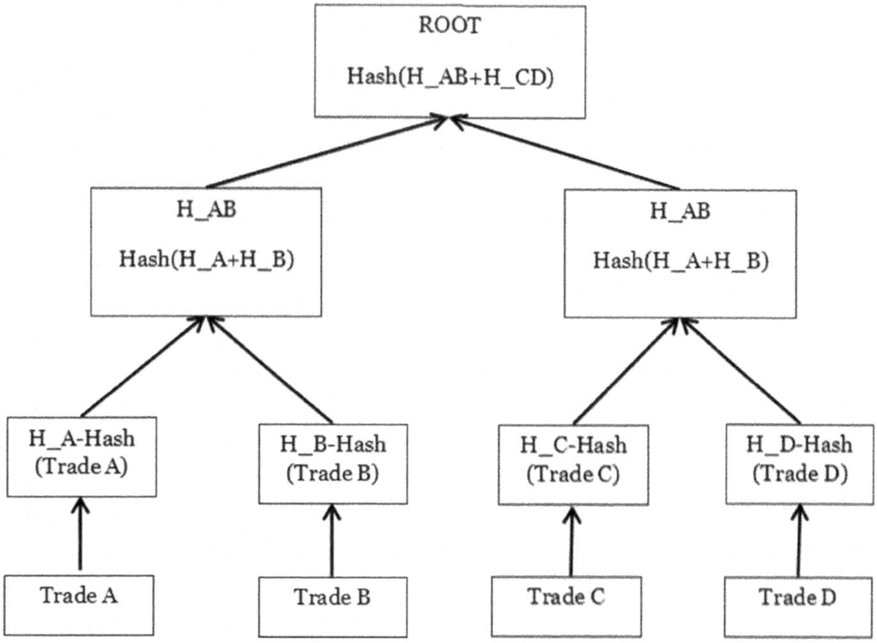

Fig. 11 Merkle tree

value of H_AB and H_CD middle nodes that do not perform hash functions straight line, H_A, and H_B as a string, H_C and H_D have strings and perform the hash function. Next, the root bump is the hash's worth by breaking the integrated string of H_AB and H_CD, the Merkle tree's root hash. Presume n has data and n-nodes shaping as a result of data freezing. Connect the nodes in pairs until the root node and the left node form $n/2$ nodes. This process using N hashes, the time complex defined as $O(n)$, and the tallness of the tree $\log(n) + 1$.

7.3 Consensus Mechanism Related to Trust

Blockchain is decentralized and does not require the support of loyal third parties to deliver valuable information effectively. The consensus system solves the problem of how Blockchain achieves stability in issued certificates. Consensus organization is a vital Blockchain technology that determines who owns the book rights and who owns the selection process's causes and rights. Different digital currencies support different balancing systems such as PoW, PoS, DPoS, and PBFT. Go and divide the work accordingly depend on how many coins in the extraction process are finding in this process, which takes longer and improves system performance is to mine.

The main feature of the load resource system is that the user has to work hard to get the result, but as a result of its consistency, the user does the results of the associated work. One of this approach's key features is asymmetry: the investigator's work is moderate and easy to verify. Employer and stock certification is a system in which users pay interest to calculate quantity and time. The PoW system requires more energy and time to find a random number that meets the conditions. The PoS system eliminates the need for multiple random number processes to save resources and speed up each block.

7.4 Smart Contract

Suppose a specific program is to implement, the intelligent program automatically evaluating and implementing. An innovative transaction that allows one to enter into a trusted transaction based on credit approval business is essential. The difference between a smart contract and a traditional contract is that there are no subjective comments from people working on the computer about sending the promised code to the participants. With smart deals, users and strangers can switch without costly transparency. Smart contracts can be implemented independently of Blockchains.

When there is a problem with a traditional contract, many agencies have to intervene and use many material and financial resources. A contract based on an intelligent Blockchain is subject to the terms and conditions of the contracting authority and automatically terminates as it does not require a third party's trust. Determine the level of motivation to choose the next step.

The decentralized concept of Blockchain knowledge is very secure. Eliminating the adverse effects of intelligent business reduces the cost of intelligent contract operations integrated into Blockchains. Simultaneously, the scheme of government machinery built using the Blockchain algorithm also helps us execute smart contracts professionally. Elegant deals are also wrong. First, the author of an elegant agreement must be rigorous, and a strict contract can be detrimental to a particular party. All Blockchain customers can find smart deals based on this Blockchain, which helps them see all the losses. Overall, a smart contract's role will surely turn out to be clear in the future [6].

8 Security and Privacy in Blockchain

Network security analyzes each node's records and their detailed data. When one node receives data from another, that node checks the IDs of the other nodes. If the check is successful, the node sends information to the network. At the same time, diversification causes problems with the transfer of data between nodes. This feature increases the transparency and efficiency of transactions can use the timeline to view and record Blockchain activity and add timeline data to the survey.

Blockchain uses asynchronous encryption to encrypt and sign data using community and secret keys connected with a smart contract ensures high security and data privacy. Blockchain-based networks contain large amounts of data, but most of this data seems to be fragmented. Traditional management and storage management mainly base on highly centralized management. Security attacks or centralized damage can lead to identity leaks or network failures.

Blockchain can prevent and improve security. Blockchain creates a distribution framework that prevents network security incidents through all processing nodes, processing errors, and centralized administration. Blockchain does not rely on centralized interventions to store or update information. Instead, each user has a "record" in which the recorded information is to write and check the Blockchain, which provides a high security level that is invariant, visible, reliable, and profitable. Additionally, Blockchain faces some challenges, including data management, privacy, IoT device permissions, connectivity, and doodle attacks. Several issues have resolves to address these issues [21].

9 Open Research Challenges

The future challenges for integrating the two technologies are listed below:

Privacy: Different ledgers organized with the security terms for real-time data collection and data analysis in Blockchain technology can lead to privacy avoidance and anxiety. Besides, IoT regularly collects personal and sensitive data from users of different sensitivities, and posting this data in open ledgers may lead to privacy protection. Data privacy ensures through private Blockchain ledgers, encryption, and restriction of access to ledgers. Such a private Blockchain platform limits the availability and influence of excessive amounts of data for AI to achieve accurate and precise decision-making analysis.

Scalability and Side Chains: Measuring Blockchain sites is a big challenge today. On the Crypto Blockchain platform, the Bitcoin Blockchain can process an average of four transactions per second, while Ethereum can process 12 transactions per second. This performance is not acceptable compared to Facebook, which handles millions of transactions per second, including complaints, messages, and comments. Lateral Blockchain acceleration uses when party activities outside the main party are terminated quickly and terminated only once a day. Many new Blockchain's are significantly improving the mining integration system. For example, sites like Al corrant and IODA work better than Ethereum and Hyper Ledger Blockchain. However, additional steps are needed to improve the comparable size of Facebook and its variants [22].

9.1 Future Research Directions

Security and Privacy: Several security issues were raised, including threats, including DDOS, and BC. The discussion about the connection of the attack is based on intelligent computers. These documents also outline specific strategies for protecting against personal harm.

Communication Protocols: Many popular communication protocols used for device-to-device communication are now widely used in IoT ecosystems. For securing the data, Blockchain uses Lightweight encryption and protocols. Ensuring safety requires creating and developing a homogeneous system in a hybrid mining environment that can modify secure protocols.

Connection and Scaling: Measurable problems solves in Blockchain. In recent works, scaling has always been an issue that requires immediate and practical solutions. Some jobs are associated with previously selected specific miners. Some other tasks show incompetence in networking, like fewer transactions per day when adding equipment. Therefore, more research needs on the level of a reliable connection without reducing the workload.

Energy consumption and Resource allocation: The basics approach is used to avoid unwanted power utilization; low-end devices are still not as efficient compared to the work they offer. High processing Blockchain nodes directly affect the system's overall consumption power consumption to increase the regression of IoT installations in some Blockchain can be maintained at a moderate level only if the extraction algorithm uses only the nozzles and reduces the complexity. It is also imperative to reduce the calculated overlaps when using different Crypto systems.

Blockchain Standardization: Offer different structures to meet their needs. A typical model of the IoT ecosystem suggests.

Optimization in Blockchain: It covers the design and improvement of several optimization techniques compatible with IoT environmental conditions. Considering all the inconsistencies and difficulties. LoraWAN complete Blockchain network created to connect to user touch portals and application servers through wireless touch networks.

10 Conclusion

Therefore, this approach allows stones to be rewarded and invested according to their categories of the work to have a hybrid encryption (encoding) mechanism to encrypt patients' electronic health records before sending to a distributed ledger that supports a decoding process that is the reverse phenomenon of the encoding procedure. We need a mechanism to have a patient's electronic health records package suitable for persisting in the Blockchain repository. This efficient search mechanism helps obtain required data from the Blockchain and manages security keys to secure communications in the system. A set of smart contracts that govern the rules and regulations from time to time. When they have to submit a high type of high investment, they are more rewarded for promoting it. This paper provided the security mechanism for locating UAVs in the network of UAVs to ensure surveillance activities. This method uses the principle of faith, inspired by the principles of the Blockchain. This paper discusses various options for the behavior of malicious hijacked UAVs. In short, the uncompromising drone has two options, which are to avoid actual observations or to emit sound through false alarms so that the actual signals are not taken seriously by degrading the system. This system considers as reliable because it assumes only minority aircraft will compromise if the uncompromising UAVs avoid actual observations. This paper provided the security mechanism to safeguard healthcare professionals' data items and healthcare units across the globe. Further attacks against the generation of misinformation explore critically.

References

1. Hurlburt, G.F. (2016). Might the blockchain outlive bitcoin?. *IT Professional, 18*, 12–16. https://doi.org/10.1109/MITP.2016.21.
2. de la Rosa, J. L., Torres-Pedrosa, V., & el Fakdi, A., et al. (2017). A survey of blockchain technologies for open Innovation. In *WOIC*, pp. 14–15.
3. Smith, T. D. (2017). The blockchain litmus test. In *Big data* (pp. 2299–2308).
4. Antonopoulos, A. M. (2014). *Mastering Bitcoin: Unlocking digital Crypto-currencies.* O'Reily Media Inc.
5. Kraft, D. (2016). Difficulty control for blockchain-based consensus systems. *Peer-to-Peer Network. Appl., 9*(2), 397–413.
6. Ma, Y., Sun, Y., Lei, Y., Qin, N., & Lu, J. (2020). A survey of blockchain technology on security, privacy, and trust in crowdsourcing services. *World Wide Web, 23*(1), 393–419.
7. Swan, M. (2015). *Blockchain: Blueprint for a new economy*. O'Reilly Media
8. Tschorsch, F., & Scheuermann, B. (2016). Bitcoin and beyond: A technical survey on decentralized digital currencies. *IEEE Communications Surveys & Tutorials, 18*(3), 2084–2123.
9. Croman, K., Decker, C., Eyal, I., Gencer, A. E., Juels, A., Kosiba, A., & Song, D. (2016, February). On scaling decentralized blockchains. In *International conference on financial cryptography and data security* (pp. 106–125). Springer.
10. He, D., Habermeier, K. F., Leckow, R. B., Haksar, V., Almeida, Y., Kashima, M., & Epes, C. V. (2016). *Virtual currencies and beyond: Initial considerations (No. 16/3)*. IMF Staff Discussion Note. International Monetary Fund.
11. Gordon, L. A., Loeb, M. P., & Zhou, L. (2016). Investing in cybersecurity: Insights from the Gordon-Loeb model. *Journal of Information Security, 7*(2), 49–59.
12. Hoch, J. J., & Shamir, A. (2008). On the strength of the concatenated hash combiner when all the hash functions are weak. In L. Aceto, I. Damgård, L. A. Goldberg, M. M Halldórsson, A. Ingólfsdóttir, & I. Walukiewicz (Eds.), *Automata, languages and programming* (pp. 616–630). Springer Berlin Heidelberg.
13. Alkhalifah, A., Ng, A., Kayes, A. S. M., Chowdhury, J., Plaza, M., & Watters, P. (2019). *A taxonomy of blockchain threats and vulnerabilities*. Preprints.
14. Loi, L., Yaron, V., Jason, T., & Prateek, S. (2017). SMARTPOOL: Practical decentralized pooled mining. *SEC'17 proceedings of the 26th USENIX conference on security symposium* (pp. 1409–1426).
15. Manoj, K. S., & Aithal, P. S. *Blockchain cyber security vulnerabilities and potential countermeasures.*

16. Krishnan, K. N., Jenu, R., Joseph, T., & Silpa, M. L. (2018, July). Blockchain-based security framework for IoT implementations. In *2018 international CET conference on control, communication, and computing (IC4)* (pp. 425–429). IEEE.
17. Shala, B., Wacht, P., Trick, U., Lehmann, A., Ghita, B., & Shiaeles, S. (2017, September). Ensuring trustworthiness for p2p-based m2m applications. In *2017 internet technologies and applications (ITA)* (pp. 58–63). IEEE.
18. Javed, M. U., Rehman, M., Javaid, N., Aldegheishem, A., Alrajeh, N., & Tahir, M. (2020). Blockchain-based secure data storage for distributed vehicular networks. *Applied Sciences, 10*(6), 2011.
19. García-Magariño, I., Lacuesta, R., Rajarajan, M., & Lloret, J. (2019). Security in networks of unmanned aerial vehicles for surveillance with an agent-based approach inspired by the principles of Blockchain. *Ad Hoc Networks, 86*, 72–82.
20. Alharby, M., & Van Moorsel, A. (2017). *Blockchain-based smart contracts: A systematic mapping study*. arXiv preprint arXiv:1710.06372
21. Shi, S., He, D., Li, L., Kumar, N., Khan, M. K., & Choo, K. K. R. (2020). Applications of Blockchain in ensuring the security and privacy of electronic health record systems: A survey. *Computers & security* (p. 101966).
22. Soltanisehat, L., Alizadeh, R., Hao, H., & Choo, K. K. R. (2020). Technical, temporal, and spatial research challenges and opportunities in Blockchain-based healthcare: A systematic literature review. *IEEE Transactions on Engineering Management*.

Industry 4.0 Challenges in e-Healthcare Applications and Emerging Technologies

Shruti Suhas Kute, Amit Kumar Tyagi, and S. U. Aswathy

1 Introduction

The ideas related to industry 4.0 and with the ongoing modern transformation that has been arising around the world are not restrictive to assembling creation measures but rather can be applied to a few zones, for example, coordination, transportation, energy, and exceptionally medical services [1]. This paper means to give a diagram of the cutting edge of late industry 4.0 applications in the medical services area and to assess the function of empowering advances in the groundbreaking cycle of the present Emergency clinic 4.0. Emergency clinic 4.0 or Shrewd Clinics can be viewed as medical services offices that plan to upgrade assets and cycles through better association of data, patients, clinical and authoritative staff [2]. Similarly, it is conceivable to discuss Brilliant Patients, for example, common individuals who buy unique gadgets equipped for checking their own medical issues and who comprise the supposed Wellbeing Internet of Things (IoT) or Shrewd Wellbeing. As Medical care keeps on turning out to be more serious, the capacity to evaluate trade-offs between asset use, administration, and working expenses fill in significance, for example, regarding arrangement access, sitting area deferrals, and telephone utility. Bendato et al., (2015), Patrone et al., (2017), and Cassettari et al., (2013) examined the utilization of stochastic recreation examination for considering and improving wellbeing measures and other complex frameworks [3–5]. The controlling component of Keen

S. S. Kute (✉) · A. K. Tyagi
School of Computing Science and Engineering, Vellore Institute of Technology, Chennai, Tamilnadu 600127, India

A. K. Tyagi
Centre for Advanced Data Science, Vellore Institute of Technology, Chennai, Tamilnadu 600127, India

S. U. Aswathy
Department of Computer Science and Engineering, Jyothi Engineering College, Thrissur, Kerala, India

A. K. Tyagi et al. (eds.), *Intelligent Interactive Multimedia Systems for e-Healthcare Applications*, https://doi.org/10.1007/978-981-16-6542-4_14

Wellbeing and, therefore, additionally of Emergency clinic 4.0 is the utilization of the Internet of Things (IoT) to medication. Notwithstanding the IoT, the utilization of prescient calculations and man-made brainpower, fit for preparing a lot of information, assume a major function in this specific circumstance [6]. The 4.0 Emergency clinics are consequently observing the introduction of another method of imagining the clinic, where the cycle of conveyance of medical care, clinical checking, lounge areas, and tasks plans change drastically to adjust and effectively serve patients and clinicians [7]. The fundamental difficulties found in medical are:

- Self-analysis frameworks for patients: patients through wearable gadgets can screen their wellbeing status and accordingly figuring out how to self analyze a decent number of infections and medical issues without going to the facility or emergency clinic.
- Tolerant checking: In the present clinics, the capacity to have persistent or irregular life boundary appraisals accessible is a key component. The extra necessity is to make the framework as space-sparing as could reasonably be expected and, from a 4.0 point of view, to ensure far-off access by specialists. The future possibility is to fabricate robotized medical clinics, in which a total imaging framework is set up when the emergency clinic is checked in.
- Computerized information chronicle: the point is to coordinate the gadgets with the advanced clinical records, to ensure a consistent and programmed update of the patient's indispensable conditions and of the consideration and treatments to which he is oppressed.
- Acknowledgements of Man-made brainpower (simulated intelligence): computer-based intelligence is starting to play an undeniably significant and pivotal function in judgments and treatments.
- Coordination and joint effort: a similar patient can regularly be dealt with and inspected by various experts, and consistent communication is consequently vital to empower the trading of valuable data. Consequently, sharing data is essential.

The qualities of a guideline of clinic modernization, put together increasingly more with respect to the steady joining of the IoT in everyday clinic errands, must be connected with a lot of dangers, primarily connected with the issue of wellbeing yet, in addition, an issue identified with the requirement for a generational change, so the innovation is something simple to utilize. The accompanying areas of the paper will give an initial fundamental presentation of Wellbeing 4.0 and progressively particular investigations are featured.

It is conceivable to discover in writing different commitments and uses of what it has been qualify with the name "Wellbeing 4.0". We chose articles utilizing ScienceDirect via looking "Wellbeing 4.0" and joined watchwords, for example, "Industry 4.0" in addition to "Medical care", "Internet of Things" in addition to "Medical services". The study gave a consequence of 46 examination articles recognized in this field. The majority of the papers dissected are as of late distributed [8]. 11 papers of the 46 explored were distributed in 2017, 17 of every 2018, meaning addition in distributions identified with such subject [9]. 6 examination articles referred to in this audit paper have been distributed in 2019. Breaking down the Branch of knowledge and Classification recognized by Scopus the Creators saw that the software engineering zone gives the top-level input of 41% in absolute exploration distributions. Notwithstanding, the general designing field contributes 35%, choice sciences and arithmetic contributing 14%, business, the board, and bookkeeping 6%; materials science 4%. We arranged the logical commitments found in the writing into eight classifications, contingent upon the kind of empowering innovation to which they allude: Digital Actual Frameworks, Internet of Things, Edge/Cloud computing, Addictive Assembling, Advanced mechanics, Artificial intelligence, Computer-generated Reality, Increased Reality. The review did make it conceivable to feature the forthcoming future improvements expected, the likely connected to innovative progression yet, in addition, the limits associated with the utilization of new empowering advances in this field.

2 Organization of the Work

Section 3 discusses literature work regarding Internet of Things based healthcare. Section 4 discusses about self-determination medicine for healthcare sector in detail. Further, the combination of Internet of Things and Big Data, i.e., Big data produced by IoT communications which can bring a major revolution in Biomedical Industry, is discussed in Sect. 5. Then, Sect. 6 discusses the importance of Data mining, i.e., as a New Hope in (for) Healthcare System. Further, Sect. 7 presents an introduction to CPS in healthcare industry. Section 8 presents several opportunities and challenges in e-Healthcare Systems in this smart era. In last, Sect. 9 concludes this work in this brief by including interesting remarks with reset to healthcare sectors for future readers (researcher and scientists).

3 Literature Review

The limited usage of Information Systems Time (IST) as a genuine weapon has been penetrated by various people for quite a while. The huge segments for the imperative use of IS by strategy for researching the multifaceted employment of IS inside the social protection setting are tried in the article discussed. Three proposals are created as:

- re-separating a decision of viable IS packages each inside and outdoors therapeutic administrations associations,
- re-creation use of the mixing thought from the composition,
- seeing locale experiences inside the human administrations venture. The article focuses on the significance and effect of industry 4.0. The aftereffect of the web associated applied sciences in the inception of significant worth conveyed for the

associations and society [10]. The article is reasonable. With the growth of web, the Internet of Things that is centre to the new modern unrest has been directed to "industry 4.0."

The article talks about hypothesis, and practices of industry 4.0. As of today, sensors are being touted as a significant capacity in essentially a wide range of uses. Explicit to medical services, wearable devices are seen as urgent in creating factual wellbeing data. This immense assortment of information is likewise named as Large Information. The part proposes an agreeable current net of components IoT structure to store and technique versatile sensor records (gigantic records) for wellbeing care packs. The data can be of respiratory nuances, coronary heartbeat, circulatory strain, plot temperature, and glucose. The tactile gadget can likewise alarm the surgeons of any change or danger [11]. Industry 4.0 which misuses digital actual frameworks and speaks to advanced change of assembling is profoundly influencing medical services just like other ordinary assembling quarters. The paper talks about the new methods of assembling in wellbeing to oblige the developing need of coordinated, flexi, and relative rates. "The proposed engineering comprises of three layers: thought, sending, and execution. The paper examines request-based medication bundling production [12]. The Internet of Things utilizes the web to impart over the world-over-contraptions. Here chart of medical care 1.0, 2.0, 3.0, and 4.0. The paper talks about the effect of haze, cloud, and IoT to limit the patient-visits to online visits. A three layered design is proposed for the patients. Edge figuring worldview is an impending innovation for cloud-based IOT applications. This can be an adjusting innovation for the IoT by lessening the load on IOT and improving the applications. The paper proposes BodyEdge, a novel structure using wearable contraptions for human-driven applications. With respect to the rising human administrations industry, a genuine usage has been tried in this unique circumstance. In BodyEdge was discovered to be a legitimate and economical answer for medical services software. In current years, there is an expansion in the utilization of Medical care 4.0-based diagnostics frameworks all through the world. In medical services 4.0, the patient's data is spared in Electronic Healthcare Record (EHR) storehouse which can be found both at a concentrated or distributed region [13]. It can help the medical care experts to section to the patient's medical services insights from anyplace and whenever. Security and protection are chief concerns while approaching it from any area.

The paper advocates a biometric-based verification plan to guarantee secure rights of passage to patient's EHR from any area [14]. Here assurance dangers and difficulties are discussed. A proposed biometric-based plan approved the Computerized Approval of Web Security Conventions and Applications device is discussed. The proposed component is assessed through a sweep the use of an example of 18 present heterogeneous logical data sources [15]. In light of the caught results, we had the option to get mindful of a measurement flexibly of obscure sort, perceiving that it was before a build weight scale. Thereafter, we were able to discover that the programming interface procedure that was once liable for social occasion data out of this information source was at one time the get Estimations() technique, while consolidating each the bodyweight scale's extraordinary and its inferred realities quality, we might need to confirm that this records source was viewed as subjective enough. By taking full advantage of shooting the pleasant of a data gracefully through estimating and relating each the measurements source's incredible itself and the phenomenal of its determined information, the proposed component gives effective outcomes, being in a situation to make certain start to finish both information sources and data quality."

The arising idea of industry 4.0 and its significance is demonstrating an effect on the economy. The article investigations the medical services gracefully chain. The creators gathered colossal information. The outcomes examined the effect of normal assets. The utilization of web was examined. An indirect economy progress determined framework was proposed. The assessment suggested that the possibility of industry 4.0 and corporate commitment can improve the social protection smoothly chains [16]. Western made success and care system is moving from a male driven clinical model to a co-coordinated and united strategy. The fourth mechanical insurgence for example industry 4.0 is changing get-together according to the motorized client change. The paper takes a gander at a continuously individual focused use of industry 4.0 capacities with respect to therapeutic organizations [17]. It presents 'Care 4.0', an early viewpoint that could change the way where individuals make modernized flourishing and care workplaces, focusing on trusted, solidified structures of affiliations, individuals, and advancements. This article presents the dataset of the human administrations structures markers of 120 nations all through 2010–2017, which is related to the investigation article "Cross-profitability evaluation inside seeing bendy measures with an application to social protection frameworks". The data is from World Bank. Dependent upon their circumstance in the overall execution of the therapeutic administrations structures, the results are arranged into input (I), output (O), and frequency measure (FM). The dataset can be used to process capability similarly as cross-viability assessment of the social protection systems using methodology, for instance, bits of knowledge envelopment examination inside seeing versatile measure.

The progression of savvy and estimations pushed advancements has pushed and made a way for recorded answer for human-driven for instance Social protection 4.0. The upward push of net of things, IoT structures, and wi-fi frameworks has capable the wellbeing care condition with a maker-new electronic change maintained by strategy for capacity of forefront work region examining and man-made thinking computations. In this, social protection related improvements have ascended as a riding power for giving persevering driven modified human administrations commitments. Counsel structures are electronic structures that infer the decisions on the possibility of a couple of real enter boundaries and basic wellbeing records amassed through the current wearable gadget innovation, implantable innovation, and various sensors. Thusly, to catch the bleeding edge airs in the human administrations' atmosphere, this paper bears an all-out audit on restorative administrations proposition advancements and the connected ideal models. This examination begins from the essential human administrations' advancement and circles nearer to the Medical services four of each an organized way. The guide from Medical care 1.0 to Medical care 4 is analyzed to focus on incredibly extraordinary age verticals helping the serious change. A significant assessment of wellbeing care recommender systems and its sorts is in like way given. Definitely, the open issues and incites related to the adaption and execution of human-driven Medical care 4 conditions are referred to. That is furnished to find the possible inquiry questions and openings all together that the contrasting plans may besides be preferable inside the closed over future.

4 Self-determination Medicine for Healthcare

Note that an efficient healthcare model could be delivered by 5G Wireless Technology. But, what does 5G mean for medical services is an inquiry worth contemplating. In spite of the fact that the 5G for a great many people implies quicker web, the effects of 5G on medical care will be increased. Clearly, 5G can't be just equal to a very quicker web, yet basically dependable web network in gigantic articles and clinical gadgets, data transfer capacity, and super inclusion and accessibility than what we see or envision in the present 4G LTE. Virtual Reality (VR) and Augmented Reality (AR) are bound to turn into the most straightforwardly profited zones and add to insight medication once 5G innovation develops. The 5G will enormously advance the incorporation of virtual and reality, which is basic for exhaustive restoration preparing, just as compact limit recovery and telemedicine because of its specialized attributes (refer Fig. 1).

Firmly identified with the VR and AR's application in medical care is limit recovery work out, including automated help for the fine engine aptitudes of the appendages, gravity pay, separately customized video preparing program. The use of VR in medical care is definitely not another innovation arising in the 5G period, all things considered, the therapeutically material innovation can be followed back in any event 20 years prior, however, it has not been completely evolved until development of 5G. A significant imperative is idleness, which was characterized as the

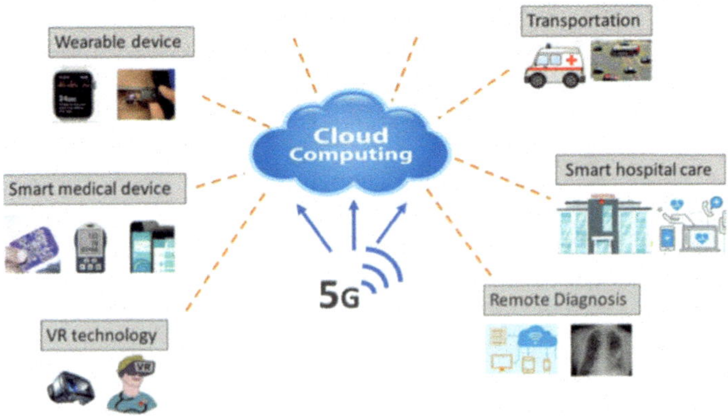

Fig. 1 Applications of 5G

reaction time between sending an information solicitation to a terminal gadget and getting the information. Contrasted and 4G LTE remote correspondence innovation, in fact, 5G can offer a 10-overlap decline in inertness, in particular from the current 20 ms (ms or msec) at 4G LTE leap to as meager as one millisecond. This advantage is critical for virtual reality (VR) innovation and telemedicine. In the 5G time, with its intrinsic high data transfer capacity and low inertness advantage, VR is required to help smooth out the whole emergency clinic, particularly in telemedicine, teleconsultation, and even far off a medical procedure [18]. The imperative signs can be spilled to clinical gear or screen screens in the clinic with right around zero inertness (<1 ms radio idleness with, 10–9 mistake rate without a doubt) during natural careful preparing or even in distant medical procedures. Clearly, the current LTE band range distributions for 4G can't adapt. The more significant point is, 5G is sufficiently amazing to help a great many clinical gadgets all the while, from sensors to mobiles, clinical gear, camcorders, and enhanced by 4 k or even 8 K super top-notch TV, or screen framework, certainly can offer web-based video with more honed, clearer and more detail content settled data past the retina.

Another advantage to be noted would be telemedicine. The 5G will extend the extent of telemedicine, and comparably, this change will happen soon. Individuals will in general connection huge information and artificial intelligence with customized medication, otherwise called individualized medication or accuracy medication. Notwithstanding, what should be unmistakably called attention to is that, without 5G's specialized help, exactness medication will be a riddle that can't be illuminated [19]. The essential restricting element has for some time been credited to transfer speed and information transmission speed. In the period of 4G, even 4G LTE-Progressed, inside a restricted transmission capacity, despite a very organization can just proposal around 50 Mbps and hypothetical constraints of 300 Mbps download speeds in reality, also the need to settle rapid real time video and picture information and effective super-low inactivity mediations. It is remarkable that here the information move speed isn't the main issue that hindered the usage of telemedicine in the 4G LTE. The central issue is data transmission and lower dormancy. This implies that gigantic clinical gadgets can interface with the focal cloud computing stage, worker or between gadget availability at the time without network blockage. These backings genuinely intensify computer-generated simulation, no defer reaction, and expanded reality applications, which can make an intuitive involvement with telemedicine. This sort of telemedicine, along with 4 k/8 k screen, and 360 degrees VR will offer a "live" experience not just for doctors accommodates quick determination and chooses therapy system, however more viable activity and ground-breaking preparing instruments for clinical staff. Past empowering fast information transmission, 5G has a progressive change in the conveyance of low inactivity transfer video, 3D high-goal clinical imaging, and strategic intercessions.

5 Internet of Things and Big Data: A Revolution in Biomedical Industry

Commonly we missed a regular check-up since we had a customer meeting or social obligations. It is fundamental to Conclusion the indications at a beginning phase so that specialists can endorse crucial medication to fix the medical problems [20]. Why not consider taking the assistance of rising innovations, for example, IoT and Big Data to remain refreshed about your present ailment? Public mists push and pull data in a shared strategy to our brilliant gadgets in routine use. Internet of Things (IoTs) associates somewhat to related industry data that is useful for clients show up at custom fitted and better choices.

- Advances like big data and machine: It helps specialist organizations to analyze and endorse suitable medication ahead of time. Complete course and customized diagnostics of medication is the current extent of AI.
- Data investigation: It gives numerous possibilities that help solid conduct. Well-being examination help medical care suppliers' interface and help patients outside the facility. Insightful apparatuses are useful for patient's conduct direction, it tracks as well as gives explicit guidelines to create and keep up wellbeing practices.

Significant advances have been made in the area of relieving and overseeing infections, broadening future, and improving general personal satisfaction. On the off chance that considers everything is acceptable, we are halfway right; indeed, new difficulties are generally advertised. Since the normal life desires for people are expanding; long haul medical issues require consistent checking and progressing therapy. These prerequisites put additional focus on effectively expanded medical care frameworks and ever-expanding rates. The expect of great importance is a response for changing and diminishing paces of medical services observing and conveyance with upgrading total quality and making it accessible and appropriate to patients. Industry specialists like Gartner foresee that in excess of 25 billion gadgets will be associated through IoT before the finish of 2020. What number of will screen or clinical gadgets? Numerous wearable gadgets, for example, track weight, pulses, quality and measure of rest, strength level of exercises; people focus on these subtleties and deal with their wellbeing vivaciously utilizing wearable gadgets [21].

Individuals going through medical problems; use modern observing gadgets to track and report level hydration, glucose, blood oxygenation, lung limit, state of mind swings, Weight, and furthermore fine bloodstream. The ability to allot, manage and control measurements of medication is currently offered as shrewd pill bottles. At last, specialists are utilizing their portable, brilliant gadgets to convey medical services and furthermore state "visit" outline that is changed to message and put away in patient computerized clinical records as a part of their clinical history [22]. Admittance to medical services improvements permits more individual to fittingly follow everyday exercises. Besides, we can control our medical problems from our home as opposed to visiting a clinic. Presently we can upgrade your personal satisfaction utilizing IoT gadgets (devices) and other shrewd advancements. Persons, as well as medical care suppliers, can expertly offer medical care administrations with these gadgets. They can follow patient's wellbeing, oversee medication and medicines from a far-off area, consequently upgrading the medical services level conveyed to numerous patients simultaneously. We can direct doctors and rundowns of release, along these lines keeping up state-of-the-art electronic wellbeing records. With the assistance of an oversaw specialist co-op to electronic change your medical services arrangements. Big Data can possibly change the Clinical Business; big data instruments assemble billions of data focuses that can be used for wellbeing the board in three fundamental zones:

- Expressive examination: It ascertains what has occurred, for example, cost, recurrence, and assets.
- Prescient investigation: It utilizes illustrative data to predicate anticipated outcomes later on.
- Prescriptive examination: It offers the capacity to settle on sure choices considering envisioning forecasts.

Uses of Big data.

- Perceive expected confined events of infection and diseases.
- Progress analytic rightness.
- Create customized treatment plans.
- Abatement contamination rates.
- Offer prevalent dynamic help.

5.1 Internet of Things and Big Data Technology for Personalized Medicine

Internet of Things (IoT) extends the freedom of people to interface, contribute and work together on things. IoT step by step created heterogeneous advances with complex conventions and calculations. It plays significant in worldwide correspondence among a great many gadgets with wired/remote sensors, electronic apparatuses like TV, Cooler, and so forth, associated with the internet. At that point it assumes an astounding function in numerous fields, for example, Horticulture, medical care, excitements, cars, sports, home, modern machines, business, and so forth. The purposes behind the fast improvement of the IoT are high exactness, minimal effort, and diminish time by anticipating the future in a superior manner. The IoT device like sensors and actuators were inserted into actual gadgets, for example, home apparatuses, vehicles, and savvy modern machines to screen and trade data utilizing remote organizations with the assistance of Bluetooth, Zigbee, IEEE 802.11 (WI-FI), WiMAX, and so forth. The sensors are implantable in the body or wearable that detects physiological states like pulse, pulse, internal heat level, pressure rate, electrocardiogram (ECG), electroencephalogram (EEG). Observing weak individuals are more agreeable for individuals who had older folks, kids alone in the home

[23]. The sensor associated with the clients, oftentimes screen the client day in and day out and gives cautions on client's changing medical issue to the family, specialists, and crisis administrations. The developing necessities of better advancements for tending to constant issues in handling bigger data without trading off security and protection require critical consideration from the worldwide examination network.

Big Data investigation arose as the great answer for the cycle of bountiful data and improves dynamic described by 6 V's: volume, assortment, speed, veracity, legitimacy, and unpredictability. The primary trademark is volume that alludes to an amount of data being utilized and investigated to get the ideal outcome. It raises a surge of data from different sources incorporates sensors, scanners, cell phones, digitizers, video, email, informal organizations, and the internet [24]. Assortment alludes to the kind of data put away, dissected, and handled. The kind of data might be content, pictures, recordings, sound, geometrics, and the blend of each sort. Veracity alludes to the exactness of data is sufficient for Big Data. Big Data likewise presents a test to store, cycle, and help the data successfully. To conquer the issues of Big Data, cloud computing arises as a key help to store and handle the assets data, gotten to from any area through the internet. Getting to assets put away in the cloud ordered into the public cloud, private cloud, and cross breed cloud. The assets of the public cloud can be gotten to, shared, and prepared by outsiders. A private cloud permits the assets got to by the association. A cross breed cloud consolidates both public and private mists, frequently used to enhance inner data with public organizations. Software as a Service (SaaS), Infrastructure as a Service (IaaS), Platform as a Service (PaaS) is the cloud administrations or assets accessible to clients on interest by means of the internet. As the data expand step by step, the huge measure of data must be gathered, examined, oversaw, and put away, in the cloud which builds the intricacy of cloud-based administrations. To address this issue, we present haze registering at the edge of the cloud for pre-preparing of produced data [25]. Haze improves productivity by diminishing the data moved to the cloud change from actual gadgets. Mist empowers a protected data exchange inside large number of gadgets associated, guarantees high versatility and even dissemination of data. Big Data examination is a voluminous data mining approach that requires both cloud globalization and mist confinement.

Among numerous self-GPS beacons, a cell phone is an easy to understand gadget that gives continuous distant medical care framework associated with clients and clinical staff. Universally, advancement and the use of cell phones have upgraded the exhibition of medical care applications by offering productive types of assistance to clients. It screens both dynamic data and everyday social exercises from inserted portable sensors. It has a pocket-sized presentation with remote organization correspondence and battery capacity to handle the equipment programming framework [26]. Cell phone wellbeing checking application includes a far-off medical care framework improved with the progression of versatile, correspondence organizations, detecting, and inserted gadgets. The portable based application advancement has cleared the conceivable path for straightforwardly getting to and examining the patient's data from the sensors associated with clients. Versatile medical care applications furnish quicker conveyance of data with decreased cost, limitless Internet-based administrations, and have proficient battery reinforcement. The principal goals of this review are diverse:

- Inspect the function of cloud computing portrays the medical services framework with general design.
- Outlining an elevated level correlation among cloud and mist registering and furnishing secure protection of patients with haze processing.
- Enlargement of the IoT medical care application with IoT-based medical care observing design.
- An attention on medical services checking framework in Big Data period.
- Intuitive medical services applications are checked on with a cell phone.
- Giving the upsides and downsides of the medical services framework took for the review.
- Investigating current difficulties in the customized medical services framework.
- Conversation on a promising answer for the continuous medical care checking issues.

5.2 *Internet of Things and Big Data Technology for Next Generation Based Healthcare*

The IoT is continually adding new, helpful, data-producing gadgets to the medical services industry's collection. Wearable gadgets are now being used for diabetes patients to follow glucose levels and even to convey insulin, movement trackers for disease patients are being utilized related to cell phones to follow patients' recuperations, and even fundamental sign screens in medical services offices are being overhauled to total, store, and examine data to hail notice signs in a speedier, more effective way [27]. "IoT is ready to impact medical caretakers' expert lives," says nursing instructor Dr. Susan Athlete in her paper, "Medical attendants Will Profit by The Internet of Things" on AdvanceWeb.com. IoT will turbocharge development in distant patient checking, telemedicine, and conduct change. It will assist with controlling avoidable costs, surface new business openings, and upgrade the administration of ongoing conditions. In 2017, the Medical care IoT is decidedly influencing three territories specifically, as indicated by the Connection Labs.com IT industry blog entry, "How IoT Clinical Gadgets Are Changing Medical care Today." These zones are:

- Eldercare—Following meandering patients, observing exercises in nursing homes, and following medication regimens.
- Understanding data gathering—Fundamental signs, EKG details, and most clinical parts intended to gather tolerant data.
- Continuous area—RFID, Bluetooth, and Wi-Fi track the two individuals and gear easily.

As more data is moved onto distant workers and simulated intelligence consistently improves, the medical services industry is starting to comprehend that clinical data will before long be moved into Big Data space. HIPAA and security concerns are easing back the cycle, yet network safety development is advancing close by Big Data and will be completely equipped for ensuring delicate clinical data. Pioneers in the nursing business, for example, Elsevier Clinical Arrangements nursing master Michelle Troseth, are preparing for proceeded with transformation of the clinical business to Big Data. “At the point when we have data, it is conceivable to benchmark and improves quality, wellbeing, and cost-adequacy of medical services,” Troseth says in a meeting with medical services tech essayist Eden Estopace in “Innovation Advancing the Function Of Attendants And The Fate Of Patient Consideration” on EnterpriseInnovation.net [28]. “Without data, it resembles tossing a dart in obscurity—we would not know precisely where things stand. By making dashboards, digitizing data, making normalized big data, and connecting it with normalized phrasing, we can take a gander at patterns in nursing and settle on choices on a nursing practice that we’ve never had the option to make.”

Later on, Big Data advancement and upgrades in data investigation will keep on profiting the medical care industry in significantly more regions. TheInnovationEnterprise.com records a few forecasts in its “Future Data Patterns in Pharma and Medical care” blog entry. Data will before long have the option to assist with clinical preliminaries by finding appropriate guineas pigs quicker and all the more productively, as indicated by the post. The Open Data development will help simulated intelligence calculations recognize warnings and likely inconsistencies in pictures by looking into a huge number of high-goal pictures. What’s more, prescient demonstrating will give medical services leaders strong, data put together proof with respect to which to base basic choices.

5.3 *Role of Artificial Intelligence in HealthCare*

At the point when a significant number of us hear the expression “artificial intelligence” (simulated intelligence), we envision robots taking care of our responsibilities, delivering individuals out of date. What’s more, since artificial intelligence driven PCs are customized to settle on choices with minimal human intercession, some keep thinking about whether machines will before long settle on the troublesome choices we currently endow to our PCPs. As indicated by David B. Agus, MD, a teacher of medication and designing at the College of Southern California Keck Institute of Medication and Viterbi School of Designing, it’s imperative to isolate certainty from sci-fi, on the grounds that artificial intelligence is now here—and its essentially evolving medication. As opposed to advanced mechanics, artificial intelligence in medical services fundamentally alludes to specialists and clinics getting to tremendous data sets of conceivably life-sparing data. This incorporates treatment techniques and their results, endurance rates, and speed of care accumulated across a great many patients, topographical areas, and endless and some of the time interconnected medical issues. New registering forces can distinguish and dissect huge and little patterns from the data and even make expectations through AI that is intended to recognize potential wellbeing results. AI utilizes measurable methods to enable PC frameworks to "learn" with approaching data and to distinguish examples and settle on choices with insignificant human heading. Outfitted with such focused-on investigation, specialists might be better ready to evaluate hazards, make right judgments, and offer patients more successful medicines, says Agus, the writer of The Fortunate Years: How to Flourish in the Exciting modern lifestyle of Wellbeing and The Finish of Sickness [29]. He trusts computer-based intelligence's capability to improve medical care is "faltering." We have heaps of data that we've been gathering over many years," he says. "Unexpectedly, figuring power permits us to utilize the data in a manner to profit patients."

5.3.1 Virtual Nurses for Monitoring the Patients

Nursing has developed in the course of recent many years. The ordinarily seen perspective on the medical caretaker at the bedside, observing a patient's crucial signs or helping doctors during adjusts, has changed. With the coming of new advanced innovations in medical care, for example, telehealth and far-off observing apparatuses, the present attendant can be for all intents and purposes virtual. Without a doubt, there is a precarious expectation to absorb information in this new virtual war room. Yet, medical caretakers have generally been the most punctual adopters of new advancements, and admittance to these instruments has improved patient consideration, but on the other hand, is changing the battleground for attendants. Here are a few different ways the "virtual" climate is changing nursing:

- Growing attendants' specialization–Telehealth medical caretakers should be technically knowledgeable, with most of their job being behind a PC screen and intensely dependent on advanced investigation. Yet, the new virtual medical attendant likewise has further information and comprehension of an assortment of clinical strengths from nervous system science, cardiology, oncology, and so on telehealth attendants are viewed as an asset for clinicians, which implies they can get all sorts of clinical inquiries that require speedy exploration and answers. It's not astounding that all telehealth attendants start within any event five years of involvement with concentrated consideration. In any case, a virtual medical caretaker's learning proceeds for a more drawn-out time.
- Filling in as a basic asset for all clinicians—An attendant might be liable for a few patients, yet when taking a shot at a solitary patient, he/she should be—and must be—centered uniquely around that tolerance. With a telehealth program, medical caretakers can feel sure that on the off chance that they're wheeling one patient down for a test and another patient requires help, a distant attendant can take care of them quickly or bring in another attendant on the floor to help give

care. Bedside nurture presently additionally approaches a doctor at the press of a catch.
- Expanding length of vocation—Nursing is an actually requesting position. Envision moving a 200-pound understanding, on a 350-pound bed, with several hundred pounds of extra observing gear required for transport. Over the long run, these actual requests become more troublesome. Telehealth gives nurture the occasion to expand their profession. It positively had its own requests—for instance, medical attendants are acquainted with zeroing in on a couple of patients, instead of overseeing bigger populaces of patients. Be that as it may, nurture currently have the choice for broadening their abilities into the later long stretches of life.

The idea of virtual medical caretakers is still new and will require the two patients and staff to change. As an ever-increasing number of patients become mindful of the advantages of telehealth, clinics around the nation are beginning to receive these projects, requiring more talented medical caretakers to oversee them. Telehealth is developing and will be a market driver for wellbeing frameworks.

5.3.2 Development of the Precision Medicine

Medical care is going through a change, and it is basic to use new advancements to produce new information and backing the appearance of Precision Medication (PM). Ongoing logical discoveries and mechanical progressions have improved our comprehension of sickness pathogenesis and changed the manner in which we analyze and treat infection prompting more exact, unsurprising, and groundbreaking medical care that is redone for the individual patient. Hereditary, genomics, and epigenetic changes seem, by all accounts, to be adding to various illnesses. Profound clinical phenotyping joined with cutting edge sub-atomic phenotypic profiling, empowers the development of causal organization models in which a genomic area is proposed to impact the degrees of records, proteins, and metabolites [30]. Phenotypic investigation bears incredible significance to elucidate the pathophysiology of organizations at the sub-atomic and cell level. Advanced biomarkers (BMs) can have a few applications past clinical preliminaries in diagnostics to distinguish patients influenced by sickness or to manage therapy. Advanced BMs present a major occasion to gauge clinical endpoints in a distant, objective, and fair-minded way. Nonetheless, the utilization of "omics" advancements and enormous example sizes have produced monstrous measures of informational indexes, and their examinations have become a significant bottleneck requiring complex computational and factual strategies. With the abundance of data for various sicknesses and its connect to inborn science, the test is presently to turn the multi-parametric ordered characterization of an illness into a better clinical dynamic by more correctly characterizing an infection. Subsequently, the huge information transformation has given an occasion to apply artificial intelligence (artificial intelligence) and AI calculations to this huge informational index. The headways in computerized wellbeing openings have likewise emerged various inquiries and worries on the eventual fate of medical services rehearse specifically with what respects the unwavering quality of simulated intelligence symptomatic instruments, the effect on clinical practice, and weakness of calculations. Artificial intelligence, AI calculations, computational science, and advanced BMs will offer an occasion to make an interpretation of new information into significant data in this way, permitting prior conclusion and exact treatment choices. A superior arrangement and cohesiveness of the various segments of the information network is an absolute necessity to completely misuse its capability.

5.3.3 Digital Consultation Chatbots

Chatbots are PC programs that impersonate discussion with individuals utilizing Normal Language Preparing (NLP) and Artificial Intelligence (AI). They can collaborate with individuals on the internet by starting a discussion. They go about as computerized associates that address inquiries with respect to explicit items or administrations. Chatbots don't should be downloaded, and along these lines needn't bother with extra room on client gadgets. They can be immediately utilized, are anything but difficult to fabricate, and, in particular, are locked in. A portion of the average use cases is addressing Frequently Asked Questions (FAQs) of clients getting to sites, produce client leads, give data on attendant services, offer help administrations (HR, IT, Money, and so forth), and furthermore give legitimate counsel to the client. Since chatbots can work 24 $\times$ 7, they offer types of assistance with no disturbance and can be gotten to whenever anyplace. Here, few Potential Benefits are:

- Whenever and anyplace access on any gadget
- Proper and moment input by gathering client data
- Decrease in ticket volume and quicker question goal
- Improved client and worker experience
- Improvement inexactness and dependability with trend setting innovations.

6 Data Mining: A New Hope in Healthcare System

Data mining holds extraordinary potential for the medical care industry to empower wellbeing frameworks to efficiently utilize data and investigation to distinguish failures and best practices that improve mind and lessen costs. A few specialists accept the occasions to improve mind and diminish costs simultaneously could apply to as much as 30% of generally speaking medical care spending. This could be mutually advantageous in general. However, because of the multifaceted nature of medical care and a slower pace of innovation appropriation, our industry lingers behind these others in executing successful data mining and logical techniques. Like investigation and business intelligence, the term data mining can mean various things to various individuals. The most fundamental meaning of data mining is the investigation of huge data sets to find examples and utilize those examples to figure or foresee the probability of future occasions.

6.1 Intelligent Heart Disease Prediction System

Any emergency clinic data frameworks are intended to help quiet charging, stock administration, and age of basic measurements. A few emergency clinics use choice emotionally supportive networks, yet they are to a great extent restricted. They can answer straightforward questions like “What is the normal time of patients who have coronary illness?”, “The number of medical procedures had brought about medical clinic remains longer than 10 days?”, “Recognize the female patients who are single, over 30 years of age, and who have been treated for malignant growth.“ Notwithstanding, they can’t answer complex inquiries like “Distinguish the significant preoperative indicators that expansion the length of medical clinic remain”, “Given patient records on disease, should therapy incorporate chemotherapy alone, radiation alone, or both chemotherapy and radiation?”, and “Given patient records, foresee the likelihood of patients getting a coronary illness.“ Clinical choices are regularly made dependent on specialists’ instinct and experience instead of on the information rich data covered up in the database. This training prompts undesirable predispositions, blunders, and unreasonable clinical costs which influence the nature of administration gave to patients. Wu, et al. recommended that joining of clinical choice help with PC based patient records could lessen clinical blunders, upgrade tolerant security, decline undesirable practice variety, and improve quiet results. This proposal is promising as data demonstrating and investigation instruments, for example, data mining, can possibly create an information rich climate that can help to fundamentally improve the nature of clinical choices.

The medical care industry gathers immense measures of medical care data which, shockingly, are not “mined” to find shrouded data for compelling dynamics. Revelation of concealed examples and connections frequently goes unexploited. Progressed data mining strategies can help cure this circumstance. This exploration has built up a model Keen Coronary illness Expectation Framework (IHDPS) utilizing data mining strategies, in particular, Choice Trees, Guileless Bayes, and Neural Organization. Results show that every method has its one-of-a-kind strength in understanding the targets of the characterized mining objectives. IHDPS can answer complex “consider the possibility that” inquiries which conventional choice emotionally supportive networks can’t. Utilizing clinical profiles, for example, age, sex, circulatory strain, and glucose it can foresee the probability of patients getting a coronary illness. It empowers critical information, for example, designs, connections between clinical components identified with coronary illness, to be set up. IHDPS is Electronic, easy to understand, adaptable, solid, and expandable. This framework is useful for people of this smart era/ intelligent stage.

6.2 Diagnosis and Prognosis of Cancer Disease

Data mining strategies can be utilized to anticipate malignant growth in a patient utilizing different side effects data from past outcomes. Important information can be found through these data mining procedures. In this paper, we are utilizing Affiliation Rule Mining (ARM) and Arrangement for finding and guess of malignant growth. Under ARM we are utilizing FP development calculation which is applied on after properties of patient data to foresee being nor malignant. There are 699 records in this database. Each record in the database has nine credits. The nine credits point by point in Table 1 is evaluated on a stretch scale from a typical condition of 1–10, with 10 being the most irregular state. Under arrangement, we are utilizing choice tree for anticipation of disease. Following is a guide to comprehend the choice tree approach. The choice tree appeared in Fig. 1 is worked from the little preparing set. In this table, each column compares to a patient record. We will allude to a line as a data occurrence. The data set contains three indicator credits, to be specific Age, Sexual orientation, Power of side effects, and one objective trait, specifically sickness whose qualities (to be anticipated from manifestations) shows if the comparing tolerant have a specific illness.

Choice tree can be utilized to order an obscure class data occasion with the assistance of the above data set given in Tables 1 and 2. The thought is to push the example down the tree, following the branches whose ascribes values coordinate the instances attribute values until the instance reaches a leaf hub, whose class name is then allotted to the occasion. For instance, the data occasion to be characterized is portrayed by the tuple (Age = 23, Gender = female, Power of manifestations = medium, Objective = ?), where "?" signifies the obscure estimation of the objective example. In this model, Sexual orientation trait is immaterial to a specific grouping task. The tree tests the power of manifestation esteem in the case. In the event that the appropriate response is medium; the occasion is pushed down through the comparing branch and arrives at the age hub. At that point, the tree tests the Age an incentive in the occasion. In

Table 1 Data set for consideration

(1) Age	Data set		
	Gender	Intensity of symptoms	Disease (goal)
25	Male	Medium	Yes
32	Male	High	Yes
24	Female	Medium	Yes
44	Female	High	Yes
30	Female	Low	No
21	Male	Low	No
18	Female	Low	No
34	Male	Medium	No
55	Male	Medium	No

Table 2 Data set for implementation

Attribute	Domain
Sample code number	Id
Clump Thickness	1–10
Uniformity of cell size	1–10
Uniformity of cell shape	1–10
Marginal adhesion	1–10
Single epithelial cell size	1–10
Bare nuclei	1–10
Bland chromatin	1–10
Normal nucleoli	1–10
Mitosis	1–10
Class	(2 for begin, 4 for maligant)

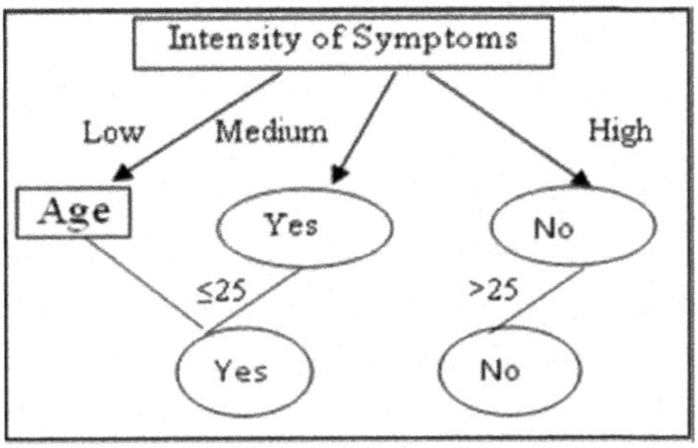

Fig. 2 Decision tree built from Table 1

the event that the appropriate response is 23, the occurrence is again pushed down through the comparing branch. Presently the example arrives at the leaf hub, where it is named yes (Fig. 2).

6.3 *Customer Relationship Management (CRM) Systems*

Client Relationship Management (CRM) is a system for dealing with all your organization's connections and co-operations with your clients and expected clients. It encourages us to improve our productivity. All the more generally, when individuals talk about CRM they are typically alluding to a CRM framework, an apparatus that assists with contact management, deals management, work process cycles, efficiency, and then some. Client Relationship Management empowers us to zero in on your association's associations with distinct individuals—regardless of whether those are clients, administration clients, partners, or providers. CRM is not only for deals. Probably the greatest additions in profitability can emerge out of moving past CRM as a deal and advertising apparatus and installing it in your business—from HR to client administrations and flexibly chain management. In the event that your business is going to last, we realize that we need a procedure for what's to come. You'll as of now have targets identifying with deals, business destinations, and productivity. Yet, getting modern, solid data on your advancement towards your objectives can be precarious. How would we interpret the numerous floods of data rolling in from deals groups, client assistance staff, advertisers, and web-based media checking into helpful business data? Utilizing a CRM framework can give us an away from your clients. We can see everything in one spot, i.e., a straightforward, customizable dashboard that can disclose to us a client's past history with you, the status of their requests, any exceptional client assistance issues, and that's only the tip of the iceberg.

We can even decide to incorporate data from their public web-based media action—their preferences, what they are stating and sharing about you. Advertisers can utilize CRM to all the more likely comprehend the pipeline of deals or forthcoming work coming in, making anticipating less difficult and more precise. You'll have away from each chance or lead, demonstrating us the make way from inquiries to deals. Furthermore, its generally been utilized as deals and showcasing apparatus, client care groups are seeing incredible advantages from CRM frameworks. The present client may bring an issue up in one station—state, Twitter—and afterward change to email or phone to determine it in private. A CRM stage empowers us to deal with the inquiry across channels without losing track.

6.4 Avoidance and Early Detection of Various Frauds in Healthcare Industry

Improper installments by protection associations or outsider payers happen in light of mistakes, misuse, and misrepresentation. The size of this issue is sufficiently enormous to focus on its issue for wellbeing frameworks. Conventional strategies for identifying medical services extortion and misuse are tedious and wasteful. Consolidating computerized strategies and factual information lead to the rise of another interdisciplinary part of science that is named Knowledge Discovery in Databases (KDD). Data mining is a center of the KDD cycle. Data mining can help outsider payers, for example, medical coverage associations to remove valuable data from a huge number of cases and distinguish a more modest subset of the cases or petitioners for additional evaluation. We explored considers that performed data mining strategies for identifying medical care extortion and misuse, utilizing directed and solo data mining draws near. Most accessible examinations have zeroed in on algorithmic data mining without an accentuation on or application to extortion recognition endeavors with regards to wellbeing administration arrangement or medical coverage strategy. More investigations are expected to associate sound and proof-based analysis and treatment approach toward false or injurious practices. At last, in light of accessible investigations, we prescribe seven general strides to data mining of medical care claims.

In conventional techniques for medical services extortion and misuse location, a couple of inspectors handle a large number of paper medical care claims. In all actuality, they possess little energy for each guarantee, zeroing in on specific qualities of a case without focusing on the exhaustive image of a supplier's conduct. This technique is tedious and wasteful. It is as yet the predominant picture in some low-pay and center pay nations. Electronic healthcare records and developing utilization of automated frameworks have prompted recently arising open doors for better discovery of extortion and misuse. Developments in AI and artificial intelligence focus on mechanized techniques for extortion identification. Joining computerized strategies and factual information prompted a recently arising interdisciplinary part of science that is named Information Revelation in Databases (KDD). Data mining is the center of the KDD cycle. Data mining can help outsider payers, for example, medical coverage associations to remove valuable information from a huge number of cases and recognize a more modest subset of the cases or inquirers for additional appraisal and investigation for extortion and misuse. Hence, the data mining approach is important for a more proficient and viable IT-based examining framework.

7 Introduction of Cyber Physical System in Healthcare Industry

Cyber Physical System (CPS) associates the virtual world with actual world. It can add more intelligence to public activity. It integrates actual gadgets, for example, sensors and cameras, with digital parts to shape a scientific framework that responds astutely to dynamic changes in genuine world scenarios. CPS can have wide running applications, such as keen clinical innovation, helped living, environmental control, and track management [31]. A significant piece of CPS is the coordination of Wireless Sensor Network (WSN) and Cloud computing. A couple of works have been done on the CPS for medical services applications CPS architectures proposed by Rajkumar et al. and Xia et al. researched different applications, for example, helped living and observing organization. Creators underscore that the CPS architectures must catch an assortment of actual information, reliable data investigation, occasion recognition, and security. General characteristics of CPSs, and its types for different applications are discussed in [32]. CPS is a promising answer for the coordination of physical and cyber-world because of a few benefits, for example, the following.

- Organization Incorporation: CPS has interoperability with WSNs and Cloud computing. This may give the compliance organizing principles. CPS involves multiple computational stages collaborating over communication organizations. CPS gives network mix qualities, for example, media access control strategies and their consequences for framework elements, middleware, and programming that give coordination over organizations, command over planning of organization exchanges, and adaption capabilities.

- Association among Human and Framework: Displaying and estimating situational mindfulness human perception of the framework and its ecological changes in boundaries are basic for dynamic. This is an outright need for unpredictable and dynamic frameworks. Some CPSs incorporate humans as a necessary piece of the framework which makes the association simpler on the grounds that normally people are hard to display utilizing independent frameworks.
- Managing Sureness: Conviction is the way toward giving verification that a plan is legitimate and dependable. Proof can remember formal verifications or comprehensive tests for re-enactments and models. CPS is intended to have the option to develop and work with new and temperamental climates. CPS can exhibit obscure framework conduct to concentrate further and develop into better framework.
- Better Framework Execution: With the nearby communication of sensors and digital framework, CPS can give better framework execution regarding input and programmed overhaul. Better computational assets and digital subsystems in CPS guarantee the presence of numerous detecting substances, different communication instruments, significant level programming language, and end-client upkeep which further guarantees the better framework execution by CPS.
- Versatility: CPS can scale the framework as per request using the properties of Cloud computing. Clients can get important frameworks without contributing extra assets. CPS is inherently heterogeneous as it joins actual elements with computational cycles. The actual area may consolidate mechanical movement control, compound cycles, organic cycles, and human involvement. The digital area may join networking framework, programming instruments, and programming demonstrating. CPS can give plan procedures and apparatuses that help those philosophies, which scale to enormous plans and advance comprehension of complex frameworks.
- Self-rule: CPS can give self-rule due to having sensor-cloud combination. Regularly, CPS is a shut circle framework, where sensors make estimations of actual elements. These estimations are supportive of cessed in the digital subsystems, which at that point drive actuators and applications that influence the actual favorable to cesses. The control methodologies in the digital subsystems are versatile and typically prescient.
- Adaptability: Present frameworks dependent on CPS supportive of vide significantly more adaptability contrasted with the prior examination endeavors in WSN and Cloud computing alone.
- Improvement. Present biomedical sensors and cloud frameworks offer huge advancements for assortment of utilizations. This ability opens the pathway for CPS to upgrade the framework in wide degree.
- Quicker Reaction Time: CPS can give quicker reaction time because of quicker handling and correspondence ability of sensors and cloud framework. Quick reaction time can encourage the early identification of far-off disappointment, appropriate usage of shared assets, for example, transmission capacity.

8 Opportunities and Challenges in e-Healthcare System in this Smart Era

The greatest test confronting healthcare is the need to improve an incentive for patients. Healthcare frameworks today are battling with increasing expenses and shifting quality. Most findings and treatment conventions are intended for normal patients. Conveyance of care is divided and is just centered on volume. Healthcare is yet to use the maximum capacity of information, and the patient experience venture stays in its outset. At Healthcare Business Worldwide (HBI) 2018 [33], top heads from Siemens Healthineers shared their contemplations about the eventual fate of healthcare and how healthcare could address these difficulties by empowering healthcare suppliers to expand esteem. Conversations were around the subjects of growing accuracy medication, changing consideration conveyance, improving patient experience, and digitalizing healthcare, driven by specialists from Siemens Healthineers.

- Changing consideration conveyance: As we take a shot at improving worth, we need to verify that the consideration conveyance model guarantees positive patient results without an expansion in expenses. This will require combination. The new consideration conveyance model should improve clinical tasks and computerize normalized work processes. Failures present inside our healthcare conveyance framework frequently influence quiet consideration. Not exclusively do these shortcomings increment costs, yet they likewise contrarily sway quiet results. Healthcare enactment is another factor that influences the effectiveness of healthcare conveyance. The fate of healthcare can be significantly better if our healthcare framework zeroed in additional on upgrading work processes, utilizing clinical choice help programming to smooth out activities, and making the correct foundation to guarantee viable conveyance of care.
- Improving patient experience: The new healthcare model will see patients as customers. Furthermore, as most shoppers, patients will likewise request an incentive from healthcare specialist co-ops. They will have desires, and they will need the option to pick and the option to settle on their own choices. The fate of healthcare will subsequently observe a more educated patient, a patient who will request better results. Healthcare suppliers can offer this benefit and improve understanding results by guaranteeing precise and very much educated conclusions, ideal treatment arranging, a steadier clinical workplace, more noteworthy straightforwardness, congruity of care, improved patient help, and associated care. Managing doctor burnout, improving coordination, and guaranteeing excellent correspondence are extra components that can assume a basic function in offering some benefit based consideration to patients. The significant thing here is to improve the principal structure of the healthcare framework to advance customized treatment and patient results.
- Digitalising healthcare: At long last, digitalization will be the new essence of healthcare later on. Artificial intelligence will turn into an essential piece of future healthcare arrangements; healthcare information will be all the more adequately

utilized with the assistance of better than ever computerized instruments, and the advanced upset will change the very idea of care conveyance and treatment of infection. The healthcare business today is confronted with the test of improving worth. It is managing maturing populaces, expanded pervasiveness of constant sicknesses, and expanded healthcare spending. There is the additional strain to convey better and more improved consideration without expanding costs. The best way to give this is by digitalizing healthcare. Advanced innovations can help the healthcare business address the issues of patients and suppliers. They can do as such by:

- Improving access for the two patients and suppliers to healthcare conveyance
- Empowering distant checking of patients
- Giving patients responsibility for wellbeing and health
- Expanding precision, normalization, and productivity in consideration conveyance
- Encouraging consistent correspondence inside the healthcare framework
- Utilizing artificial intelligence to all the more likely coordinate and dissect healthcare information.

Hence, readers (including future researchers) are suggested to read various applications of AI in current era in [34], also open issues, challenges in IoT-based Applications in [34–36] and issues, critical challenges in AI based solutions (in current and for next decade) in [37].

9 Conclusion

Healthcare modernization is being driven by various patterns including rising healthcare costs, a maturing populace, and the developing occurrence of ongoing conditions that will require long haul care, (for example, diabetes and heart infections). The eventual fate of healthcare will settle upon three columns: an advanced methodology, information knowledge, and a patient-driven culture. IT will be at the focal point of this change, assisting with reducing expenses, drive profitability gains and reveal new economies of scale for more prominent proficiency and better patient consideration. Past that, IT can likewise upset the present frameworks and in a general sense change healthcare conveyance through customized medication and associated care. Prescient Investigation and the Internet of Things (IoT) will shape the fate of numerous enterprises, including healthcare. Nonetheless, before these new advancements can genuinely convey an incentive to patients, for example, expanding survivability and future or giving prescient and prescriptive markers to illnesses, healthcare associations should initially get their information procedure right. This incorporates recording of information, sparing crude information and keeping it free from any and all harm, and utilizing it for more noteworthy patient experiences. Dell EMC's Arising Innovations Division gives the base advancements that assemble Information

Lakes (multi-convention, versatile information holders that store this crude information and give examination motors to deal with this information) that will direct that adjustment in the healthcare frameworks. Information Lakes dispose of information storehouses inside the healthcare environment and fuse advances such a cloud, enormous information, portable and social to enable healthcare associations to use continuous information at the purpose of care.

References

1. Oztemel, E., & Gursev, S., (2020, January). Literature review of Industry 4.0 and related technologies. *Journal of Intelligent Manufacturing, 31*(4). https://doi.org/10.1007/s10845-018-1433-8
2. Kang, et al. (2020). Artificial intelligence algorithm to predict the need for critical care in prehospital emergency medical services. *Scandinavian Journal of Trauma, Resuscitation and Emergency Medicine, 28*, 17. https://doi.org/10.1186/s13049-020-0713-4
3. Bendato, et al. (2015). New markets forecast and dynamic production redesign through stochastic simulation. *International Journal of Simulation Modelling, 14*(3), 485–498. https://doi.org/10.2507/ijsimm14(3)10.307
4. Patrone, et al. (2017, March). Optimization of lean surgical route through POCT acquisition. *International MultiConference of Engineers and Computer Scientists* (Vol II). IMECS.
5. Cassettari, et al. (2013). *A system dynamics study of an emergency department impact on the management of hospital's surgery activities*.https://doi.org/10.5220/0004617205970604
6. Rajesh, E., et al. (2020). Different dimensions on healthcare using internet of things (IoT): Health monitoring. *Journal of Critical Reviews, 7*(9), 638–641. https://doi.org/10.31838/jcr.07.09.125
7. Knowles, E., et al. (2018). Exploring variation in how ambulance services address non-conveyance: a qualitative interview study. *BMJ Open, 8*(11). https://doi.org/10.1136/bmjopen-2018-024228
8. Aceto, G., Persico, V., & Pescapè, A. (2018, February 15). The role of information and communication technologies in healthcare: Taxonomies, perspectives, and challenges. *Journal of Network and Computer Applications*. https://doi.org/10.1016/j.jnca.2018.02.008
9. Dash, S., et al. (2019). Big data in healthcare: management, analysis and future prospects. *Journal of Big Data, 6*, Article number: 54.
10. Rejikumar, G., et al. (2019, July). Industry 4.0: key findings and analysis from the literature arena. *Benchmarking an International Journal*. https://doi.org/10.1108/BIJ-09-2018-0281
11. Ashwin, M., et al. (2018, April). Heart life: A heart beat monitoring system using IoT. *International Research Journal of Engineering and Technology (IRJET), 05*(04), ISSN: 2395–0056.
12. Ocen, G. G., et al. (2020). Exponential disruptive technologies and the required skills of industry 4.0. *Journal of Engineering, 2020*, ID 4280156. https://doi.org/10.1155/2020/428015
13. Lee Ventola, C. (2014, May). Mobile devices and apps for health care professionals: Uses and benefits. *P & T: A Peer-reviewed Journal for Formulary Management, 39*(5), 356–364.
14. Enrique, A., et al. (2010, October). Biometrics for Electronic Health Records. *Journal of Medical Systems, 34*(5):975–83.https://doi.org/10.1007/s10916-009-9313-6
15. Jayabalan, M., & O'Daniel, T. (2019). A study on authentication factors in electronic health records. *Journal of Applied Technology and Innovation* (e-ISSN: 2600–7304), *3*(1).
16. Nagy, J., et al. (2018). The role and impact of industry 4.0 and the internet of things on the business strategy of the value chain—The case of Hungary. *Sustainability, 10*, 3491. https://doi.org/10.3390/su10103491

17. Sima, V., et al. (2020). Influences of the industry 4.0 revolution on the human capital development and consumer behavior: A systematic review. *Sustainability, 12*, 4035. https://doi.org/10.3390/su12104035
18. https://towardsdatascience.com/the-power-of-artificial-intelligence-ai-virtual-and-augmented-reality-vr-and-ar-on-medical-4949c7a6fd72
19. Li, J. -P. O., et al. Digital technology, tele-medicine and artificial artificial intelligence in ophthalmology: A global perspective. *Elsevier Public Health Emergency Collection*. https://doi.org/10.1016/j.preteyeres.2020.100900
20. Nass, S. (2015, September). *Improving diagnosis in health care*. National Academies Press, ISBN: 978-0-309-37769-0. https://doi.org/10.17226/21794
21. Hossain, M., et al. (2018, May). *An internet of things-based health prescription assistant and its security system design. Future Generation Computer Systems, 82*. https://doi.org/10.1016/j.future.2017.11.020
22. Blowers, M., et al. (2016, October). *The future internet of things and security of its control systems*. https://www.researchgate.net/publication/308915644_The_Future_Internet_of_Things_and_Security_of_its_Control_Systems
23. Ramya, G., Sai Lohitha, N. (2019, December). The role and advancements of IOT technology in smart farming for agribusiness. *Journal of the Gujarat Research Society, 21*(16), ISSN: 0374–8588.
24. Banerjee, S., & Badr, Y. (2018, January). Evaluating decision analytics from mobile big data using rough set based Ant Colony. https://doi.org/10.1007/978-3-319-67925-9_9
25. Vaishnnave, M. P., Suganya Devi, K., & Srinivasan, P (2019). A survey on cloud computing and hybrid cloud. *International Journal of Applied Engineering Research,* 14(2), 429–434, ISSN 0973–4562.
26. Behmann, F., & Wu, K. *Collaborative internet of things (C-IOT): For future smart connected life and business. Wiley Online Library*. ISBN: 9781118913741. https://doi.org/10.1002/9781118913734
27. Bruen, D., et al. (2017, August 12) Glucose sensing for diabetes monitoring: recent developments. *Sensors (Basel)*.https://doi.org/10.3390/s17081866
28. Thuemmler, C., & Bai, C. *Health 4.0: How virtualization and big data are revolutionizing healthcare*. https://link.springer.com/book/10.1007%2F978-3-319-47617-9
29. Kashyap, R. (2019, January). Machine learning for internet of things. *Next-generation wireless networks meet advanced machine learning applications* (pp. 57–83). https://doi.org/10.4018/978-1-5225-7458-3.ch003
30. Ginsburg, G. S., & Phillips, K. A. (2018, May). *Precision medicine: From science to value. 37*(5), 694–701. https://doi.org/10.1377/hlthaff.2017.1624
31. Mizanoor Rahman, S. M. (2018). Cyber-physical-social system between a humanoid robot and a virtual human through a shared platform for adaptive agent ecology. *IEEE/CAA Journal of Automatica Sinica, 5*(1), 190–203.
32. Tyagi, A. K. (2016, March). Cyber physical systems (CPSs)—Opportunities and challenges for improving cyber security. *International Journal of Computer Applications, 137*(14):19–27, Published by Foundation of Computer Science (FCS), NY, USA.
33. Robidoux, R., et al. (2019). *An analysis of pay-for-performance schemes and their potential impacts on health systems and outcomes for patients. 2019*, Article ID 8943972. https://doi.org/10.1155/2019/8943972
34. Tyagi, A. K., Nair, M. M., Niladhuri, S., & Abraham, A. (2020). Security, privacy research issues in various computing platforms: A survey and the road ahead. Journal of Information Assurance & Security, 15(1), p1–16, 16p.
35. Tyagi, A. K., & Goyal, D. (2020). A survey of privacy leakage and security vulnerabilities in the internet of things. *2020 5th International conference on communication and electronics systems (ICCES)* (pp. 386–394), Coimbatore, India. https://doi.org/10.1109/ICCES48766.2020.9137886
36. Shamila, M., Vinuthna, K., & Tyagi, A. (2019). *A review on several critical issues and challenges in IoT based e-Healthcare system*. 1036–1043. https://doi.org/10.1109/ICCS45141.2019.9065831.

37. Pramod, A., Naicker, H. S., & Tyagi, A. K. (2020). Machine learning and deep learning: Open issues and future research directions for next Ten Years. In *Computational analysis and understanding of deep learning for medical care: Principles, methods, and applications*. Wiley Scrivener.

Security, Privacy and Trust Issues in Internet of Things and Machine Learning Based e-Healthcare

Shruti Suhas Kute, Amit Kumar Tyagi, and S. U. Aswathy

1 Introduction—Internet of Things (IoT) and Machine Learning in e-Healthcare

In the IoT, healthcare is a significant application zone, since it assists with lessening costs and improves administration quality. Likewise, biomedical gadgets or sensors are utilized in the IoT to screen biomedical factors, for example, pulse, blood glucose level, circulatory strain, and internal heat level [1]. The IoT's present impact on healthcare is principal because of the advances that have been made regarding correspondences, sensors, and innovations for data preparing, and specifically, the appearance of wearables (convenient body sensors) for continuous observation of boundaries or biomedical factors. The day by day exercises of individuals with constant ailments and handicaps are simpler gratitude to help living conditions, which give assorted healthcare administrations to patients since they have sensors with more noteworthy limits and productivity to handle data progressively. The IoT offers a few advantages for healthcare, for example, the capacity to acquire biomedical factors from the patient through an organization of keen gadgets connected to biomedical gadgets, the utilization of cloud administrations for the preparing and capacity of data, and the pervasive trade of information between wellbeing experts [2]. Nevertheless, IoT keen gadgets have restricted assets, so it is important to think about different choices to examine information, for example, machine learning. Machine

S. S. Kute (✉) · A. K. Tyagi
School of Computing Science and Engineering, Vellore Institute of Technology, Chennai, Tamilnadu 600127, India

A. K. Tyagi
Centre for Advanced Data Science, Vellore Institute of Technology, Chennai, Tamilnadu 600127, India

S. U. Aswathy
Department of Computer Science and Engineering, Jyothi Engineering College, Thrissur, Kerala, India

A. K. Tyagi et al. (eds.), *Intelligent Interactive Multimedia Systems for e-Healthcare Applications*, https://doi.org/10.1007/978-981-16-6542-4_15

learning is a subset of man-made brainpower that comprises examining the calculations and measurable models utilized in PC frameworks to accomplish explicit targets viably, in view of examples and deductions. In this specific circumstance, there are a few difficulties in the wellbeing area that give territories of occasion to the IoT and machine learning to give arrangements or options that add to improving the healthcare or personal satisfaction of patients. This work presents PISIoT: a machine learning and IoT-based savvy wellbeing stage for the avoidance, identification, treatment, and control of overweight and heftiness, and different sicknesses or medical issues from these conditions. Machine learning strategies are basic in this work because of the need to arrange patients dependent on their biomedical factors and conduct to give the most suitable proposals to improve their wellbeing [3].

Presently, the Internet of Things (IoT) has gotten perhaps the most blazing point among analysts and specialists. It is viewed as a general presence that permits all items/things in our current circumstance to be associated over the web with the capability to interconnect with one another without human intercession. The IoT includes an assortment of articles that can be associated with utilizing either remote or wired organizations [4]. These articles have an exceptional tending to conspire that permits them to interface and help out one another to make novel applications and administrations, for example, keen homes, shrewd transportation, associated vehicles, savvy lattices, brilliant urban communities, brilliant traffic lights and others. The social acknowledgement of IoT applications and administrations is firmly relying upon the dependability of data and the insurance of private information. Since the IoT is a mind boggling, conveyed and heterogeneous framework in nature, it faces a few difficulties with respect to security and protection. Presently, building a powerful and solid security procedure is probably the most noteworthy need to consider. Albeit various analysts have acquainted a few arrangements with the security and protection issues, a solid security method for the IoT is as yet sought after to fulfil prerequisites of information secrecy, uprightness, protection and trust.

Also, the IoT wellbeing is viewed as perhaps the most elevated criticality to keep the IoT and its components from delivering actual harm or bothersome danger and shield the general climate from such harm. Building the IoT framework with inserted security and dependability highlights should be considered to make new plan designs that give a protected and solid framework climate. Furthermore, there is a need to build up a moral structure that guarantees the IoT is utilized to benefit humankind and not the reverse way around. A solid moral standard will spur organizations to plan more brilliant and all the more comprehensive items to dodge algorithmic issues and guarantee worldwide availability. The fundamental goal of this section is to give an outline of IoT security, privacy, wellbeing and morals. It begins by examining the engineering and basic characteristics of the IoT framework. This is trailed by researching IoT security by featuring security prerequisites, security by plan, security attacks and security difficulties of the IoT framework. IoT security with exploring protection dangers and recommended solutions are likewise talked about. Additionally, IoT security and morals are researched by featuring the requirement for moral plan and morals challenges in the IoT framework [5]. Eventually, a contextual analysis of the shrewd city is acquainted with talk about security dangers and proposed arrangements in the savvy city setting.

Organization of the work: Sect. 2 discusses background work of IoT applications in healthcare in previous century. Further, Sect. 3 discusses IoMT as Future of healthcare. Then, Sect. 4 presents the Development of Personalized Medicine using Internet of Things and Machine Learning. Internet of Things in Healthcare Industry including Internet of Things uses for all sectors is discussed in Sect. 5. Further, Sect. 6 discusses several applications (best uses) of machine learning in (for) healthcare industry. Then, popular Security and Privacy Issues of Internet of Things and Machine Learning in e-healthcare are discussed in Sect. 7. Further, popular attacks (in recent year or in near future) on healthcare Systems is discussed in Sect. 8. Further, Sect. 9 provides explanation of existing methods to tackle security and privacy issues in healthcare industry. In last, we conclude this work in brief by including several interesting future remarks for future researchers in Sect. 10. Note that in this work, terms 'smart devices', 'Internet of Things' and 'internet connecting things' have been used interchangeably.

2 Background Study

The utilization of Internet of Things based gadgets is changing individuals' ways of life, especially in exercises identified with healthcare. In this sense, IoT-based gadgets screen, dissect, analyse, and add to the age of clinical suggestions for different ailments, for example, overweight and corpulence. Consequently, this theme has become the focal point of much consideration in late examination. In this segment, we present a survey of the cutting edge of exploration including the IoT in healthcare, especially concerning overweight, corpulence, and ongoing degenerative infections. Vazquez et al. [6] proposed "mhealth", a wellbeing stage that adds to improving youngster nourishment by checking admission and sends warnings and instructive messages dependent on the decision of food. What's more, Vilallonga et al. introduced an examination led on a gathering of fat patients having gone through a medical procedure, who thought that it was propelling them to notice, effectively and rapidly, a steady realistic portrayal of their exercises [7]. Mun-Lee and Ouyang introduced an investigation that tried to distinguish connections between the dangers of building up specific infections and utilized healthcare gadgets with regards to the IoT. Conversely, Zaragoza et al. [8] introduced a stage that utilizes intercommunication sensors to screen the exercises of kids with stoutness issues.

Further, Mun-Lee and Ouyang [9] proposed a cooperative convention to send hazard warnings to brilliant gadgets utilized in the IoT, alongside another help application calculation that was utilized in gadgets connected to patients with circulatory strain issues, heftiness, and diabetes. Hiremath et al. [10] introduced a proposition for the conceptualization of Wearable IoT (WIoT) regarding applications, capacities, and plans. Furthermore, they proposed a framework for WIoT that suggests new bearings with respect to clinical and usable techniques. In like manner, Vázquez et al. proposed new portable wellbeing engineering to forestall youth corpulence through smart dieting recommendations utilizing versatile wellbeing options [11]. What's more, they thought about messages and notices for a solid eating routine for grown-ups. Kim et al. [12] introduced the iN Touch versatile application to screen the everyday exercises of oppressed youngsters with overweight and stoutness who partook in a wellbeing apprenticeship program. Alloghani et al. [13] introduced a versatile application to expand youngsters' and guardians' familiarity with the results of being overweight and hefty while giving data on the best way to continue a sound and adjusted eating routine. On the other hand, Wibisono and Astawa [14] proposed a website page and a portable application for the treatment of weight decrease through Machine-to-Machine (M2M) data trade or correspondence, in which a particular extent of loads was utilized to accomplish a solid eating regimen. Dobbins et al. [15] proposed a technique to acquire physiological information from gadgets connected to triaxial accelerometers and a pulse screen, to distinguish actual work. Moreover, they assessed the exhibition of the classifiers comparable to the proactive tasks of the patients. Also, Shin et al. [16] characterized another idea of IoT-learning, with which a wellbeing application was created utilizing a mix of the IoT and engineering upheld by the IoT. Similarly, they proposed a patient-centred treatment utilizing IoT-learning to look after weight.

Now we will discuss background work of IoT used in healthcare. Liu et al. in 2012, [17] proposed secure clinical administrative techniques being applied to the organizational climate of the clinical association data framework in order to keep away from the outer or inner data security occasions, permit the clinical framework to work easily and securely that benefits the patients, yet in addition permit the specialists to utilize it all the more advantageously, and further advance the general clinical quality. The targets could be accomplished by keeping from unlawful attack or clinical data being taken, ensuring the fulfilment and security of clinical data, dodging the administrative mix-ups of the interior data framework in clinical associations, and giving the exceptionally dependable clinical data framework. Paschou et al. [18] in 2013 uses the Internet of Things ideas in the area of wellness and doesn't come without additional information and subsequently an information move costs overheads. To manage these overheads, novel measurements, and strategies are acquainted in an endeavour to augment the abilities and extend acknowledgement/utilization given by the Internet of Things. Without losing its over-simplification, the strategy talked about is tentatively assessed in the worldview of the Wellbeing area. The attention is on the requirement for a diagram of accessible information configurations and transmission strategies and determination of the ideal blend, which can result in decrease/minimization of expenses. A logical technique is introduced sponsored with hypothetical measurements and assessed tentatively. Ziegeldorf et al. [19] in 2013 dissects the security issues in the Internet of Things in detail. To this end, this work initially talks about the developing highlights and patterns in the Internet of Things with the objective of examining their security suggestions. Second, this work grouped and analysed the security dangers in this new setting, bringing up the moves that should be defeated to guarantee that the Internet of Things turns into a reality.

Further, Sawand et al. [20] in 2015 introduced an engineering structure to portray the whole observing life cycle also, feature the basic help segments. More nitty gritty conversations are then dedicated to {em information collection} at the tolerant side, which we contend that fills in as a key premise in accomplishing strong, effective, and secure wellbeing checking. Thus, a significant conversation of the security dangers focusing on eHealth observing frameworks is introduced, and the significant constraints of the current arrangements are investigated and broadly talked about. At last, a bunch of configuration challenges is distinguished to accomplish high calibre and secure patient-driven checking plans, alongside some possible arrangements. Gope et al. [21] in 2016 features the significant security necessities in BSN-based current medical care framework. Therefore, this work proposed a protected IoT-based medical services framework utilizing BSN, called BSN-Care, which can productively achieve those prerequisites. Benssalah. M. et al. [22] in 2016 featured the weaknesses of the latest proposed convention for TMIS in the writing and proposed attacks dependent on the shortcomings identified with the abuse of the timestamp procedure, the figuring of the perused solicitation and label reaction messages utilizing the single direction hash work, which are not mindfully investigated. Second, this work proposed a proficient double RFID-TMIS versatile verification convention with high productivity and security for medical care frameworks. Their proposition is an improvement and augmentation of the convention of Li et al. [23], where they have proposed to connect the RFID innovation with TMIS in a similar validation framework to take favourable circumstances of both these two promising advances. The presentation examination shows that our improved convention could settle security shortcomings of the considered convention and give versatility, proficiency and is appropriate for TMIS selection in distant territories and low populace thickness.

3 Internet of Medical Things (IoMT): Future of Healthcare

Past the developing business sector for healthcare IoT, the COVID-19 pandemic has prodded discussions around the eventual fate of IoT in healthcare and how it can securely associate healthcare experts and patients. Emergency clinics and centres had to rapidly assess telehealth to keep on treating a few patients without expanding their danger of contamination by bringing them into care offices. Medical clinics are additionally compelled to recognize approaches to decrease costs. Wearable gadgets that empower a few patients to be dealt with and checked at home could lessen the quantity of assets required at the healthcare office. Another innovation adding to the fate of IoT in healthcare is the presentation of 5G organizations, which give multiple times quicker speeds to availability than customary 4G organizations. IoT gadgets depend on availability to impart and move information among patients and care suppliers. Quicker cell information move gives IoT adaptability regarding the volumes of information it can trade and at a lot quicker rate. With these upgrades, new healthcare IoT utilizes incorporate gadgets that help patients with their medicine adherence at home; rest checking gadgets that can follow pulse, oxygen levels and developments for high-hazard patients; distant temperature observing apparatuses; and ceaseless glucose checking sensors that associate with cell phones and ready patients and clinicians to changing glucose levels. This new pandemic experience joined with the advancement and ongoing headways will expand the selection of IoT and support the individuals who may have in any case disregarded the innovation in the past to jump aboard [24].

With the expanding utilization of cloud, administrations joined with AI, IoT gadgets are getting more brilliant and are going past communicating information from patient to healthcare proficient. For instance, IoT gadgets that utilize cloud administrations for information investigation are the savvy glucose observing framework and smart insulin pen. These two advances persistently catch data with respect to glucose levels yet in addition transfer the information to a cloud administration or a portable application to be examined. In view of the result of the examination, the insulin siphon would then be able to infuse the patient with the fitting measurement of insulin. Another model is the utilization of brilliant caretaker cameras for checking older patients. These shrewd cameras perceive when schedules stray from the standard, for example, if an older individual goes into the restroom yet doesn't come out after a brief timeframe. Another utilization of the camera is for fall location, which would then alarm crisis administrations or parental figures. Different employments of IoT that will start to drift later on incorporate the utilization of bots or virtual specialists to cooperate with patients. By consolidating sensor data gathered by various IoT gadgets and sensors and utilizing voice-empowered speakers, seniors can approach an individual remote helper to remind them to take their prescription, review them for any important data that identifies with their wellbeing or agony levels, and respond to any gathered data from their gadgets, for example, glucose levels, fall location or oxygen levels.

Past wearables and patient-explicit connections, healthcare associations will receive IoT in offices for stock administration and hardware following. This innovation—for the most part, alluded to as continuous area frameworks—keeps on improving due to progressions in remote innovation and the size of the sensors. By following the development of gear and general use, medical clinics will improve perceivability of potential hardware deficiencies and who may have interacted with the hardware. This is particularly significant for forestalling the spread of disease, for example, how the COVID-19 pandemic constrained emergency clinics to follow hardware and staff who interacted with contaminated patients.

4 Development of Personalized Medicine Using Internet of Things and Machine Learning

As of late, the Internet of Things (IoT) is arising as another worldview in data innovation pointed toward developing a unique worldwide organization framework by associating an assortment of physical and virtual 'things' with the developing versatile and sensors. IoT was at first proposed to allude to extraordinarily recognizable items (things) and their virtual portrayals in an internet-like structure, by means of utilizing Radio Frequency Identification (RFID) innovation. Later on, the idea of IoT has been reached out to cover more sort of 'things' with an assortment of sensors, for example, actuators, Global Positioning System (GPS) gadgets and cell phones. The consistent joining and compelling outfit of these sensors in a stage related to the Internet have raised a ton of exploration issues, from framework design, information preparing to applications. These days, IoT innovation has been quickly making strides as a need for multidisciplinary research in numerous scholastic and modern orders, particularly in medical care.

The underlying vision of IoT was to broaden the term 'Internet' into this present reality grasping ordinary actual items by methods for Radio Frequency Identification (RFID) innovation. Before long, as quick advances in detecting advances, more heterogeneous sensors, for example, accelerometers, whirligigs, altimeters and other compact ease gadgets are equipped for being associated in an IoT climate [25]. Driven by the outstanding development of business wearable gadgets and versatile applications, the idea of IoT-based PHS is set up and turn out to be progressively well known. These medical care frameworks utilize a bunch of interconnected gadgets to make an IoT network for performing medical services exercises, for example, conclusion, checking and distant medical procedures. Regarding a notable meaning of four layers, IoT framework engineering has been discussed in [26]. Various common studies in an IoT empowered PHS will be sorted by detecting, systems administration, handling and application, appeared in Table 1. The detecting layer for PHS intends to plan and create novel sensors or detecting advancements for viably and effectively gathering an assortment of sorts of customized wellbeing and clinical data in an IoT climate. Existing sensors and wearable gadgets, for example, inertial sensors, GPS (Global Positioning System), ECG (Electrocardiogram), EEG (Electroencephalogram) are fit for noticing and recording numerous sort wellbeing information, including weight, area, pulse, circulatory strain and client setting data. Additionally, numerous examinations start to utilize cell phones to gather human feelings and conduct information by explicit versatile applications. Up until now, these tangible procedures are generally actually and practically refined in physically controlled conditions. Be that as it may, planning savvy and non-intrusive wearable gadgets is requesting and testing. Numerous explores spotlight building up some novel precise, solid practical and non-obtrusive detecting procedures for a programmed assortment of human wellbeing information in IoT-based uncontrolled conditions.

The systems administration layer for PHS is dependable to associate all gadgets in tangible layers together and permit customized wellbeing information to be gathered, put away, sent, shared and collected under IoT frameworks. Additionally, it gives interoperability and security required with regards to IoT for medical services. Islam et al. [27] have surveyed a cutting edge of IoT medical care network with three issues: geography, engineering and stage. Each issue has gotten one of the imperative exploration sub-stream in the IoT empowered PHS. Customary IoT geography for PHS alludes to the portrayal, design and arrangement of various wellbeing sensor components in an IoT medical services organization, for example, P2P, Star and Mesh. As the development of associated gadgets and sub-organizations, one key exploration issue of IoT geography for PHS is the means by which to move

Table 1 Studies on PHS

Sensing layer		Network layer	Processing layer				Application	Assessment	
Device specification	Placed position	Network	Methods	Users	Subjects	Accuracy		Advantages	Limitations
1 ACC	Back	Chipcom CC243D transceiver	Self-defined Thresholds	Young healthy people	Walk, fast walk, ascend stairs, etc	91.5–100%	Recognition and monitoring elder people at home. [3]	Low-cost simple algorithms; adaptive	Short time monitoring; uncontrolled environment
ACOR + kinematic system	day: belt; night: chest	Bluetooth	DT	Patients, healthy people	Postures, walk, read, exercises	77–94%	COPD patients monitoring. [4]	Simple device and algorithm	The model only useful for COPD patients
Multi-channel sensors module (EEC respiration)	Head	Bluetooth	SVM	Twenty mentally healthy people	Awake, drowsy, etc	93.5 ± 1.4%	Lifelogging mental fatigue monitoring [5]	Real-time feedback on mobile device	Multiple sensors may increase the cost and simplicity
ACC and pressure sensors;	Feet	Bluetooth	SVM	Young, mid-aged healthy people	Postures, walk, step, sweep, cycle, jog	92–98%	Reduce Energy and memory on smart phone [6]	Energy efficient; real-rime feedback	Smart shoes are non-universal; no mention of feasibility
Wearable device	Wrist	Not mentioned	Multivariate analysis	16 elder people	Sleep, wake	Not mentioned	Monitoring elderly health and sleep patterns [7]	Real-life environment: high targetedsubjects	No obvious disadvantages

(continued)

Table 1 (continued)

Sensing layer		Network layer	Processing layer				Application	Assessment	
Device specification	Placed position	Network	Methods	Users	Subjects	Accuracy		Advantages	Limitations
SHIM-MER's ECC and GSR	Wrist	Bluetooth	DT, Bayesian Network. SVM. R-Means	20 people	Baseline, stressed	92.4%	Continuous human stress monitoring for interventions [8]	Inclusive of PA impact on the stress; long-term monitoring	Patients are not considered and tested
1 3D ACC, 1 wearable camera	ACC on The belly; Camera hung over neck	ZigBee, Wi-Fi, Bluetooth	SVM	Not mentioned	Run, go downstairs, go upstairs, take an elevator, walk, etc	90–99%	Lifelogging health monitoring in context-aware environment [9]	The approach could recognise movement directions	Lack of privacy; inconvenience in daily lives; limited subject categories
Mobile phone	No strict position	Bluetooth, GSM, Wi-Fi	HMM. DT	16 healthy people (8 F, 8 M. ages 20–45)	Still, walk, run, cycle, motor	87.9–96.2%	Lifelogging healthcare monitoring personal transportation [10]	No needs for phone's 6DOF; fine grained activity categories	Not mentioned whether the model is useful for elderly or patients
1 gyro on shoe	Feet, knee	Not mentioned	Knowledge-based	10 people, 6 people with impaired gait	Walk on level ground, walk up and down a steep, etc	>96%	A system of controlling the gair cycle of a neuroprosthesis for walking in real time [11]	Identify transitions in gait phase; present walking and non-walking activities	No obvious disadvantages

(continued)

Table 1 (continued)

Sensing layer		Network layer	Processing layer				Application	Assessment	
Device specification	Placed position	Network	Methods	Users	Subjects	Accuracy		Advantages	Limitations
1 3D ACC 1 3D gyro. 1 3D magnetic sensor	Upper and lower limb	Bluetooth	Kinematic modeling	8 healthy male people (24–40 years old)	circular, rectangular motion, reach, elevation, etc	95–98%	Home-based stroke rehabilitation [12]	Low-cost, real-time robust in different motion circumstances	No obvious disadvantages

the heterogeneous static and cell phones into cross breed figuring frameworks. As to models for PHS, numerous past examinations have utilized IPv6 or 6LoWPAN frameworks as a premise IoT structure, which can upgrade the nature of information transmission and expand the scope of medical care administrations with versatility and adaptability. Presently, to help more principles for interoperation, the Software Oriented Architecture (SOA) has been proposed and approved by numerous specialists as a promising arrangement in IoT empowered PHS. Under SOA, various guidelines have been worked to help the requirements of interoperability, as Extensible Markup Language (XML), Simple Object Access Protocol (SOAP), and so forth A few examinations research the issues of cost, danger and benefit in actualizing SOA for huge scope IoT empowered medical care frameworks. Aside from over two issues in systems administration layers, originators likewise need to address factors, for example, network the board advancements for heterogeneous organizations, (for example, fixed, remote, versatile, and so forth), energy effectiveness in organizations, QoS prerequisites, administration revelation and recovery, information and sign handling, security, and protection. Especially, since customized wellbeing data is generally delicate for clients, any improper revelation may disregard client protection. The work in reading security and protection for IoT empowered PHS has set off numerous arrangements, such as solid directing, cryptographic plan, security safeguarding wellbeing information conglomeration.

The handling layer of IoT empowered PHS focuses on planning helpful computational approaches for preparing an assortment of complex wellbeing related information with pointing quality. The early work in versatile wellbeing centres around creating explicit calculations for certain illness related information as opposed to general strategies dealing with both wellbeing and clinical information. For example, Acampora et al. [28] explored various encompassing knowledge calculations in medical services with respect to five applications: action acknowledgement, standard of conduct revelation, irregularity recognition, and choice help. However, presently in the IoT empowered PHS, the critical function of explicit application is generally arranged into the application layer, the examination focal point of information preparing layer here has moved to conventional calculations to improve the exactness and legitimacy of wellbeing information and additionally new information insightful devices to encourage versatile, assessable and feasible information structure. So, this paper will sum up information handling calculations for IoT empowered PHS into three key parts: information driven methodologies, information-based methodologies and half breed draws near. All the more explicitly, information driven methodologies contain directed learning, semi-managed learning and solo learning strategies; information-based techniques cover demonstrating and semantic thinking draws near; half breed approaches are a blend of over two kinds of approaches by incorporating AI into information thinking.

The function of the use layer in IoT empowered PHS is to offer top notch types of assistance and simple-to-utilize interfaces to end clients. As referenced previously, past portable wellbeing investigates don't think about application as an individual layer in medical services, and join the interface or ease of use into the calculation layer. So, their exploration centres around assessing if the whole framework or new calculations have functional impact or help on clinical consideration. In the IoT climate, PHSs are utilized by an enormous scope populace with the goal that the extent of exploration in application layer has ventured into all the more wide territories, including medical care administration disclosure, medical services administration arrangement, medical services stage API, human–PC communication in medical services, and so forth additionally, investigations of utilization layer in IoT empowered PHS likewise cover various types of medical care applications in scholarly community and industry, as nonstop checking, helped living, treatment and restoration, convincing prosperity, passionate prosperity and brilliant emergency clinics, and so on [29].

Versatile advancements these days assume basic functions in medical care checking and benefits. These innovations incorporate mobile telephones, Personal Digital Assistant (PDAs), versatile cameras (e.g. SenseCam), keen watches, and so on. As the greater parts of cell phones are inserted an assortment of inertial sensors (e.g. accelerometer, gyrators, and so on) and biomedical sensors (skin temperature, pulse, and so forth), they are intended for giving customized and consistent considerations to clients. For instance, numerous versatile items (e.g. Fitbit) and applications (e.g. Moves) have been delivered for the drawn-out record and assortment of individual lifelogging active work. A few gadgets include in patient's self-administration and mediation. Different applications that utilize inertial sensors are fit for recognizing falling and accordingly dodge bothersome outcomes [30].

5 Applications of Internet of Things in Healthcare Industry: Internet of Things for All

Internet of Things uses is increasing year by year by many sectors. Till now, many industries have implemented IoT-based production or IoT-based communication to do everyday tasks or do a task. From Agriculture to military applications, transportation, smart city, smart home, to wearable devices, IoT devices have improved the way the communication, i.e. have enhanced every sector to a better level. Further, we mention few applications of IoT in healthcare sector/some of the use cases of IoT in healthcare as:

(a) **Far off Patient Care**: In numerous pieces of the world, occupants live miles from the closest emergency clinic. In that capacity, when there is a crisis, it takes effort for them to arrive at the medical services offices. Essentially, for medical services suppliers, it gets hard to visit patients with ongoing conditions often. The issue with tedious drive can be tackled with far off patient consideration controlled by the IoT. The availability can permit medical care experts to help patients with solutions, medicine, and furthermore measure their biometrics utilizing sensors and distant gear. For example, patients can associate any wearable or convenient gadget to the cloud and update the information progressively. A portion of the IoT gadgets can likewise encourage vis-à-vis talk over the internet. This can give medical care experts the vital data to get ready consideration plans while the patients are headed to the emergency clinic. Or on the other hand, even without them expecting to visit the medical clinic in any case! For persistent patients, this makes a program of the patients' day-to-date wellbeing update. The gathered information can frame graphs and outlines to be handily imagined by medical services experts. Live video and sound real time can be utilized to screen patients' current condition without the requirement for the drive.

(b) **Crisis Care**: Crisis care yields depend on the time, precision, and accessibility of logical data. Besides, it additionally relies upon the nature of the information got during the crisis call and the data gathered while the patient is being moved for sure fire care at the medical care offices. Additionally, the whole cycle of gathering, putting away, preparing, and recovering the information during that time is relentless and tedious. IoT can help in gathering information precisely, which can be gotten to by crisis care staff, for example, paramedics or staff in the ER for speedy and better clinical help. This information can likewise be communicated to ER staff continuously while the patient is headed to the medical clinic—permitting the medical clinics to be more ready for consideration.

(c) **Following of Inventory, Staff, and Patients**: Medical services associations are tied in with expanding the efficiencies of their labour force and decreasing operational expenses. This is valid for both little and huge establishments that incorporate a few staff individuals, patients, and stock. Utilizing IoT gadgets as remote ID cards, medical clinics can oversee affirmations, increment the security, and measure the general exhibition of the staff. Bluetooth Low Energy (BLE) guides and RFID labels can be utilized to follow the area of the stock and furthermore follow the staff individuals if there should be an occurrence of any desperation. Also, IoT and RTLS (Real Time Location Systems) together can encourage resource following. This is one of the most economical approaches to monitor the gear, medications, and free assets, who would then be able to invest more energy on patient consideration.

(d) **Increasing Surgeries**: With regards to medical care, IoT has infiltrated working rooms too. Consider associated mechanical gadgets, which are fuelled by Artificial Intelligence and are utilized to do different medical procedures. These tasks are about expanded exactness delivered by robot-helped specialists. Additionally, associated gadgets and IoT applications can consummately smooth out the exercises of the clinical staff at both pre and post-working stages. In the two cases, IoT sensors can be utilized to gather, send information, and investigate it. These aides record the littlest subtleties and along these lines are valuable in forestalling careful confusions.

(e) **Virtual Monitoring of Critical Hardware**: It is a given that all the advanced medical services offices require best in class equipment and programming to work. When these are not dealt with in the most ideal way, the equipment can present different dangers and dangers. Consider power blackouts, framework disappointments, or even digital attacks. Since no medical care association would need these disasters to happen, they settle on the best IoT driven arrangements. A valid example is that of e-Alert by Philips, which can practically screen basic clinical equipment. In the event that there is an irregularity in any gear, the arrangement alarms the emergency clinic staff, so a disappointment can be kept away from by preventive upkeep.

(f) **Drug Store Management**: The drug store business is worth a huge number of dollars and is very confused. Since there are a few stages in moving and dealing with the medications from plant to storerooms in an emergency clinic, there are a few protection benefits that might be related to them. IoT can help join the best security draws near and the most recent innovation to guarantee quicker medication conveyance, more secure tasks, and better patient consideration. For example, take the case of shrewd refrigerators, which can be utilized to store antibodies and shield them from getting harmed during taking care of, capacity or move. IoT empowered drug stores can guarantee more prominent efficiencies and viability in tasks, mistake free clinical apportioning, security, and generally improved patient fulfilment.

(g) **Wearables Devices**: IoT gadgets, as wearables, can let the consideration groups gather various information focuses on the patient's rest designs, action, pulse, temperature, etc. These wearables can offer constant data to parental figures and patients. Think about a circumstance in which a heart tolerant has a raised pulse. The wearable will promptly send the sign to the nursing staff and permit them to give quick and opportune help to the patient. This can likewise help in distant wellbeing checking of older patients who are outside the medical clinic premises yet need consistent observing. IoT in medical care has huge potential and can end up being tremendously useful for medical services suppliers and patients. It is set to change quiet minds and hierarchical efficiencies. A few emergency clinics around the globe have just utilized the intensity of IoT under their keen emergency clinic activities.

(h) **Internet of Things for Doctors**: By utilizing wearables and other home observing gear inserted with IoT, specialists can monitor patients' wellbeing all the more successfully. They can follow patients' adherence to therapy plans or any requirement for guaranteed clinical consideration. IoT empowers medical care experts to be more vigilant and interface with the patients proactively. Information gathered from IoT gadgets can assist doctors with distinguishing the best treatment measure for patients and arrive at the normal results.

(i) **Internet of Things for Patients**: Gadgets as wearables like wellness groups and other remotely associated gadgets like pulse and pulse observing sleeves, glucometer and so on give patients admittance to customized consideration. These gadgets can be tuned to remind carbohydrate level, practice check, arrangements, pulse varieties and considerably more. IoT has transformed people, particularly old patients, by empowering steady following of medical issues. This majorly affects individuals living alone and their families. On any aggravation or changes in the normal exercises of an individual, ready instrument imparts signs to relatives and concerned wellbeing suppliers.

(j) **Internet of Things for Hospitals**: Aside from checking patients' wellbeing, there are numerous different territories where IoT gadgets are helpful in emergency clinics. IoT gadgets labelled with sensors are utilized for following continuous areas of clinical hardware like wheelchairs, defibrillators, nebulizers, oxygen siphons and other checking gear. Arrangement of clinical staff in various areas can likewise be dissected continuously. The spread of contaminations is a significant issue for patients in medical applications/clinics. IoT empowered cleanliness checking gadgets help in keeping patients from getting contaminated. IoT gadgets additionally help in resourcing the executives like drug store stock control, and ecological observing, for example, checking cooler temperature, and dampness and temperature control.

In summary, few disadvantages of IoT and Machine Learning in healthcare can be listed as: A few disadvantages that join the huge usage of the IoT in medical care include:

- Protection can be conceivably sabotaged. As we have just referenced, frameworks get hacked. Loads of consideration should be centred on information security, which requires huge extra expenditures.
- Unapproved admittance to centralization. Quite possibly deceptive intruders may get to concentrated frameworks and understand some remorseless expectations.
- Worldwide medical care guidelines. Worldwide wellbeing organizations are as of now giving rules that should be carefully trailed by administrative clinical foundations incorporating the IoT in their work process. These may confine potential abilities somewhat.

Hence, this section about Internet of Things used in healthcare industry and applications of Internet of Things for All, i.e. in popular applications. In last, this section discusses few disadvantages of IoT in healthcare. Now, the next section will discuss the application of machine learning in healthcare industry in detail.

6 Application of Machine Learning in Healthcare Industry

The expansion in the quantity of AI applications permits us to investigate the future where medical care suppliers will utilize information and examination to offer better types of assistance, improve measures, and mechanize assignments. Before long, AI based applications working with continuous patient information will become typical, expanding the productivity of treatment choices and driving the expense of medical services below.

(a) **Taking Care of Managerial Errands with Common Language Preparing**: Probably the best weight doctors experience today is the association and execution of managerial errands. Via mechanizing them, medical care organizations could help take care of the issue and permit doctors to do what they excel at:

invest more energy with patients. Here's an illustration of how AI and Regular Language Handling can help:

- An enormous segment of managerial errands includes surveying and refreshing electronic wellbeing records. Virtually every medical clinic in the US uses quite a bound together framework, and most facilities do too.
- Organizations could execute NLP-controlled devices that would utilize calculations to recognize and arrange words and expressions to permit doctors to direct notes straightforwardly to the framework during persistent visits. Thereafter, specialists could survey the graphs and synopses aggregated by the apparatus as opposed to perusing all the notes and test results to comprehend the general soundness of a patient.
- The device would help doctors invest less energy keeping up the patient records, accordingly permitting them to convey better medical care administrations to patients.

(b) **Instruments for Hazard ID**: Medical care suppliers are presently exploiting computerized arrangements based on top of AI models that utilize inconsistent location calculations to anticipate occasions, for example, strokes, cardiovascular failures, sepsis, and other genuine inconveniences. These instruments pull information from authentic patient records, day by day assessments, and continuous estimation of crucial signs, for example, the pulse or circulatory strain. The devices can make staff aware of inescapable patient dangers and permit them to make preventive moves.

(c) **Analysis and Sickness Distinguishing Proof**: One of the main utilizations of AI calculations in medical care is identified with the distinguishing proof and determination of sicknesses that are viewed as difficult to analyse. This can incorporate tumours that are hard to distinguish during their underlying phases of hereditary illnesses. An illustration of such an application is IBM Watson Genomics, which coordinates intellectual figuring with genome-based tumour sequencing to help doctors in making a quick finding. There are likewise apparatuses that exploit man-made brainpower to create helpful medicines in territories like oncology. The thought here is building up a financially reasonable approach to analyse and give treatment in clinical conditions via robotizing the cycle however much as could be expected.

(d) **Finding New Medications with Unaided Learning**: The beginning phase drug disclosure measure is another zone that can profit a great deal from AI. It's as of now overwhelmed by research and development innovations, for example, accuracy medication and cutting edge sequencing, which are utilized to discover elective ways for treatment of multifactorial sicknesses. Since AI procedures depend on solo picking up (distinguishing designs in information without giving any forecasts), they can be extremely valuable for finding new medications as well as customizing drug mixes for explicit cases.

(e) **Clinical Imaging Diagnostics:** AI and deep learning brought us advancement innovation called PC vision. Numerous tech organizations around the globe are presently bustling creating devices that give diagnostics to picture investigation for doctors. As AI calculations become broader and fill in their ability, we will see an expanding number of information sources from different clinical symbolism. For instance, one of the main applications we have seen so far is the examination of skin pictures that plan to recognize skin malignancy. In a few examinations, such devices were demonstrated to be more exact than doctors—they arrived at 87–95% exactness while dermatologists have 65% to 85% precision rate in identifying melanomas.

(f) **Customized Medication**: Medicines are best when they're joined with singular wellbeing factors. That is the reason AI and its prescient investigation segment can assume quite a colossal function in customized medicines. Right now, doctors can browse a restricted arrangement of findings or gauge the danger to their patients based on their suggestive history and accessible hereditary data. Later on, AI instruments will have the option to use quiet clinical history to create different treatment alternatives. We are additionally going to see more gadgets and biosensors with cutting edge wellbeing estimation abilities show up available. They will consider information to turn out to be promptly accessible for ML-based innovations.

(g) **Smart Healthcare Records**: Keeping up and refreshing wellbeing records is a tedious and costly cycle. The facts demonstrate that innovation has assumed a fundamental part in encouraging the information passage measure. Nonetheless, most cycles actually set aside a great deal of effort to finish since they should be done physically. This is the place where AI applications in medical care come in. It vows to save time, cash, and exertion. For example, record characterization strategies that utilization vector machines and AI based OCR acknowledgement are currently showing up available. An illustration of that is Google Cloud Vision Programming interface or Matlab AI based penmanship acknowledgement innovation. Different foundations are currently building up the novel and upcoming age of brilliant wellbeing records that will consolidate ML devices from the beginning to help in the clinical treatment proposals and conclusions.

7 Security and Privacy Issues of Internet of Things and Machine Learning in e-Healthcare

In the past decades, several researchers and scientists have listed or identified several serious issues with Internet of Things or IoT devices [26, 31–37] like security, privacy, limited battery, standardization of IoT gadgets, etc. Now in this section, few other issues in healthcare [34, 38, 39,] can be listed as:

(a) **Dangers of Cyber Attacks on Protection**: Cyber attacks can infuse bogus information into a framework, causing basic harm in IoT applications. It is crucial to give a sufficient degree of insurance against cyber attacks in savvy home applications for the impaired. Notwithstanding, the asset compelling nature of a significant number of IoT gadgets present in a keen home climate doesn't permit actualizing the standard security arrangements. Tajer et al. [40], proposed a structure that ensures location of the cyber attacks and recuperating from them. Diverse controlling specialists, conveyed across the organization, establish the attack location subsystem. Framework recuperation includes iterative nearby handling and message passing. Nguyen et al. [41] proposed another appropriated cyber attack identification calculation, in view of the choice cost minimization methodology. It is indicated that is an appropriate answer for the location of both known and obscure cyber attacks.

(b) **Information Snooping and Information Classification**: For the most part, the wellbeing information of patients, including the handicapped, are held under the lawful commitments of classification, and made accessible just to the approved guardians. It is imperative to keep taking information from capacity or snooping on them while they stream over the remote connections. For instance, a famous IoT-based handicapped glucose checking and insulin conveyance framework uses remote correspondence joins, which are much of the time used to dispatch security attacks. Information listening may harm the patient by penetrating the patient's protection. Li et al. [23] propose moving code cryptographic conventions and body-coupled correspondence moderate the listening in on patient's wellbeing information. Miaou et al. [42] propose a bi-polar numerous base information counselling procedure for pictures, where a pixel esteem distinction between a unique picture and its default JPEG lossy decompressed picture is taken as the number transformation base. The calculation permits stowing away, for example, specialists' advanced seals and PHR inside a still picture. (The specialists' advanced seals are fundamental to the verification of PHR). The still picture could be a logo of a medical clinic distinguishing where the PHR comes from. A demonstrative report and a biomedical sign, for example, an electrocardiogram (ECG), can likewise be covered up in a picture. The proposed approach permits concealing various information types in a similar picture. All this information can be isolated and re-established consummately by the proposed clients. Information privacy can be improved by utilizing Public Key Infrastructure (PKI). PKI makes a viable way to deal with information encryption as it can give significant levels of certainty to trading data in an uncertain climate. Atzori et al. [43] present a calculated plan and a model execution of a framework dependent on IoT passages that total wellbeing sensor information and resolve protection issues through computerized endorsements and PKI information encryption.

(c) **Personality Dangers and Protection of Put away Information**: Loss of a patient's protection, particularly her character information may bring about critical physical, monetary, and enthusiastic mischief to the patient. Slamanig and Stingle present systems for forestalling revelation attacks.

(d) **Location Security**: Location security is worried about area protection dangers and snooping on a client's area. Area protection in WSNs, explicitly concealing the message sender's area, can be accomplished through steering to a haphazardly chosen middle hub. Snooping and following of bundles can be forestalled by the Location Privacy Routing (LPR) convention, which consistently disseminates the bearings of approaching and active traffic at sensor hubs. Apparition single-way steering makes guarantees that bundles arrive at the Base Station (BS) following various ways so that each parcel made by a source follows an alternate irregular way toward the BS.

8 Popular Attacks on Healthcare Systems

Several serious attacks have been identified/mitigated on IoTs and its variant in the previous decade. Few of the attacks (popular) are listed here as:

(a) **Denial of Service Attack (DoS)**: A Denial of Service (DoS) attack is an attack intended to close down a machine or organization, making it blocked off to its expected clients. DoS attacks achieve this by flooding the objective with traffic or sending it data that triggers an accident. In the two examples, the DoS attack denies real clients (for example workers, individuals, or record holders) of the administration or asset they anticipated. Casualties of DoS attacks frequently target web workers of prominent associations, for example, banking, business, and media organizations, or government and exchange associations. Despite the fact that DoS attacks don't normally bring about the robbery or loss of critical data or different resources, they can cost the casualty a lot of time and cash to deal with. Note that there are two general techniques for DoS attacks: flooding administrations or smashing administrations. Flood attacks happen when the framework gets a lot of traffic for the worker to cushion, making them delayed down and ultimately stop [44]. Well known flood attacks include:

- Cushion flood attacks—the most widely recognized DoS attack. The idea is to send more traffic to an organization address than the software engineers have constructed the framework to deal with. It incorporates the attacks recorded underneath, notwithstanding others that are intended to abuse bugs explicit to specific applications or organizations.
- ICMP flood—influences misconfigured network gadgets by sending satirize bundles that ping each PC on the focused organization, rather than only one explicit machine. The organization is then set off to enhance the traffic. This attack is otherwise called the smurf attack or ping of death.
- SYN flood—sends a solicitation to associate with a worker, yet never finishes the handshake. Proceeds until all open ports are soaked with solicitations and none are accessible for authentic clients to associate with.

(b) **Permanent Denial of Service (PDoS)**: A Permanent Denial of Service attack, or a PDoS attack, is forswearing of administration through equipment damage. One strategy for directing a PDoS attack is regularly alluded to as phlashing. During such an attack, an assailant blocks a gadget or annihilates firmware, delivering the gadget or a whole framework pointless. In this situation, the casualty has no other choice than to fix the gadget or purchase another one to reestablish activities. PDoS attacks have been a known opportunity for quite a while, yet these strategies haven't yet picked up footing with programmers. Our accomplice Radware, a main online protection firm, predicts in their 2017 Global Application and Network Security Report that this kind of attack will be on the ascent this year. PDoS attacks can be completed by transferring undermined BIOS to a gadget, or by means of far off organization of the administration interface as a rule. One strategy is to abuse weaknesses to supplant a gadget's essential programming with a bad firmware picture. This technique is the thing that is known as phlashing. PDoS attacks are additionally led actually. For example, an article on Help Net Security highlighted a USB stick alluded to as USB Killer 2.0. This noxious instrument can be connected to any gadget that has a USB interface, including switches, workers and modems. The USB stick utilizes a voltage converter to charge the gadget's capacitors to 220 V and discharges a negative electric flood into the USB port. These floods proceed until the gadget can at this point don't draw power, and certain segments should be supplanted before the gadget can be operable once more. There is a developing worry in the business about the capacity to utilize malware and bots to distantly overheat gadgets, harming them and in any event, setting them ablaze. An aggressor might cost an organization millions by completing a PDoS attack to crash a couple of switches or workers, making their administrations inaccessible until those gadgets could be fixed or supplanted.

(c) **Fingerprint and Timing-based Snooping (FATS)**: Fingerprint and Timing-based Snooping (FATS) attack in which private inhabitant data is gathered from the remote transmissions of sensors in a home, in any event, when the entirety of the transmissions are encoded. This attack would already be able to be completed on a huge number of homes today and will turn out to be more significant as omnipresent processing conditions become more predominant. We address this issue utilizing a setup of security arrangements and contend that protection of observed people should be tended to in all plan layers in future digital actual frameworks.

(d) **Trust Issues in Internet of Things and Machine Learning Applications in Healthcare**: One of the main difficulties looked at by IoT is Data Security and Privacy. IoT empowered cell phones catch information progressively; however, the majority of them need adherence to information conventions and guidelines. There is critical equivocalness with respect to information proprietorship and guidelines. Henceforth, the information put away inside IoT empowered gadgets are inclined to information burglaries and it makes the information more vulnerable to cybercriminals that can hack into the framework to bargain individual wellbeing data. A few instances of abuse of IoT gadget information are deceitful wellbeing claims and the production of phony IDs for purchasing and selling drugs. Because of the non-constancy of information and correspondence conventions, it is hard to total information for fundamental experiences and investigation. IoT gathers information in mass and for legitimate information investigation; the information should be isolated in pieces without over-burdening with exact precision for better outcomes. Over-burdening of information may influence the dynamic cycle in the cordiality area in the more drawn-out run.

(e) **Cyber Physical System (CPS) Involvement in Healthcare**: Cyber Physical System (CPS) is pulling in a ton of consideration lately and is being considered as an arising innovation. It joins calculation and correspondence capacities with the actual world. CPS was recognized as a key examination zone in 2008 by the US National Science Foundation (NSF) and was recorded as the main exploration need by the US President's Council of Advisors on Science and Technology. CPS depends on detecting, preparing, and organizing. The new advances in Wireless Sensor Network (WSN), clinical sensors, and Cloud Computing are making CPS an incredible contender for medical services applications remembering for clinic and in-home patient consideration. These advances guarantee to give CPS the capacity to notice tolerant conditions distantly and make moves paying little heed to the patient's area. Significant examination is being led on clinical sensors. These sensors can gather indispensable patient data containing wellbeing information. Gathered information is shipped off a passage through the remote correspondence medium. Wired sensors can likewise be utilized; nonetheless, remote sensors give greater adaptability and solace to both the parental figure and the patients. The information gathered by the sensors can be put away in a worker and made available to clinicians.

(f) **Medjacking**: In near future, a popular attack on healthcare is medjacking. This attack will be a big threat to healthcare industry in near future, hackers can control hospitals or healthcare devices or machines remotely and as result this attack can cause someone's life. In general, Medjacking is a digital attack on clinical gadgets or the commandeering of biomedical gadgets to make secondary passages in medical clinic organizations to get to programming in the gadget. Numerous clinical gadgets are remote or associated with the web, which makes them especially alluring focuses for programmers. While the Food and Drug Administration (FDA) gives criticism concerning network safety weaknesses of clinical gadgets that are looking for FDA endorsement. Utilizing tainted messages, or malware containing memory sticks in life uphold hardware, programmers access weak clinical gadgets [45]. A demonstrated countermeasure against the medjacking of IoMT and other organization associated gadgets is to send a reason assembled security layer to:

- Distinguish each and every gadget on the arrange and allocate it a personality profile. This makes a forward-thinking and extensive information base or stock of 100% of the biomedical gadgets and hardware.
- Installed each clinical gadget safely utilizing basic components in its profile. This conveys a substantially more granular and secures technique for MAC confirmation to build up and uphold access advantages and limitations.
- Screen the organization to identify any gadget showing unique conduct. Endpoint profiling gives nonstop observation, which is basic to recognize and foil an attack in advancement.

- Authorizing access limitations varying to ruin an endeavoured penetrate. Endpoint and IoMT association security frameworks give a decision of manual and programmed authorization choices to boost clinical gadget security.

Hence, security is an indispensable (or serious) issue here as patient information is secret from lawful and moral perspectives. So, while planning CPS design for medical services applications, uncommon considerations should be paid to guarantee information security. There are additionally various other significant issues to consider, for instance, the prerequisite to store and deal with the enormous volume of information gathered from a large number of clinical sensors. In this manner, information base administration frameworks should be productive and dependable. As clinical information can give valuable understanding into activities (therapies) important to save a patient's life, all information should be promptly accessible and open to approved clinical faculty whenever from any place. What's more, medical care applications require enormous processing assets for canny dynamics dependent on the gigantic patient information. Notwithstanding, the organizations of remote sensors gathering the patient information are seriously compelled in energy, preparation, and capacity limits. They neither have the ability to store huge measures of information nor have the assets needed to handle the information. As CPS innovation is as yet thought to be new, numerous issues are open for future exploration. Ongoing handling, information questions, stockpiling, and security are among those issues. Thus, one of the points of this paper is to show some unanswered inquiries in CPS for medical services, for example, culmination, proficient correspondence, and exact caution age.

9 Existing Methods to Address Security and Privacy Issues

As discussed above sections and in [32, 46, 47], we have reached a statement that Security, Privacy, Trust, etc., issues are a critical issue of IoT, IoMT, and its variant. These issues become more dangerous when they are attached to someone's (human being) personal life. This section discusses several methods that how these serious issues can be overcome or tackle against serious breaches/attacks. Few solutions/methods are discussed here:

(a) **Encryption of Data**: Healthcare information encryption has become a mainstream choice for securing delicate clinical data. Wellbeing information encryption happens when information is changed over into encoded and confused content to make the data distant without an unscrambling key. Encryption ensures quiet wellbeing data when it's sent starting with one client then onto the next. PHI has become an objective of programmers lately, and this information should be protected from unapproved people. In huge associations that license specialists to utilize cell phones and tablets, encryption is a significant method for keeping information secure.

- It permits us to effortlessly follow HIPAA (Health Insurance Portability and Accountability Act) specialized shields for wellbeing information security.
- Encryption makes information safer, regardless of whether it's being moved or very still.
- Encrypted information holds its trustworthiness. In any event, when a programmer attempts to modify it on the way, the beneficiary will realize that it has been undermined.
- It shields patients' private and individual data from burglary.
- It ensures information when clients need to utilize various kinds of gadgets. It tends to be joined with cutting edge confirmation to make the information safer.
- Encryption forestalls exorbitant information breaks. On the off chance that hoodlums access a removable gadget, cell phone, or PC that has touchy data, your office might be punished with gigantic fines.

(b) **Anonymization of Data**: Anonymization of information, additionally called de-distinguishing proof, is a basic bit of the medical services puzzle. It is an information preparing procedure that eliminates or changes actually recognizable data that outcomes in anonymized information that cannot be related to any one person. It allows the sharing of information for auxiliary purposes. Optional reasons for existing are by and large purposes that are not identified with giving patient consideration like examination, general wellbeing, affirmation or accreditation, and showcasing and so on Each contextual analysis was chosen to feature a particular procedure or to disclose how to manage a specific sort of informational index. They depend on our encounters anonymizing several informational indexes, to give expansive inclusion of that region. Anonymization is a cycle that eliminates the relationship between the distinguishing information and the information subject. This is accomplished through veiling and de-ID. There are two unique ways to deal with anonymization

- Masking (no insightful utility): Decreasing the danger of distinguishing an information subject to a little level by applying a bunch of information change procedures with no worry for the insightful utility of the information.
- De-identification (preserving scientific utility): Lessening the danger of distinguishing information subject to a little level by applying a bunch of information change methods with the end goal that the subsequent information holds high scientific utility.

(c) **Access Control Systems**: Access control frameworks in medical services are novel in that they should be fit for confining admittance to delicate territories, forestalling the spread of illness, following and forestalling the robbery of essential medical care gear and medicates, and securing both staff and patients. Accordingly, the sort of emergency clinic access control framework and the particular highlights chosen should address these security concerns. About upholding decides to guarantee that lone approved clients gain admittance to assets in a framework. In medical care frameworks, this implies securing tolerant protection. To forestall the spread of infection, an emergency clinic access control arrangement ought to decrease the quantity of "touch focuses" in an office. Contact focuses are purposes of access where a staff part should genuinely connect with an item to traverse, for example, a handle, push bar. With the beginning of new advances, access control frameworks for emergency clinics presently don't need many touch focuses. Entryway peruses‘ which pursue and confirm an accreditation from a good way eliminate the requirement for contacting keys or keypads. Accreditations could be introduced as a brilliant card that can be utilized for various passageways and can be perused without contact. Medical clinic access control frameworks may likewise be utilized to follow medications and hardware as they are moved from area to area inside a clinic so when a bit of gear is required in a rush, the entrance control framework has, in any event, an unpleasant gauge of its area so clinic staff can discover it rapidly.

10 Conclusion

The IoT can be absolutely an insurgency in the field as significant on the worldwide scale as medical services. There are as yet numerous challenges, characteristics, and innovative obstructions to survive. What's more, despite the fact that there are, as of now, disadvantages just as points of interest to the idea, things appear to go very well for this mechanical development. We are pretty certain that in the event that we get some information about their assessment regarding the matter, they will say that full IoMT joining and variation is the lone sensible method of improvement for cutting edge medication of things to come. As there is tremendous development done in the advances, a few patients are getting more mindful and engaged with the medical care measure. Such upgrades in medical care will prompt making it more usable and secure. A few medical care suppliers can utilize these high likely advances, to upgrade the experience of medical services. And furthermore, it will lessen a few expenses ready and would make them champs in the serious medical care area. Particularly innovations, IoT and ML would make the medical services industry run all the more precisely and without any problem. It assists with making a superior encounter of the patients, likewise with such innovations in medical care. Taking everything into account, everybody would be given legitimate medical care offices. Likewise, it will lessen the immense number of fakes occurring in medical services since all the clinical information would be put away safely. In summary, this work discussed several serious issues like security, privacy and trust in Internet of Things (IoTs) and Machine Learning (ML) based e-healthcare and invite researchers, scientists to work on such issues (or overcome such issues) to make patient/human life's easier and hassle free (privacy preserved, secured and trusted).

References

1. Baker, S., Xiang, W., & Atkinson, I. M. *Internet of things for smart healthcare: Technologies, challenges, and opportunities.* http://www.ieee.org/publications_standards/publications/rights/index.html
2. Riazul Islam, S. M., et al. *The internet of things for health care: A comprehensive survey.* http://www.ieee.org/publications_standards/publications/rights/index.html
3. Darling-Hammond, L., Flook, L., Cook-Harvey, C., & Barron, B. *Implications for educational practice of the science of learning and development.* https://doi.org/10.1080/10888691.2018.1537791
4. Motlagh, N. H., Mohammadrezaei, M., Hunt, J., & Zakeri, B. *Internet of things (IoT) and the energy sector.* IEEE Access 2017.https://doi.org/10.3390/en13020494
5. Atlam, H. F., & Wills, G. *IoT security, privacy, safety and ethics.* Springer Nature Switzerland AG 2020. https://doi.org/10.1007/978-3-030-18732
6. Vazquez et al. (2012). Mhealth—A proposal for using the internet of things concept to increase children's health awareness. *IEEE 2012 22nd international conference on electrical communications and computers (CONIELECOMP)* (pp. 168–172). https://doi.org/10.1109/CONIELECOMP.2012.6189903
7. Vilallonga et al. Transforming a surgical department during the outbreak of new coronavirus pandemic. *Clinical Implications, Langenbeck's Archives of Surgery, 405*(6), 867–875. https://doi.org/10.1007/s00423-020-01931-x
8. Zaragoza et al. (2015). Projected growth of the adult congenital heart disease population in the United States to 2050: An integrative systems modeling approach. *Population Health Metrics, 13*(1), 29. https://doi.org/10.1186/s12963-015-0063-z
9. Lee, B. M., & Ouyang, J. (2014). Intelligent healthcare service by using collaborations between IoT personal health devices. *International Journal of Bio-Science and Bio-Technology, 6*(1), 155–164.
10. Hiremath et al. (2014, January). Wearable internet of things: Concept, architectural components and promises for person-centered healthcare. *International conference on wireless mobile communication and healthcare—Transforming healthcare through innovations in mobile and wireless technologies.* https://doi.org/10.4108/icst.mobihealth.2014.257440
11. Vázquez, et al. (2007). Comparison of body mass index, waist circumference, and waist/hip ratio in predicting incident diabetes: A meta-analysis. PMID: 17494056. *Epidemiologic Reviews, 29*(1), 115–128. https://doi.org/10.1093/epirev/mxm008
12. Kim, et al. (2015). Youth-centered design and usage results of the iN Touch mobile self-management program for overweight/obesity. *Personal and Ubiquitous Computing, 9*, 59–68.
13. Alloghani et al. (2016, April 21–23). A mobile health monitoring application for obesity management and control using the internet-of-things. *Sixth international conference on digital information processing and communications (ICDIPC)* (pp. 19–24).
14. Wibisono, G., & Astawa, I. G. B. (2016). Designing machine-to-machine (M2M) prototype system for weight loss program for obesity and overweight patients. *IEEE 2016 7th international conference on intelligent systems, modelling and simulation (ISMS)* (pp. 138–143). https://doi.org/10.1109/ISMS.2016.5
15. Dobbins et al. (2017). Detecting physical activity within lifelogs towards preventing obesity and aiding ambient assisted living. *Neurocomputing, 230*, 110–132. https://doi.org/10.1016/j.neucom.2016.02.088
16. Shin et al. (2017). Empirical study of the IoT-learning for obese patients that require personal training. *Advances in Computer Science and Ubiquitous Computing, 421*, 1005–1012.
17. Liu, C.-H., et al. (2012). The enhancement of security in healthcare information systems. *Journal of Medical System, 36*, 1673–1688.
18. Paschou, M., et al. (2013). *Health Internet of Things: metrics and methods for efficient data transfer. Simulation Modelling Practice and Theory Elsevier*, 1569–190X.
19. Ziegeldorf, et al. (2014). Privacy in the internet of things: Threats and challenges. *Security and Communication Networks, 7*(12), 2728–2742. https://doi.org/10.1002/sec.795

20. Sawand, et al. (2015). Toward energy-efficient and trustworthy eHealth monitoring system. *China Communications, 12*(1), 46–65. https://doi.org/10.1109/CC.2015.708438
21. Gope et al. (2015). BSN-Care: A Secure IoT-based modern healthcare system using body sensor network. *IEEE Sensors Journal*, 1–1. https://doi.org/10.1109/JSEN.2015.2502401
22. Benssalah, et al. (2016). Dual cooperative RFID-telecare medicine information system authentication protocol for healthcare environments. *Security and Communication Networks*. https://doi.org/10.1002/sec.1665
23. Li et al. (2015). A secure RFID tag authentication protocol with privacy preserving in telecare medicine information system. *Journal of Medical Systems, 39*(8), 77. https://doi.org/10.1007/s10916-015-0260-0
24. Karjagi, R., & Jindal, M. (2016, July). Medical internet of things and big data in healthcare. *Healthcare Informatics Research, 22*(3), 156–163. Published online 2016, July 31. https://doi.org/10.4258/hir.2016.22.3.156
25. Landaluce, H., et al. (2020, May). A review of IoT sensing applications and challenges using RFID and wireless sensor networks. *Sensors (Basel), 20*(9), 2495. Published online 2020 April 28. https://doi.org/10.3390/s20092495
26. Tyagi, A. K., Nair, M. M. (2020). Internet of Everything (IoE) and Internet of Things (IoTs): Threat Analyses, Possible Opportunities for Future. *Journal of Information Assurance & Security (JIAS), 15*(4).
27. Islam, R., et al. (2015). *The internet of things for health care: A comprehensive survey*. IEEE Access, 3, 678–708. https://doi.org/10.1109/ACCESS.2015.2437951
28. Acampora, et al. (2013). A survey on ambient intelligence in healthcare. *Proceedings of the IEEE, 101*(12), 2470–2494. https://doi.org/10.1109/JPROC.2013.2262913
29. Sethi, P., Sarangi, S. R. (2017). Internet of things: Architectures, protocols, and applications. *Journal of Electrical and Computer Engineering*. Article Id: 9324035.
30. Ali, S., et al.(2014, December). Sensors and mobile phones: Evolution and state-of-the-art. *Journal of Science, 66*(4),386–400.
31. Tyagi, A. K., Rekha, G., & Sreenath, N. (2020). Beyond the hype: Internet of things concepts, security and privacy concerns. In S. Satapathy, K. Raju, K. Shyamala, D. Krishna, & M. Favorskaya (Eds.) *Advances in decision sciences, image processing, security and computer vision* (Vol. 3). ICETE 2019. Learning and Analytics in Intelligent Systems. Springer. https://doi.org/10.1007/978-3-030-24322-7_50
32. Siddharth, M. N., Ramesh, V. & Tyagi, A. K. (2021). Issues and challenges (Privacy, security, and trust) in blockchain-based applications. In *Opportunities and challenges for blockchain technology in autonomous vehicles* (p. 14). https://doi.org/10.4018/978-1-7998-3295-9.ch012
33. Reddy, K. S., Agarwal, K., Tyagi, A. K. (2021). Beyond Things: A Systematic Study of Internet of Everything. In: A. Abraham, M. Panda, S. Pradhan, L. Garcia-Hernandez, K. Ma (Eds.) *Innovations in Bio-Inspired Computing and Applications*. IBICA 2019. Advances in Intelligent Systems and Computing, vol 1180. Springer, Cham. https://doi.org/10.1007/978-3-030-49339-4_23.
34. Goyal, D., & Tyagi, A. (2020). A Look at Top 35 Problems in the Computer Science Field for the Next Decade. https://doi.org/10.1201/9781003052098-40.
35. Tyagi, A. K., & Goyal, D. (2020). A Survey of Privacy Leakage and Security Vulnerabilities in the Internet of Things. *In 2020 5th International Conference on Communication and Electronics Systems (ICCES)*, pp. 386–394, https://doi.org/10.1109/ICCES48766.2020.9137886.
36. Tyagi, A. K., & Shamila, M. (March 20, 2019). Spy in the Crowd: How user's privacy is getting affected with the integration of internet of thing's devices. *In Proceedings of International Conference on Sustainable Computing in Science, Technology and Management (SUSCOM), Amity University Rajasthan, Jaipur - India*, February 26–28, 2019.
37. Nair, M. M., Tyagi, A. K., & Sreenath, N. (2021). The Future with Industry 4.0 at the Core of Society 5.0: Open Issues, Future Opportunities and Challenges. *In 2021 International Conference on Computer Communication and Informatics (ICCCI)*, pp. 1–7, https://doi.org/10.1109/ICCCI50826.2021.9402498.

38. Aupetit, M., Fernandez-Luque, L., Singh, M., & Srivastava, J. (2017, June 22–24). Visualization of wearable data and biometrics for analysis and recommendations in childhood obesity. In *Proceedings of the 2017 IEEE 30th international symposium on computer-based medical systems (CBMS)* (pp. 678–679), Thessaloniki, Greece.
39. Nair, M. M., Kumari, S., Tyagi, A. K., & Sravanthi, K. (2021). Deep learning for medical image recognition: open issues and a way to forward. In D. Goyal, A. K. Gupta, V. Piuri, M. Ganzha, & M. Paprzycki (Eds.) *Proceedings of the second international conference on information management and machine intelligence* (Vol. 166). Lecture Notes in Networks and Systems. Springer, Singapore. https://doi.org/10.1007/978-981-15-9689-6_38
40. Tajer, et al. (2019). Non-linear state recovery in power system under bad data and cyber-attacks. *Journal of Modern Power Systems and Clean Energy*. https://doi.org/10.1007/s40565-019-0561-2
41. Nguyen, et al. (2008). A survey of techniques for internet traffic classification using machine learning. *IEEE Communications Surveys & Tutorials, 10*, 56–76.
42. Miaou, S. G., et al. (2000). A secure data hiding technique with heterogeneous data-combining capability or electronic patient records. *Proceeding of the 22nd annual EMBS international conference* (Vol. 1, pp. 280–283).
43. Atzori, et al. (2012). The social internet of things (SIoT)—when social networks meet the internet of things: Concept, architecture and network characterization. *Computer Networks, 56*(16), 3594–3608.
44. Carl, G., et al. (2006, January–February). Denial-of-service attack-detection techniques. *IEEE Internet Computing, 10*(1), 82–89. https://doi.org/10.1109/MIC.2006.5
45. Adashi, E. Y., & Thomasian, N. M. (2020). Medical devices in Harm's Way: Medjacking. *JAMA Health Forum*. https://doi.org/10.1001/jamahealthforum.2020.0007
46. Shamila, M., Vinuthna, K., & Tyagi, A. (2019). *A review on several critical issues and challenges in IoT based e-healthcare system*. 1036–1043. https://doi.org/10.1109/ICCS45141.2019.9065831
47. Tyagi, A. K., Nair, M. M., Niladhuri, S., & Abraham, A. (2020). Security, privacy research issues in various computing platforms: A survey and the road ahead. *Journal of Information Assurance & Security*, *15*(1), 1–16, 16p.

Future of Intelligent System in Healthcare and Other Sectors

Industry 4.0: A Revolution in Healthcare Sector via Cloud, Fog Technologies

Gillala Rekha and Jasti Yashaswini

Objective: The main objective of this paper is to provide cutting-edge technologies for addressing the problems encountered in healthcare sector.

Motivation: This paper provides a detail study on various technologies such as Internet of things (IoT), cloud computing, fog computing and big data facilitating health sector.

1 Introduction

Health care is now becoming one of the world's tedious social as well as economic hurdles. There is a pressure on healthcare sectors due to the increase in world's population and for a better quality of life. This led to advanced technological applications where the information and communication systems (ICTs) have shown a positive impact on healthcare mechanisms [1]. Since then, the word eHealth (application of ICTs to healthcare) came into wide usage and brought in huge investments for its development. Recently, the proposed Industry 4.0 manifests the fourth industrial revolution that integrates with data processing intelligence with a focus on consumer requirements and control over the product lifecycle. The word "Industry 4.0" originated in Germany in 2011 [2, 3].

In healthcare sectors, ideas of Industry 4.0 comprise of automation of manual processes and data, clinical trial digitization. However, these facilities still present challenges. If we look into the technological view of Industry 4.0, the emphasis is on the notion of cyber-physical systems or CPS and counts on three technology classes (pillars) [4]: The model of the Internet of things (IoT) (unique handling of

G. Rekha (✉) · J. Yashaswini
Department of Computer Science and Engineering, Koneru Lakshmaiah Educational Foundation, Hyderabad, India
e-mail: gillala.rekha@klh.edu.in

A. K. Tyagi et al. (eds.), *Intelligent Interactive Multimedia Systems for e-Healthcare Applications*, https://doi.org/10.1007/978-981-16-6542-4_16

collaborating artifacts with devices, such as cell phones, sensors, and actuators); cloud and fog computing (providing virtually big data analytics to derive value from complicated volumes of data); limitless processing, storage, and communication services as utilities, i.e., on-demand and pay-per-use. The worldwide efforts and technological developments tell us that healthcare industry is growing and eHealth is moving to healthcare [5]. Health 4.0 enables real-time technologies that maximize resources and reduce deterioration of patient health. These are becoming pertinent accounting safety management impacts. To meet the needs of consumers, Health 4.0 opens up opportunities for collaboration with stakeholders sharing delivery and development strategies in an agile and effective way.

This paper structure is as follows. Section 2 incorporates the introduction of health sector and its convergence with Healthcare 4.0. Brief description of each pillar is with its contributions to HC4.0 in Sect. 3. Reviewing of major application use cases by HC4.0 in Sect. 4. Challenges of the ICT pillars for HC4.0 in Sect. 5. Section 6 draws the conclusions.

2 Health Sector-Industry Technologies 4.0

The health sector has been impelled to a great extent by various technical advancements. Various practices of medical and public health assisted by smart mobile devices, intelligent healthcare, and medical services using information technology can be observed in the literature ranges [6, 7]. Innovative actives like robots, sensors, and many more are identified to be the best medical services as they offer alternatives to the medical support. Some of the developments are related to the Internet of things (IoT) and cloud computing (CC) [8]. Additionally, they will interconnect with cyber-physical frameworks and sensors, communication and processing tools and technologies that fetch in decision-making to deliver reliable and prominent data.

With the interconnection of hospitals, optimized time, individuals and structures have real complexities and are self-sorted out concerning the state of the patient. New ideal models for occupational wellbeing and security management can be set up by Industry 4.0 developments as more secure hardware is needed for working and workplaces and activities with better monitoring and management. In [7], the author proposed computational intelligence that involves simulations of genes and proteins linked to cancer growth and immunity, which is another technology that can advance the disclosure of regions that cannot be easily reached by regular methods for medication. In addition, classification 4.0 utilizations the adaptability of innovation as a method of activity.

3 ICT Pillars for Healthcare 4.0 (HC4.0)

In developing nations, the unavoidable presence of remote and versatile innovations, the accessibility of low cost, advance remote sensors, and the cost-efficient services by hardware infrastructures have permitted new medical care offices, or new norms of value and cost-adequacy in the foundation. The increasing accessibility and nature of clinical programming applications are models driven by the fuse of mobile devices into clinical applications. The meaning of P4 medicine [9], predictive, preventive, personalized, and participatory, is an image of the basic move in medication by these new technological advancements. Rather than clustering patients into care classes, this technique is executed to significantly reduce worldwide health costs, for example, diminishing hospitalization and dispensing with the unnecessary or exorbitant use of medications and procedures.

These advances originate from the enormous scope of ICTs, and we will focus on three basic empowering influences among them in this section, which we name Healthcare 4.0 pillars for their noteworthiness: IoT, cloud computing, fog computing, and big data. Of these, the 5G environment, whose necessities and innovative solutions are as yet being set up and explored widely, plays a significant role. Figure 1 presents the four ICT pillars for Healthcare 4.0.

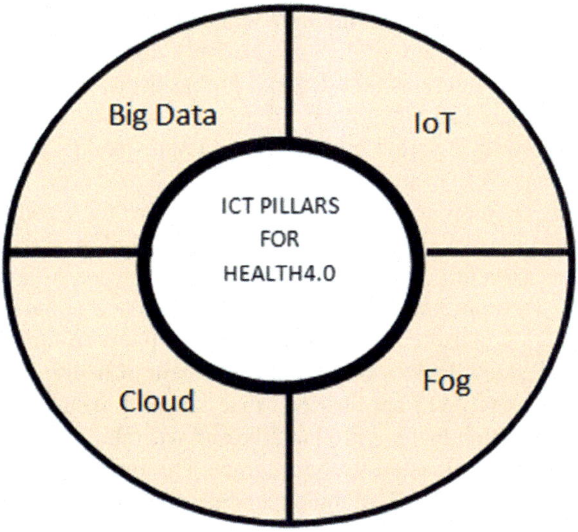

Fig. 1 Four important ICT pillars for Health 4.0

3.1 HC4.0 and Internet of Things

International Telecommunication Union (ITU) provides a general vision of the IoT as the transition from anywhere connectivity for anything that initially concentrates on digital identification and machine-to-machine (M2 M) communications.

IoT-based objects like RFID and wireless sensor networks (WSNs) that share some strict details regarding adaptability, power utilization, and processing abilities [6, 10, 11] have a large scope of understandings especially in medical care. Wireless body area networks (WBANs) comprise of wireless instruments (sensors and actuators) associated with the human body. The new IoT vision, when applied to industry (e.g. creation measures), covers altogether with Industry 4.0. Indeed, this can be viewed beyond IoT, either by including various architectures with logistics and production subtleties or, alternately, by adding IoT advances to previously existing ones. The robotized strategies came up, because of an assortment of emerging challenges and opportunities.

Healthcare has been demonstrated to be one of the most alluring IoT application domains. With various technical, economic, and social prospects, IoT is helping modern healthcare reshape the progress of the model that contributes in overall decrease in the cost and increases patient outcomes. Advancement in wireless technologies with efficient enhancements supports tracking of physiological parameters, thereby promoting uninterrupted chronic disease treatment and early diagnosis along with the emergency medical management. Sensor gadgets for clinical, diagnostic, and imaging are vital to productively utilize IoT in the health sector. IoT helps in various situations that demand proper decision making where in smart devices can communicate with others to get new information and understand both users and the world. Inspired by the IoT paradigms and its peculiarities, wearable Internet of things (WIoT) aims to include telehealth to achieve automated treatments. Additionally, to improve the quality of life of individuals, body-worn sensors of WIoT can be used to track data on a regular basis and link it to the patient's records and medical infrastructure.

The combination of cell phones is the basis of the Internet of health things (IoHT) [12]. A sensored medical device in support of applications, wearable's and other embedded devices help in improvement of health, whereas the Internet of Medical Things (IoMT) applications that can be linked to our gadgets like cell phone or smartwatch that are implantable and wearable. These gadgets act as a private hub as they are connected to the Internet. The Internet of nanothings (IoNT) involves the application of IoT in nanomedicine, the usage of proactive observation, preventive health, and chronic disease management and thereby fetches in personalizing the surveillance, diagnosis, and treatment mechanisms. A networking model is envisaged by the Internet of mobile health things (m-IoT) [13]. Between low-power individual zone organizations and rising 4G network, focusing on the special qualities that are characteristic for worldwide versatility.

3.2 HC4.0 and Cloud and Fog Computing

"Cloud computing" (or "Cloud") is an idea that permits "utility computing" with minimal interaction with the provider, for example, renting of computing resources in real time. Cloud thus simplifies operation because it does not entail careful dimensioning and planning of the necessary resources, allowing short-term pay-per-use billing without the user's immediate commitment [14]. Users are able to either exploit or offer anything as a service with the help of varied number of on-demand tools. Few such services are: Infrastructure, Network, or Software-as-a-Service (IaaS, PaaS, and SaaS, respectively), with additional variants such as Function-as-a-Service (also known as "serverless computing").

Specifically, to satisfy various IoT needs to the extent that it is proposed; cloud plays a vital role as it is also in the upper layers of IoT. The ongoing migration to cloud services is motivated by a trend that has emerged in the last decade: That is, the expansion of features embedded in field devices that have provided them more information and versatility [15]. This permits those capacities to be moved to the cloud, with the related adaptability and responsiveness (and inevitably economic) gains.

Many challenges and shortcomings have arisen over the years relating to connectivity between the end computer and the cloud service hosting datacenter. Latency, bandwidth, cost, and link availability all contribute to limiting the number of uses in cloud computing. This phenomenon has further improved the emergence of ubiquitous mobile devices, strongly threatening the cloud model. Indeed, the cloud does not fulfill all the requirements of several applications in many contexts, especially for healthcare, resulting in the need for a new architecture. For the solutions, various ideas, words, and expressions have been coined [16].

Fog computing on the other hand recommends that some cloud computing assets be moved to the edge network, close to client gadgets and most likely halfway dependent on them also. Device resources for users, thereby sharing the load between end devices and conventional cloud datacenters, offering local-term stability, low latency rates and faster responsiveness, among other, helping to increase the entire system's performance scalability [17]. Cloud-related problems like cost overheads, delay, and jitter when moving information to the cloud can be mitigated to a great extent with the use of fog computing. Moreover, it also increases on-time services. Aspects like user versatility, heterogeneity of resources, interfaces, and distributed data analytics are supported by fog computing that helps in meeting the requirements of low latency distributed applications. To achieve the decentralized and smart processing of unparalleled IoT sensor data volumes deployed to integrate physical data, fog computing serves as a powerful paradigm.

In this sense, Carnegie Mellon University introduced the concept of cloudlet [18], referring to a middle level (between the mobile computer and the conventional cloud): the cloudlet is a self-managed "datacenter in a box," a minicloud with ample resources to simultaneously host workloads for a handful of mobile users.

Suppressing integration costs and maximizing the resources are the major advantages of cloud computing. In the sense of health care, the introduction of cloud technology has been called Healthcare-as-a-Service (HaaS). In addition to the general applications, HaaS applications have advantages of scalable, on-demand, and practically unlimited computing, storage, and networking paradigm as they are integrated with the cloud facilities. Additionally, features like ease of data sharing, ease of data collection and integration and, in some cases, improved performance, usability, reliability, and security are very important. Cloud and fog computing enhance the use of mobile and PC technology by helping to handle digital data development and requests for medical services anywhere and anytime. Usability and communication latency can be serious problems can be a huge problem as many smart devices and artifacts are increasingly part of the everyday life of patients and physicians. The change in quality of service can also be observed with the change in impact predictability, interrupt decision-making processes, and potentially undermine the provision of healthcare services.

User-friendly and customized services and adaptive service management efficiency can be achieved by mobile cloud that can also solve the above problems. Summing up, cloud, fog, and mobile edge computing play a huge part in Healthcare 4.0, with positive effects on the headway of both medical services exploration and administrations, thereby improving proficiency, making them open for a more extensive number of individuals than presently conceivable, and improving patient results.

3.3 HC4.0 and Big Data

The word big data has a much wider scope and meaning lot more extensive degree and significance. Over the time, the accentuation has moved from the attributes of datasets corresponding to current technologies (datasets that, as per the necessary scope, couldn't be recorded, taken care of and handled by broad PCs inside a sensible scope). Apache Hadoop technology intends to extract data economically from exceptionally enormous amounts by permitting fast recording, discovery, or analysis [19]. The biggest and most normal arrangement of big data-related properties depend on five Vs. (I) volume (increments in information scale); (ii) speed (assortment and examination are liable as far as possible); (iii) assortment (information comprises of various structures, for example, organized, unstructured, and semi-organized information); (iv) veracity (information has fluctuating degrees of reliability dependent on provenance, the board and handling); (v) esteem (entire engineering of information) [20]. This 5-V portrayal illustrates big data's strong context-dependent existence, which is inherently characterized according to specific applications.

Over the most recent years, these particular requests that challenge the available advancements in technologies by recognizing big data have prodded significant development over data processing strategies and resources. We refer to [21] for a generally technological analysis of the advancement of big data in Industry 4.0.

Generally, big data and related ideas are inferred in various points of view and enormously being used for Healthcare 4.0 applications. It is absolutely essential to know about the broad scope of accessible data sources to comprehend the use of big data applied to Healthcare 4.0. In a perspective, all of Industry 4.0 can be viewed as an endeavor to advance such ideal contribution back into the design–production–delivery cycle from data collection. Social media are reshaping the essence of health-related experiences for what is exclusively worried about the health domain, moving the manner in which medical services experts' survey.

The increasing access to social networking sites and feeds, social media and online discussion forums brought in a huge change in the medical practice. Business data is emerging its significance in Industry 4.0. High volumes of data are already generated and handled by businesses: in addition to internal accounting, employee data, and internal communications. There are additionally rules on data custody specifications that extend out to medical care, and this kind of data enriches the scope of potential sources empowering research that does not solely cover biological and medical angles. This is just expected to increase in Industry 4.0, because of the focus on far-reaching information stream control, upgraded information sources, and metadata. This would add to outer information originating from outside the association (e.g., from outside the area), requesting increasingly more reception and progression of big data innovation from sold merchandise, purchasers, and from providers/accomplices. The advancement of innovation has gotten further increment information. In actuality, stream preparing frameworks track the wellbeing status of individuals progressively, delivering huge volumes of organized and unstructured streamed information on account of the quick and significant market infiltration of individual gadgets and the achievement of portable contact and remote sensors innovation.

Additionally, clinical studies, photographs, and explanations from doctors add to clinical patient data, which is assembled by documents that may take different forms and categories, for example, electronic health records (EHR); electronic medical records (EMR); personal health records (PHR). EHR is intended to report scenes of treatment through different organizations conveying care. EMRs are real-time patient health records with access to evidence-based decision support assets, likely used to help decision-making clinicians. PHR is a justifiable, lifetime strategy for handling explicit health information, empowering wellbeing maintenance, and assisting with controlling chronic diseases and is typically taken care of uniquely in contrast to EHR and EMR by means of patients.

Furthermore, scientific literature is still an important source of biomedical knowledge [22] (although there is a growing availability of organized resources). User search and retrieve-related publications can be made fast and more efficient with the help of dedicated web text mining software for indexing and cataloguing. Immense amounts of biological data in different forms like genomics and microbiomics are currently produced and collected, thereby making it possible to classify this data into four levels, namely molecular-level data, tissue-level data, patient-level data, and population-level data.

4 Use Cases: HC4.0 Application Scenarios

One of the sectors supporting the vision of Industry 4.0 is healthcare. In reality, IoT is leveraged in all its facets for remote monitoring, thus enabling the implementation of health care in different contexts, ranging from long-term elderly treatment to home security for urgent care [15, 23]. New technologies are required to extract the volumes of data being generated. IoT, cloud and fog technologies and big data are helping in new strategies providing good results reducing long-term care. They offer architectures that perform discovery and analysis to tackle and renew healthcare practices. In this section, the important application scenarios in healthcare allowed by these three ICT pillars and their integration are discussed.

4.1 Physiological and Pathological Signs Tracking

The study indicates how the IoT paradigm, along with the accessibility of on-request cloud and fog services with big data innovations, upholds the advancement made in mobile communication technologies just as wearable's and sensing gadgets to help inescapable monitoring applications[24]. The resulting system encourages the compilation of health data and potentially offers statistical information on health problems. The provision of new forms of cloud services that can supplement or complement existing hospital information systems. This form of automated approach means that the probability of errors is significantly reduced as compared to approaches requiring manual intervention [25].

(i) sensing and data collection hardware's to collect physiological and movement data; (ii) communication hardware and data transfer software to a remote center; (iii) data analysis techniques to extract physiological and movement data from clinically relevant information are the major three components that contribute in the remote monitoring systems for patients.

Continuous tracking of patient's psychological and physical conditions can be achieved by adopting advanced medical and environmental sensors like accelerometers and gyroscopes, temperature and humidity sensors, as well as sensors for ECG, glucose, blood pressure, and gas. This information can be sent to far-off and remote data centers by IoT devices, where information incorporation can be performed to exploit apparently infinite storage, scalable computing power, and high accessibility of services offered by cloud automation.

Besides, this strategy needs a protected network interface for remote storage processing and recovery of cloud clinical records. In fact, health monitoring is the one recorded under super-reliable communication necessities among the significant situations driving 5 G communication infrastructure development.

Fog computing uses smart gateways to provide services such as embedded data mining, distributed storage, and notification to overcome these obstacles to enhance health monitoring systems [26]. Network edge service will mitigate the challenges of implementing remote cloud services. In order to strengthen and restore human functions such as pacemakers to activate the heart muscle, deep brain stimulation system [27, 28]. Fog-based designs are needed to pave a path to assist medical devices with being embedded in human bodies.

4.2 *Self-management, Tracking of Wellbeing, and Prevention*

Self-management solutions are supported by Healthcare 4.0 in a significant manner. Big data innovations are also facilitating a change from cure to prevention [29], which is likewise one of the characteristics presented by P4 medication. Solutions that incorporate algorithms to help in the prevention of diseases by identifying modifiable risk factors and strategy development to enhance healthy behavior have been made to build intelligent services beyond basic tasks that can provide individuals with an effective input based on the observations of the researchers.

Another most significant example is self-help for wellbeing in chronic disease. For instance, these structures may provide guidelines for teaching and motivating healthy dietary habits [30, 31] and organizing exercise programs with regard to the management and prevention of diabetes and obesity.

4.3 *Monitoring of Drug Intake and Smart Pharmaceuticals*

On account of cognitive disorders, resistance to medication is predominant in elderly and chronically disabled individuals and will exasperate. Additionally, these programs are a significant strategy for disease management physicians since they offer a quantitative method to measure the achievement of treatment. Various smartphone applications are available with advanced features like alert scheduling, prescription notification, and dosage guidelines based on delivery timing in drug treatment and also consumption tracking to achieve maximum efficacy and reduce unfavorable impacts.

Advanced innovations are frequently provided, e.g., comprising of wearable or ingestible sensors, just as coordinated IoT communication and insight [32]. In this specific circumstance, smart pharmaceuticals are classified as smart value-added electronic packages, distribution frameworks or pills (e.g., through wireless connection with a web empowered PC or direct web communication allows communication to a remote machine with an ability to compile, store, and analyze the data). An assortment of micro- and macro-level metadata skilled to give new insights of knowledge into sickness, help administration plan, and to advance customized medical care by future smart drugs/pharmaceuticals.

4.4 Healthcare Customization

The aim of personalized healthcare is to be user-centered, i.e., to make patient-specific decisions (rather than stratifying patients into traditional treatment groups) [33]. It is important to collect data from different sources (e.g., from both patients and the environment), as similar data collection promotes decision-making and delivery of health and social care.

Typical sources of sensors or therapy delivery systems may be wearable (or even implantable micro- and nanotechnologies), such as fall alarms, implantable insulin pumps, and defibrillator vests. These features are characteristic of the Industry 4.0 vision (namely, user centrality and data convergence from various heterogeneous sources, including wearable devices, to deliver highly customized services). They clearly characterize Healthcare 4.0 when viewed under the framework of P4 medicine, which depends mainly on each individual's genetic knowledge. Big data analytics is therefore essential for the introduction of personalized healthcare, both at the level of the individual and the population [34].

4.5 Health Information Systems Based on the Cloud

In order to enhance the improvement and simplification of design, creation, and implementation of information systems for medical record collection, processing, and sharing hospital administrative information, or medical images, cloud architecture has been adopted on a larger scale.

These architectures help to strengthen the process of data collection. Additionally, it is also useful to share across various medical structures. Many formats of data can be incorporate into these systems. However, in few scenarios queries relating to machine efficiency are taken into consideration. The design of these systems also focuses on issues of security and privacy, both of which are regarded as important.

4.6 Telepathology, Telemedicine, and Control of Illnesses

The first significant attempts at functional telepathology like the remote collection, transmission, and examination of pathology specimens, which are from the early 1980s, when robotic microscopy, video imaging, databases, and broadband telecommunications were incorporated. As many contributions are accessible today [35, 36], this pledge has proved real, demonstrating how ICTs help a multitude of various applications related to telemedicine, telepathology, and disease monitoring. The research can be divided into two categories: (i) generic structures, applicable to the vast majority of cases; (ii) studies focusing on particular diseases, such as cancer detection, cardiovascular disease, diabetes, Parkinson's, and Alzheimer's.

In turn, these tracking systems can be implemented both to feed large-scale trials and to advise interventions customized to the particular individual's outcomes (as in the P4 medicine approach). Surgery, too, is expected to become more straightforward in the future. Indeed, for open surgery, video cameras are also built into operating room lighting. The surgical operation thus becomes theoretically noticeable to a huge number of observers. These instruments allow for teleconsultation to bypass the consultant's physical presence. Telepresence can take place if an active camera holder is used during a surgery. The final result of this application scenario is telesurgery, where the surgeon and surgeon's cockpit are geographically separate from the operations room.

The accessibility to restricted virtual paths to fog networks at the edge will facilitate in filling this void, as best-effort Internet connections are not adequate to accommodate many types of applications. For example, it may allow remote federated sites to collaborate on non-trivial diagnoses, such as providing software to unload complex image processing and data mining tasks without experiencing greater delays in accessing the cloud.

5 Challenges

5.1 IoT

Energy: In simple terms, IoT in the medical services domain and health sector is in its early stages. Taking into account that IoT comprises of interconnected smart objects, the engineering of both smart devices and communication technology is mainly concerned with issues. A significant technological challenge is energy. Surely, research on energy harvesting, energy storage, energy utilization is needed to plan and fabricate zero-entropy frameworks that separate energy from the environment and don't waste any energy in operations.

Scalability: Another serious issue to be handled is adaptability, which is intensified by the specific area. Certainly, interconnected curios would outnumber those that make up the traditional Internet by numerous significant orders and medical care services are ordinarily portrayed by popularity. Consequently, architecture versatility is among the drastic acceleration of the associated gadgets and devices.

Security: Likewise, more exploration is expected to create and design suitable projects. IoT security solutions, for example, natives that are resistant to runtime attacks and adaptable security protocols. As of today, IoT frameworks, especially while tending to adaptability prerequisites, are not adequately upgraded to meet the necessary functional necessities and endure security and protection hazards. Current security advancements are lacking as they do not scale with restricted resources and real-time requirements to broad networks of heterogeneous gadgets and cyber-physical frameworks. Likewise, enormous data is constantly delivered as sensors monitor health signals (regularly taking care of important applications), steady and efficient frameworks are required for organizations in Industry 4.0 to deal with big data.

Scientific literature demonstrates how a comprehensive cybersecurity architecture covering all abstraction layers of heterogeneous systems and across platform boundaries needs to protect IoT [37]. Additionally, connected healthcare devices (e.g., wearables) are developed that may be at risk of hacking and which will require safe management of uniqueness and authentication. Therefore, it is an important necessity to develop lightweight algorithms to secure data as resource-constrained devices commonly adopted in the healthcare sectors.

5.2 Cloud and Fog Computing

One of the key cloud issues is urgent to its tendency: It offers alluring costs to its as-a-service facilities by veiling the real framework, sparing the cloud client from dealing with cloud resource-related tasks information, and offering economies of scale grade costs.

Cloudiness of the infrastructure: The insignificance of technology may become a constraint even though they are the desired properties of cloud computing when efficiency is concerned. In reality, computing performance, communication protocol efficiency, network latency (e.g., due to low bandwidth and volatile latencies when large traffic volumes are transferred) are still barriers [38].

Performance monitoring: Additionally, while cloud technologies are considered to be scalable, the scalability of the deployed solutions is a common for an overview of problems and strategies in cloud status and performance management; accordingly, research has also focused on the performance of public cloud networks with the growing adoption of systems deployed through public clouds. According to the above considerations, co-design approaches involving various stakeholders, particularly those in network / performance engineering positions, must be taken into account in the handling and troubleshooting of service performance when dealing with data-intensive applications.

Data privacy: More extensively, cloud and fog computing solutions permit applications to deal with information from clients on third-party hardware and software, due to which data privacy concerns. These issues originate from the problem of losing control of information because of the restricted trust in the supplier liable for putting away exceptionally sensitive data in its framework. Some suggestions for addressing these problems have recently been suggested, e.g., [39] proposes an identity management architecture that enables selected recipients to have patient-controlled partial EHR disclosure, thereby making this an open and hot area of study.

Infrastructure availability: However, the solutions offered are increasingly taking advantage of external resources as a substitute for in-house solutions, as the former are often fitted with sophisticated security settings (e.g., they implement proper encryption algorithm). In addition, these services provide improved flexibility, helping to provide minimal downtime for uninterrupted delivery.

5.3 Big Data

The gigantic measure of healthcare-related data meets the standards (with respect to volume, speed, and variety) to be considered as big data because of its qualities. One of the main difficulties for Healthcare 4.0 is the variability of sources, designs; information attributes (a case of the huge data variety) among its peculiarities.

Jirkovsky et al. [40] concentrated on heterogeneity in semantics and suggested a structure to facilitate interoperability. Tracking is of the utmost importance in many medical conditions has increased the speed of mounting data, in regard to the traditional data. Additionally, the volume is increasing and demanding suitable solutions to store huge and larger volumes of data. Considering that the results of big data analytics do not have error and are precise, these techniques give a problem of opacity that is most important when we take into consideration health, decisions that are related to life and social issues, due to the new use of machine-learning algorithms on unknown quantities of healthcare data.

6 Conclusion

This paper focuses on providing an overview of the healthcare sector pertinent to Industry 4.0. The concepts of Industry 4.0 leading to health innovations such as data digitization, effective databases, and health should be enacted in the healthcare sector. Cloud computing, big data, and IoT facilitate connectivity between devices and health services. Additionally, health practitioners trying to better understand Health 4.0-related meanings and principles are also presenting a report on the subject to researchers and stakeholders. The Elucidation of the results was concentrated and important, structured, as far as possible. This is done to understand Industry 4.0, given its relevance and relevance in the healthcare sector, which is necessary for the integration of hospitals, people, and systems to provide real dynamics with time getting optimal and self-organized in relation to the patient conditions.

References

1. Chatterjee, S., Chakraborty, S., Sarker, S., Sarker, S., & Lau, F. Y. (2009). Examining the success factors for mobile work in healthcare: A deductive study. *Decision Support Systems, 46*(3), 620–633.
2. Aceto, G., Persico, V., & Pescapé, A. (2020). Industry 4.0 and health: Internet of things, big data, and cloud computing for healthcare 4.0. *Journal of Industrial Information Integration, 18*, 100129.
3. Xu, L. D., Xu, E. L., & Li, L. (2018). Industry 4.0: State of the art and future trends. *International Journal of Production Research, 56*(8), 2941–2962.

4. Kim, J. H. (2017). A review of cyber-physical system research relevant to the emerging IT trends: Industry 4.0, IoT, big data, and cloud computing. *Journal of Industrial Integration and Management, 2*(03), 1750011.
5. Elhoseny, M., Abdelaziz, A., Salama, A. S., Riad, A. M., Muhammad, K., & Sangaiah, A. K. (2018). A hybrid model of internet of things and cloud computing to manage big data in health services applications. *Future generation computer systems, 86*, 1383–1394.
6. Elhoseny, M., Ramírez-González, G., Abu-Elnasr, O. M., Shawkat, S. A., Arunkumar, N., & Farouk, A. (2018). Secure medical data transmission model for IoT-based healthcare systems. *IEEE Access, 6*, 20596–20608.
7. Farahani, B., Firouzi, F., Chang, V., Badaroglu, M., Constant, N., & Mankodiya, K. (2018). Towards fog-driven IoT eHealth: Promises and challenges of IoT in medicine and healthcare. *Future Generation Computer Systems, 78*, 659–676.
8. Maguluri, L. P., Srinivasarao, T., Syamala, M., Ragupathy, R., & Nalini, N. (2018). Efficient smart emergency response system for fire hazards using IoT. *International Journal of Advanced Computer Science and Applications (IJACSA), 9*(1), 314–320.
9. Hood, L., & Flores, M. (2012). A personal view on systems medicine and the emergence of proactive P4 medicine: Predictive, preventive, personalized and participatory. *New Biotechnology, 29*(6), 613–624.
10. Wu, T., Wu, F., Redoute, J. M., & Yuce, M. R. (2017). An autonomous wireless body area network implementation towards IoT connected healthcare applications. *IEEE access, 5*, 11413–11422.
11. Achanta, S. D. M., & Karthikeyan, T. (2019). A wireless IOT system towards gait detection technique using FSR sensor and wearable IOT devices. *International Journal of Intelligent Unmanned Systems.*
12. Rodrigues, J. J., Segundo, D. B. D. R., Junqueira, H. A., Sabino, M. H., Prince, R. M., Al-Muhtadi, J., & De Albuquerque, V. H. C. (2018). Enabling technologies for the internet of health things. *IEEE Access, 6*, 13129–13141.
13. AlMotiri, S. H., Khan, M. A., & Alghamdi, M. A. (2016). August. Mobile health (m-health) system in the context of IoT. In *2016 IEEE 4th International Conference on Future Internet of Things and Cloud Workshops (FiCloudW)* (pp. 39–42). IEEE.
14. Kuo, M. H. (2011). Opportunities and challenges of cloud computing to improve health care services. *Journal of medical Internet research, 13*(3), e67.
15. Soumya, I., Zia Ur Rahman, M., Rama Koti Reddy, D. V., & Lay-Ekuakille, A. (2015). Efficient block processing of long duration biotelemetric brain data for health care monitoring. *Review of Scientific Instruments, 86*(3), 035003.
16. Rolim, C. O., Koch, F. L., Westphall, C. B., Werner, J., Fracalossi, A., Salvador, G. S. (2010). A cloud computing solution for patient's data collection in health care institutions. In *2010 Second International Conference on eHealth, Telemedicine, and Social Medicine* (pp. 95–99). IEEE.
17. Rahmani, A. M., Gia, T. N., Negash, B., Anzanpour, A., Azimi, I., Jiang, M., & Liljeberg, P. (2018). Exploiting smart e-Health gateways at the edge of healthcare Internet-of-Things: A fog computing approach. *Future Generation Computer Systems, 78*, 641–658.
18. Satyanarayanan, M. (2013) Cloudlets: At the leading edge of cloud-mobile convergence. In *Proceedings of the 9th International ACM Sigsoft Conference on Quality of Software Architectures* (pp. 1–2).
19. Raghupathi, W., & Raghupathi, V. (2014). Big data analytics in healthcare: Promise and potential. *Health information science and systems, 2*(1), 3.
20. Lohr, S. (2012). The age of big data. New York Times, 11.
21. Lee, J., Kao, H. A., & Yang, S. (2014). Service innovation and smart analytics for industry 4.0 and big data environment. *Procedia Cirp, 16*(1), 3–8.
22. Walsh, K., & Wroe, C. (2020). Mobilising computable biomedical knowledge: challenges for clinical decision support from a medical knowledge provider. *BMJ Health & Care Informatics, 27*(2), e100121.

23. Salman, M. N., Rao, P. T., & Rahman, M. Z. U. (2017). Cardiac signal enhancement using normalised variable step algorithm for remote healthcare monitoring systems. *International Journal of Medical Engineering and Informatics, 9*(2), 145–161.
24. Habib, C., Makhoul, A., Darazi, R., & Salim, C. (2016). Self-adaptive data collection and fusion for health monitoring based on body sensor networks. *IEEE Transactions on Industrial Informatics, 12*(6).
25. Yuehong, Y., Zeng, Y., Chen, X., & Fan, Y. (2016). The internet of things in healthcare: An overview. *Journal of Industrial Information Integration, 1.*
26. Jovanov, E., & Milenkovic, A. (2011). Body area networks for ubiquitous healthcare applications: opportunities and challenges. *Journal of Medical Systems, 35*(5).
27. Barua, M., Liang, X., Lu, R., & Shen, X. (2011). Espac: Enabling security and patientcentric access control for ehealth in cloud computing. *International Journal of Security and Networks, 6*(2–3).
28. Kulkarni, P., & Ozturk, Y. (2011). mphasis: Mobile patient healthcare and sensor information system. *Journal of Network and Computer Applications, 34*(1).
29. Ramesh, D., Suraj, P., & Saini, L. (2016). Big data analytics in healthcare: A survey approach. In 2016 *International Conference on Microelectronics, Computing and Communications (MicroCom).* IEEE.
30. Vicini, S., Bellini, S., Rosi, A., & Sanna, A. (2012). An internet of things enabled interactive totem for children in a living lab setting. In *2012 18th International ICE Conference on Engineering, Technology and Innovation*, June 2012.
31. Vazquez-Briseno, M., Navarro-Cota, C., Nieto-Hipolito, J. I., Jimenez-Garcia, E., & Sanchez-Lopez, J. D. (2012). A proposal for using the internet of things concept to increase children's health awareness. In *CONIELECOMP 2012, 22nd International Conference on Electrical Communications and Computers*, Feb 2012.
32. Moh, M., Ho, L., Walker, Z., & Moh, T.-S. (2008). A prototype on rfid and sensor networks for elder health care. In *RFID handbook: Applications, technology, security, and privacy*, 17.
33. Viceconti, M., Hunter, P., & Hose, R. (2015). Big data, big knowledge: Big data for personalized healthcare. *IEEE Journal of Biomedical and Health Informatics, 19*(4).
34. Issa, N. T., Byers, S. W., & Dakshanamurthy, S. (2014). Big data: The next frontier for innovation in therapeutics and healthcare. *Expert Review of Clinical Pharmacology, 7*(3).
35. Chawla, N. V., & Davis, D. A. (2013). Bringing big data to personalized healthcare: A patient-centered framework. *Journal of General Internal Medicine, 28*(3).
36. Chen, D., Chen, Y., Brownlow, B. N., Kanjamala, P. P., Arredondo, C. A. G., Radspinner, B. L., & Raveling, M. A. (2017). Real-time or near real-time persisting daily healthcare data into hdfs and elasticsearch index inside a big data platform. *IEEE Transactions on Industrial Informatics, 13*(2).
37. Sadeghi, A.-R., Wachsmann, C., & Waidner, M. (2015). Security and privacy challenges in industrial internet of things. In *2015 52nd ACM/EDAC/IEEE on Design Automation Conference (DAC).* IEEE.
38. Balakrishna, G., & Moparthi, N. R. (2019). ESBL: Design and implement a cloud integrated framework for IoT load balancing. *International Journal of Computers Communications & Control, 14*(4), 459–474.
39. S´anchez-Guerrero, R., Mendoza, F.A., D´ıaz-S´anchez, D., Cabarcos, P. A., & L´opez, A. M. (2017). Collaborative ehealth meets security: Privacy-enhancing patient profile management. *IEEE Journal of Biomedical and Health Informatics, 21*(6).
40. Jirkovsky, V., Obitko, M., & Marik, V. (2016). Understanding data heterogeneity in the context of cyber-physical systems integration. *IEEE Transactions on Industrial Informatics*, 99.

Blockchain Technology for Securing Cyber-Infrastructure and Internet of Things Networks

Ishani Tibrewal, Manas Srivastava, and Amit Kumar Tyagi

1 Introduction

Today's Internet of things is mostly used smart devices in many applications. Internet of things when integrates together, they create a network of smart devices called computing infrastructure. This computing infrastructure needs to be properly maintained and secure against many available beaches or critical attacks. Internet of things is an emerging collaborative research environment for today's researchers, because it creates/provides many other benefits like building cyber physical system and autonomous cars. But, when these devices are being used on a large scale and generate a lot of data, and this data is stored at cloud (public, private and hybrid). This data needs to be protected against many serious attacks, and this task can be fulfilled by "Blockchain technology". Blockchain technology concept in 2008–2009 by anonymous user/group of users in cryptocurrency [1], and this concept has been introduced in many applications [2] like finance, manufacturing, medical care, agriculture and autonomous cars.

The Internet of things (IoT) will connect not only computers and mobile devices, but it will also interconnect smart buildings, homes and cities, as well as electrical grids, gas and water networks, automobiles, airplanes, etc. IoT will lead to the development of a wide range of advanced information services that need to be processed in real-time and require data centres with large storage and computing power. The integration of IoT with cloud and fog computing [3, 4] can bring not only the required computational power and storage capacity, but they enable IoT services to be pervasive, cost-effective and can be accessed from anywhere using any device (mobile or

I. Tibrewal · M. Srivastava · A. K. Tyagi (✉)
School of Computing Science and Engineering, Vellore Institute of Technology, Chennai Campus, Chennai, Tamilnadu 600127, India

A. K. Tyagi
Centre for Advanced Data Science, Vellore Institute of Technology, Chennai, Tamilnadu 600127, India

A. K. Tyagi et al. (eds.), *Intelligent Interactive Multimedia Systems for e-Healthcare Applications*, https://doi.org/10.1007/978-981-16-6542-4_17

stationary). However, IoT infrastructures and services will introduce grand security challenges due to the significant increase in the attack surface, complexity, heterogeneity and number of resources. Some of the examples of IoT technology usage and major implications during cyber-attacks are:

(a) Maritime shipping: There are multiple usage of IoT technology in Maritime shipping as the shipping companies have equipped their fleets with a variety of sensors to monitor critical vessel systems, weather and sea conditions, and cargo. The Marine industry can be impacted cyber-attack [5] on terminal computer system, navigation system and point of sale system. Possible consequences are business interruption, damage to data, theft of property through alternation of shipping contacts, bodily injury and property damage.
(b) Aviation: There are several usage of IoT in both commercial and military aviation [6]. Connecting IoT to aviation will help to access real-time data for engine performance improvement, accurate weather forecast and pilot monitoring. The cyber risk in aviation may allow hackers to gain access to some sensitive data such as the location of troops or detailed mission plans for IoT-connected military planes. There could be remote terrorism acts where the hacker could gain access to an aircraft's control system and weaponry, similar to drone hacks, and use it against the enemy.
(c) Smart City: A Smart City [7] can be equipped with IoT platform has multiple usages such as smart parking, public safety and traffic balancing. Smart grid is one of the examples which are implemented in Smart City to realize great cost savings and efficient troubleshooting. If there is no effective cyber security maintained, Hacker can gain access to such public infrastructure from his computer to shut down an entire city's electrical supply.
(d) Critical infrastructure: Because of the networked nature of IoT, i.e. that each connected object uses data from other connected objects–there is also the risk that a malfunction could lead to catastrophic system failure. The critical infrastructure like dams, bridges embedded with censors to monitor structural integrity as well as environmental conditions are vulnerable to cyber threats. Malfunctioning of these sensors may bring risk of a catastrophe if those objects fail and could lead to massive property damage or even loss of life.

Amit and Shamila [8] discussed some more examples, where Internet of things devices can be enhanced/used in everyday examples.

On another side, such infrastructure requires secure cyber security mechanisms, i.e. no more breaches/attacks on public networks. This chapter has provided introduction of Industry 4.0/smart manufacturing using IoT [9] while mapping the relevant security and privacy challenges, threats, risks and attack scenarios. This chapter presents an IoT security framework for smart infrastructures such as smart homes (SH) and smart buildings (SB) [10]. *Also, it presents a general threat model that can be used to develop a security protection methodology for IoT services against cyber-attacks (known or unknown) with provisioning several issues and challenges in respective IoT-based cyber-infrastructure.* The vast diffusion of connected devices in the IoT has created enormous demand for robust security in response to the growing demand of millions or perhaps billions of connected devices and services worldwide. The number of threats is rising daily, and attacks have been on the increase in both number and complexity. Not only is the number of potential attackers along with the size of networks growing, but the tools available to potential attackers are also becoming more sophisticated, efficient and effective.

Cyber-infrastructure is a word commonly used but lacking a single, precise definition. One recognizes intuitively the analogy with infrastructure, and the use of cyber to refer to thinking or computing but what exactly is cyber-infrastructure as opposed to information technology infrastructure? [11] propose definition of cyber-infrastructure as: "cyber-infrastructure consists of computing systems, data storage systems, advanced instruments and data repositories, visualization environments, and people, all linked together by software and high-performance networks to improve research productivity and enable breakthroughs not otherwise possible". In this chapter, we discuss the origin of the term cyber-infrastructure based on the history of the root word infrastructure, discuss several terms related to cyber-infrastructure and provide several examples of cyber-infrastructure. Cyber security is a necessary task in building and proposing an attack-free infrastructure (using by public users). Note that some elements of cyber security are application security, information security, network security, disaster recovery/business continuity planning, operational security, end-user education. Also, some benefits of using/requirement of cyber security to secure an infrastructure:

- Business protection against malware, ransomware, phishing and social engineering.
- Protection for data and networks.
- Prevention of unauthorized users.
- Improves recovery time after a breach.
- Protection for end-users.
- Improved confidence in the product for both developers and customers.

Internet of things (IoT) is an emerging concept describing a wide ecosystem where interconnected devices and services collect, exchange and process data in order to adapt dynamically to a context. IoT is tightly bound to cyber physical systems and in this respect is an enabler of smart infrastructures by enhancing their quality of service provisioning. Cyber physical systems and autonomous applications are IoT-based application development, major development/invention of the previous decade. Both the IoT critical Infrastructures and cloud are subject to cyber-attacks [12]. Cloud environments experience the same threats (at a high level) as traditional data centre environments; the threat picture is the same. That is, cloud computing runs software, software has vulnerabilities, and adversaries try to exploit those vulnerabilities. However, unlike information technology systems in a traditional data centre, in cloud computing, responsibility for mitigating the risks that result from these software vulnerabilities is shared between the cloud service provider (CSP) and the cloud consumer. A secure cyber-infrastructure is need of many organization/research communities (especially computer science) around the world. Hence now, the remaining part of this chapter is organized as (in further sections):

- Sect. 2 discusses work related to Blockchain used to secure Internet of things (IoTs)-based cyber-infrastructure smart contact, i.e. evolution of smart contract with Blockchain technology's growth.
- Sect. 3 discusses motivation behind this work, i.e. intention behind choosing area related to Blockchain-enabled and IoT-based cyber-infrastructure.
- Sect. 4 discusses necessity of secure cyber-infrastructure today and tomorrow, i.e. in current century.
- Sect. 5 discusses tools or mechanisms available for securing a cyber-infrastructure and Internet of things-based infrastructure
- Sect. 6 discusses many issues, problems and challenges in using Blockchain technology during securing respective (cyber) infrastructure.
- Sect. 7 discusses opportunities for future researchers and computer science community.
- Finally, this chapter is concluded in Sect. 8 with some future research directions (including some research gaps).

2 Related Work

Internet of things (IoT) as a technological term is around 16 years old, but the actual idea of connected devices had been around longer, at least since the 70 s and at that time it was referred to as "embedded Internet" or more as to say "pervasive computing". The coining of the actual term "Internet of things" was done by Kevin Ashton during his work at P&G in the late 20 s. Kevin used to manage supply chain optimization and wanted to attract senior management's attention to a new exciting technology called RFID, now as because the Internet was one among the burning trends during the late 20 s so it somehow made sense, he called his presentation "Internet of things" and thus giving a new identity to the technology. By the year 2010, the Internet of things (IoT) started gaining popularity because of the leakage of information of Google took people into guesses that it might be Google one of the new strategies to index not only the Internet but also the entities in the physical world. Followed by this, in the consecutive years the technology took off after which different countries, market research companies and many other organizations took over it very seriously and started researching into this particular emerging new phenomenon and now it is predicted that by the end of 2020, IoT would have gained a huge stake over the market. Currently, the technology has outgrown to such an extent that there has been mass-market awareness. From dominance motivation behind the present, a critical number of the establishments that help and oversee current lives, social requests and work practices will appear to be dull, level and still. The more settled the establishment, the more certified this feels: we consider boulevards until we can drive impact on them, and thereafter in a flash neglect (until induced by setbacks, advancement and vehicle over-burdens to re-examine). We drink from the city water supply until we cannot, and a short time later examine water. Once here, amazing establishments appear as everlasting, unsuspected, even regular features of contemporary life. This sort of naturalization and disregarding is critical to the ampleness and significant estimation of establishment and is to be certain maybe the most raised want. Be that as it may, it in like manner makes it attempting to audit what is being referred to with establishment (which winds up being an extensive sum) or to plot the methodology by which systems create and change. This is an insightful issue for capable understudies of history and social scientists; for would-be makers of a system, it is something more. Computerized establishment was developed with the arrangement to help customers with winning through our high IT aptitudes and to get new work open entryways in India and help in the country's social improvement. CIS continues creating at a pace of 300% consistently. Advanced structure continues developing its assortment of organizations and advancement portfolio to get new markets and spaces. Advanced establishment encounters critical improvements with respect to structure, bunch size and overall reach.

Hence, this section discusses work related to Internet of things, cyber-infrastructure, also Blockchain role in IoT-based applications in detail. In next section, we will discuss motivation behind this work in brief.

3 Motivation

Internets of things (IoTs) are used in building cyber physical systems, i.e. large-scale cyber-infrastructure. For that, we require proper rules and cyber security to prevent from any breaches/attacks. In general terms, cyber security is safeguarding the Internet-connected systems, including hardware and software data, from cyber-attacks, whereas information security, which is devised to preserve the confidentiality, integrity and availability (CIA) of data, is a fragment of cyber security. There are many cyber threats like malware, ransomware, social engineering and phishing on existed infrastructure (build by integration of IoT/smart devices). Such infrastructure requires strong and secure mechanism/algorithms to provide reliable and efficient services to end-users. As we have discussed many popular attacks have been mitigated (in the past decade) like Stuxnet [13], this attack has downgraded many Nuclear facilities in Iran in 2010. Further, [14, 15, 16] have discussed many examples of cyber-crime in their work. But, due to getting rapid growth in innovation, we need Blockchain type of solution to secure an infrastructure. Hence, Blockchain technology has been started using in many applications for protecting critical system/infrastructure. Providing efficient and reliable services to end-users and more security to the same users is our higher (main) priority. Blockchain [17] concept fulfilled this goal in this current era. So, we started to write some important work on Blockchain, which can play an essential role in IoT-based cloud infrastructure or IoT-based infrastructure in making a secure cyber-infrastructure. Hence, this section discusses motivation behind this work, and it provides answer to many questions, i.e. related to topic of interest and how this work will be useful to society or researchers/readers. Now, next section will discuss the necessity of cyber-infrastructure or IoT-based cyber-based physical systems in current century.

4 Necessity of Cyber-Infrastructure in Current Century

There exists a positive national framework for the general public for its smooth working and thus making it powerful. The significance of these is generally comprehended and has since quite a while ago perceived the requirement for interest in their creation and upkeep. Such frameworks will, in general, give widespread administrations, range national and universal limits and are inherently depended upon by people and associations. The need for the digital framework is difficult to disparage, and even generally minor disappointments can affect huge quantities of individuals. Disappointments can bring about genuine ramifications for the working of society, and this has additionally been perceived by assailants who have focused on these national frameworks as a method for disturbing enormous quantities of individuals generally effectively. While the profoundly interconnected nature of pc frameworks can experience challenges related to frameworks security, it can likewise be utilized as a method for upgrading it as well. A considerable lot of the techniques and advantages that identify with the utilization of processing for the basic foundation have as of late gone to the fore. Organized frameworks can give expanded vigour against both focused on assaults and incidental disappointment. These incorporate perception procedures to give mindfulness and displaying capacities; frameworks of frameworks security to all the more likely comprehend the security results of associations between numerous frameworks. Utilizing these methods in a bound together manner will give benefits as far as better seeing, ongoing mindfulness and the improvement of security strategies customized to assurance against disappointment and assault of basic framework frameworks. The genuine advantage to be picked up from combining the strategies digital foundation is to give procedures that length innovative limits. cyber-infrastructure that help our general public are produced using an accumulation of frameworks and systems worked over registering advancements and data frameworks. cyber-infrastructure are going under expanding dangers, the insurance of basic foundations requires a superior comprehension of how the control should be structured to cover all the parts of these frameworks.

Hence, this section discusses "why we require cyber-infrastructure in today's era"? Now, next section will discuss several tools available for securing cyber-infrastructure/IoT-based infrastructure in detail.

5 Tools Available for Securing Cyber-Infrastructure and Internet of Things-Based Infrastructure

There is a great significance of tools that are being developed to secure cyber-infrastructure; Blockchain is one of them. Risks, vulnerabilities, threats, cyber-crimes and frauds are increasing exponentially with the world being digitalized. To get a shield from these potential threats, Blockchain is gaining tradition today but still, significant phases of the world are unaware of it. Critical infrastructure in many countries will soon become vulnerable to cyber terrorism. Ingenious uses for Blockchain technology are already becoming incorporated of fields other than cryptocurrencies [18] and can be exclusively useful to boost cyber security. Several security techniques and approaches have been developed using Blockchain that plays a major role in securing many IoT applications. A Blockchain system depends upon the participation of allocated nodes to build a loyal chain-connected network, in which every decision is made based on the consent. The required system is proposed to have specific major components such as Blockchain-based distributed data repository and verification platform, Internet of things (IoT)-based noticeable environment and cloud-based versatile assistance delivery system. The parts sum up together to develop an infrastructure and a dynamic functional operational environment for overall entities in generation, transmission and delivery. As IoT is an ordinary result of the sensing technology and wireless sensor network, IoT technology will in future enter into each segment of the energy system and connects with other components of the cyber-infrastructure (Blockchain and cloud).

Blockchain takes the involvement of very basic technologies into IoT to make it secure. First of all, it decentralizes the data storage which is its backbone and uses consensus mechanism, this structure ensures data is not traceable nor even tamper able thus as a result giving a no-point fault system so that it can be used in the upper-level application. The connection between the blocks of data is done with a smart contract which is based on contrasting application logic. The information in Blockchain is transferred on a trusted mechanism that verifies and authorizes the user based on agreements, intellectual property rights and so on. In summary, Blockchain along with IoT in phases of cloud coordinated can work together to form a guarded, effective, service-oriented environment, which can strongly support various applications in various domains. Blockchain has promising applications across the domain of network security. IoT can contribute to big data at any level of abstraction, data acquisition could be applied at any level but the main point of data security lies in hands of Blockchain. The complete infrastructure has complete reliability and dependency on its security parameters which should be fault-tolerant, which can be smoothly accomplished through Blockchain. The monitor, control and coordination of units of the cyber-infrastructure should be supported by a dynamic cyber physical system. In any of the proposed cyber-infrastructure model, the cyber-infrastructure is mainly the backboned level of abstraction and security achieved. Under reliable supervision of IoT through Blockchain could help us in attaining a better cyber-infrastructure for a better tomorrow.

We see that Blockchain has made a Digital Ownership Revolution in previous decade (and for today's applications). This section discusses many useful tools/mechanisms which used to protect/secured a cyber-infrastructure and cloud-based IoT-enabled infrastructure. Now, next section will discuss many raised issues, problems or challenges in securing an infrastructure using Blockchain technology.

6 Issues, Problems and Challenges in Using Blockchain Technology During Securing Respective Infrastructure

Blockchain has major impact on the world, which is extraordinary and significant over other existing technologies or mechanism for protecting infrastructure. As discussed above, first time Blockchain was used in Bitcoin in 2008–2009 [18], so most people confuse it with bitcoin and Blockchain. Note that Bitcoin is not Blockchain, Blockchain is a concept used in Bitcoin (a cryptocurrency). Today's Blockchain is used in many applications (i.e. beyond cryptocurrencies) like digital copies of your health records, land records [2], and these records are saved digitally on cloud using Blockchain, called smart contract, such records/contracts no one can pirate/tamper or copy. Indeed, Blockchain has a lot of advantages still it holds a lot of consequences on the other side of its face. Here are some of the problems and challenges described in brief (also depicted in Fig. 1) which are important to overcome. Note that these challenges are facing by industries/organizations in solving everyday problems.

- Cost: The endorsement of Blockchain technology guarantees long-period benefits but initially it is pricey to put it in place. The software required by institutions and industries to implement Blockchain technology in the systems should be archetypally developed for a specific organization structure and thus leading to inflation of cost, adopting it or developing it individually. Along with it, organization structure may have to acquire specialized hardware for use with the software.

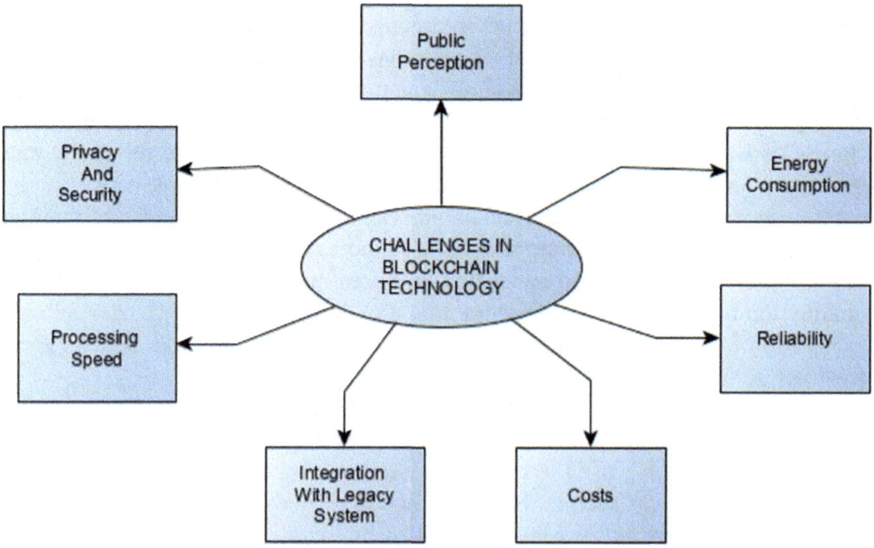

Fig. 1 Diagram depicting various issues and challenges faced in blockchain technology

- Lack of skilled/intelligent people: Apart from dealing with the cost of the technology, there is need of heavy intelligence in order to operate the technology too. This problem even more elongates as there is lack of such engineers even who can deal with it and thus leading to huge demands of these engineers in the organizations. Inferring to most small or even medium-sized businesses, due to involvement of high setup rate in setting up of even complete or partial Blockchain system it becomes out of reach for them.
- Integration with Legacy System: Now coming to integration part, since setting up of Blockchain requires completely different software so organizations should either try integrating with their existing systems or should mend their previous systems. Changes in the system should accordingly be made in order to have smooth transition as initially it will be difficult to implement Blockchain technology. Further, this process will require lot of human resource that is time, effort and money. Due to high cost of this technology, there are organization who are resistant to move towards Blockchain solution.
- Energy Consumption: Energy consumption is other challenging issue that needs to be taken into consideration. The mechanism of validating transactions on Blockchain technology is complex, also computing these complexes mathematical problems (including side by side verifying), for that network (which is secured) requires a lot of energy. Being in a place where climate change is one of the main factors, such massive use of energy does not seem sustainable. So the corporations are looking for more sustainable business methods.
- Lack of Public Awareness: Public awareness is other main challenge. The knowledge of Blockchain technology and its benefits is dampened to the industries who are involved in this technology space and to the organizations who are implementing this distributed ledger technology. So, public awareness must be done first in order to mainstream Blockchain technology. Also, people often confuse Blockchain with Bitcoin, which are two different things and the differences between them should be well understood by people so that full utilization of this technology can be done.
- Security: Blockchain technology is made in such a way that it is publicly visible. This creates a major concern for government as they have to protect the data and have to restrict the access due to very obvious reasons. This results that implementation of Blockchain technology cannot be done in places where the data is sensitive.

Hence, this section discusses many useful components like problems, and major issues and challenges faced/mitigated in securing infrastructures related to todays' requirements (needs). Now, next section will discuss several opportunities towards Blockchain, cyber and IoT-based infrastructure for research communities.

7 Opportunities for Blockchain, Cyber and Computer Security Community

Blockchain technology (in near future) will attract attention from several research communities and can be used in the following areas like Internet-connected things, banking, retail and health care. Such applications are requiring Blockchain, due to the property of distributed digital data (encrypted form, using Hash Keys). Many applications or future uses of Blockchain have been included in Fig. 2. Such functionality in Blockchain is provided by distributed ledger. Using Blockchain technology (a decentralized technology), in respective application, we can secure/store data safely with efficient authentic mechanism at remote location (also in form of Cloud). Data stores at remote location are in inconvertible and immutable using Blockchain/distributed ledger in it.

Blockchain technology has its powerful use in business domain, insurance being one of the prime commercial commodities. The trend of Blockchain within insurance will help in transforming insurance into Insurtech (i.e. Insurance + Technology). One of the many examples where Blockchain can help is in Travel Insurance, i.e. delays and cancellation of flights, can be prevented by Travel Agencies using Blockchain. Blockchain, which was just a virtual ledger, is spreading like a wave across extensive number of industries. Also, businesses are expected to spend colossal amount of money on this powerful technology in this year. From Insurance to gaming to cannabis, almost all industries are looking to develop and apply Blockchain technology, there is hardly any domain not looking for Blockchain applications because this technology is more likely to transform the industries.

Since Blockchain technology does not hold any central supervision and acts on decentralized platform, it has made Blockchain having a prominent feature of being resistant to fraud.

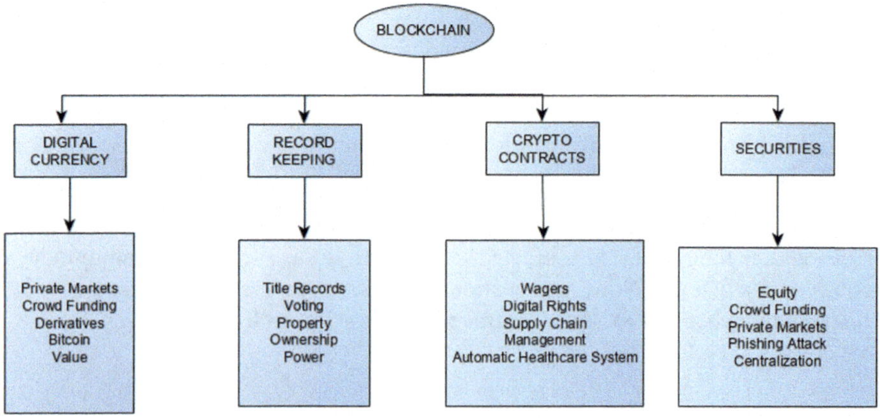

Fig. 2 Use of blockchain in near future

Companies are striving hard to implement Blockchain technology as it will provide veracity to the stored digital data information. Here are many other industries who are mobilizing the power of Blockchain technology:

- Speculative Funds: With a vast range of Numerai, systems have started adopting hedge fund model with a firm support included by First Round Capital and Union Square Ventures, it involves employment of a group of stockbrokers and quants and then regionalizing it. The distribution of data through Numerai is done when it sends its numerous quants to various distinct locations, encrypts the datasets and then is preceded by building protective models and the one among with best of them is awarded with Numerai token known as Numeraire [19]. Further, the strategy is to strategize and develop a meta-model to make trades.
- Medical Management: The medical reports associated with a person are one of the vital parameters of an individual's security, preserving this data is sole responsibility of the organization whosoever beholds it. While sharing the data among different platforms, the data may get leaked which may lead to some unavoidable circumstances. So in order to prevent this data to falling into dangerous hands, Blockchain technology allows hospitals [20], other institutions/organizations and payers to split access to their networks without compromising or suspecting data security and integrity.
- Public Mobility: Due to increase in use of public transport of vehicles, it becomes difficult for government in cities to know the status of public transportation being used, so on implementing Blockchain technology will help the cities to know and understand that how the public mobility is being used by their residents and how can they develop some different options for transportation.
- Track of Credit History: On the basis of past records, lenders tend to reduce the risk that is posed by lines of credit or loans to small ventures which also makes credit bureau to have all powers in terms of loans. It also works as a trusted platform where business owners can build a trusted network.
- Charity: Using Blockchain technology in charity institution or organization will help donators to track where their donations are going and who is going to use it. Blockchain will provide transparency and security to all the financial records and will give a greater visibility to the donors.

As mentioned above, there are many other similar industries that have great potential future with implementation of Blockchain in them like loyalty programs, natural resource management, education, advertisement, public assistance, publishing, gaming, travelling and even more. Moreover this, some other opportunities with Blockchain in near future are summarized (also included in Fig. 3) here as:

- Improve social media functionalities
- Digital ownership revolution
- Keeping our ID (Identification) and personal information secure
- Keep your identity safe and location privacy safe.

Blockchain provides digital freedom by using smart contracts: It means that the system is not governed by any central authority so that any kind of manipulation

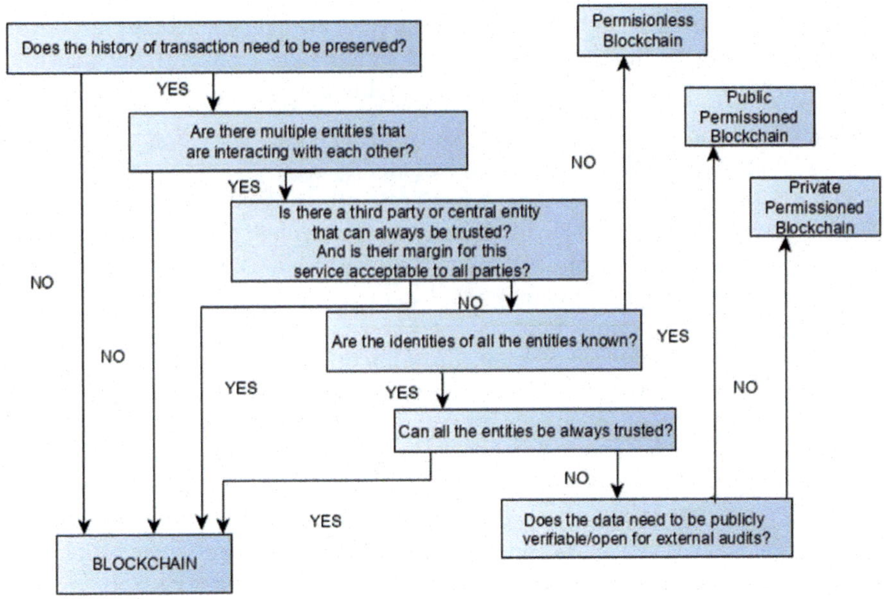

Fig. 3 Opportunities and possibilities with blockchain technology

cannot be done by them. Note that Blockchain is more popular in mortgage industry, i.e. with its transparent system, speed (when compared to the typical mortgage underwriting process) and immutability that will secure your home for as long as you own it. Hence, this section discusses several opportunities for future readers and research communities. Now, next section will wrap up this work (including some research gaps) in brief.

8 Summary

Blockchain is the necessity of the future in building trust among peers and providing more privacy-preserving too many applications (like location-based services, etc.), also security to computing environments. This concept is enhancing everyday with its uses in many applications. Today's Blockchain is the most trusted technology among all existing mechanisms (for protecting an infrastructure). Generally, Blockchain technology allows distribution of digital information in decentralized manner, but not duplicated. Blockchain also allows us to own digital assets, goods and data through its novel concept. Similarly, we face several cyber-crimes and attacks on many critical or cyber-infrastructure, [21] discussed several privacy issues), for that we suggested Blockchain to be used for the same infrastructure for providing sufficient level of security layers. This chapter has discussed several interesting components of Blockchain with Internet of things-based infrastructure and other cyber-infrastructure. We also discuss several benefits, disadvantages, issues and challenges (including opportunities) of Blockchain in securing an infrastructure, and this information will help future researchers/scientists or readers in continuing their research work in near future. In near future, some possible changes are possible with Blockchain are "Distributed Web (new Internet with Blockchain)", "Decentralized Autonomous Blockchain" and "Blockchain-based Cloud". For providing more efficient services, *the world is watching and waiting for more innovations in technologies.*

References

1. Koblitz, N., & Menezes, J. (2016). *Cryptocash, cryptocurrencies, and cryptocontracts.* Springer.
2. Sawal, N. Y., Anjali, T., Amit, T., Sreenath, N., & Rekha,G. (2016). Necessity of blockchain for building trust in today's applications: An useful explanation from user's perspective. *SSRN.*
3. Risteska Stojkoska, B. L., & Trivodaliev, K. V. (2017). A review of Internet of Things for smart home: Challenges and solutions. *Journal of Cleaner Production, 140*, 1454–1464.
4. Rekha, G., Tyagi, A.K., & Anuradha, N. (2019). Integration of fog computing and internet of things: an useful overview, 8–9 March, 2019. In *The 2nd International Conference on Recent Innovations in Computing (ICRIC), Central University of Jammu, J & K, India, Lecture Notes in Electrical Engineering (LNEE)*, Springer, ISSN: 1876-1100.
5. Andrew, E. (2016). Cyber risks in the marine transportation system. Springer, pp 113–131.
6. Cao, L., Zheng, G., & Shen, Y. (2016). Research on design of military ammunition container monitoring system based on IoT. *IEEE.*
7. Kim, T., Ramos, C., & Mohammed, S. (2017). Smart city and IoT. *Future Generation Computer Systems, 76*, 159–162.
8. Amit, T., & Shamila, M. (2019). Spy in the crowd: How user's privacy is getting affected with the Integration of Internet of Thing's Devices. Elsevier.
9. Shrouf, F., Ordieres, J., & Miragliotta, G. (2014). Smart factories in Industry 4.0: A review of the concept and of energy management approached in production based on the Internet of Things paradigm. *IEEE.*
10. Ghayvat, H., Mukhopadhyay, S., Gui, X., & Suryadevara, N. (2015). WSN-and IoT-based smart homes and their extension to smart buildings. *Sensors, 15*(5), 10350–10379.
11. Stewart, C. A., Simms, S., Plale, B., Link, M., Hancock, D. Y., & Fox, G. C. (2010). What is cyber-infrastructure. In *Proceedings of the 38th Annual Fall Conference on SIGUCCS—SIGUCCS'10.*
12. Abomhara, M., & Kien, G. M. (2015). Cyber security and the internet of things: vulnerabilities, threats, intruders and attacks. *Journal of Cyber Security and Mobility, 4*(1), 65–88.
13. Lindsay, J. R. (2013). Stuxnet and the limits of cyber warfare. *Security Studies, 22*(3), 365–404.
14. Zhang, Y., Xiao, Y., Ghaboosi, K., Zhang, J., & Deng, H. (2011). A survey of cybercrimes. *Security and Communication Networks, 5*(4), 422–437.
15. Tyagi, A. K. (2016). Cyber Physical Systems (CPSs) â [euro]" opportunities and challenges for improving cyber security. *International Journal of Computer Applications, 137*(14).
16. Tabansky, L. (2011). Critical infrastructure protection against cyber threats. *Military and Strategic Affairs, 3.*

17. Zheng, Z., Xie, S., Dai, H., Chen, X., & Wang, H. (2017). An overview of blockchain technology: architecture, consensus, and future trends. In *2017 IEEE International Congress on Big Data.*
18. Bonneau, J., Miller, A., Clark, J., Narayanan, A., Kroll, J. A., & Felten, E. W. (2015). SoK: Research perspectives and challenges for bitcoin and cryptocurrencies. In *2015 IEEE Symposium on Security and Privacy.*
19. Li, J., & Mann, W. (2018). Initial coin offering and platform building. *SSRN Electronic Journal.*
20. Mettler, M. (2016). Blockchain technology in healthcare: The revolution starts here. In *2016 IEEE 18th International Conference on e-Health Networking, Applications and Services (Healthcom).*
21. Amit, T., & Sreenath, N. (2015). Future challenging issues in location based services. *International Journal of Computer Applications, 114*(5).

AI Approach Based on Deep Learning for Classification of White Blood Cells as a for e-Healthcare Solution

Ana Carolina Borges Monteiro, Reinaldo Padilha França, Rangel Arthur, and Yuzo Iano

1 Introduction

Deep learning is based on a compilation of algorithms and digital learning techniques combined with a large volume of data to facilitate decision making, making it possible to cross the clinical data of patients with the references obtained and formulate several hypotheses about a clinical event. This means that the use of deep learning in health will provide more accurate conclusions than if it was analyzed in isolation, bringing more security to the health professional when making decisions for the patient [1].

The technology, both in the field of digitization and information technology (IT), has finally met the standards required for digital pathology, in terms of software and network maturity, and computational and storage capacity. Allowing more efficient workflows, considering that the diagnosis of computational pathology will take the field a step further, allowing health professionals to use digital medical images in more varied and efficient ways, using intelligent image recognition algorithms which can help to simplify workflows and help them focus on more important things [2, 3].

A. C. B. Monteiro (✉) · R. P. França (✉) · Y. Iano
School of Electrical and Computer Engineering (FEEC), University of Campinas (UNICAMP), Av. Albert Einstein, 400, Campinas—SP, Barão Geraldo, Brazil
e-mail: monteiro@decom.fee.unicamp.br

R. P. França
e-mail: padilha@decom.fee.unicamp.br

Y. Iano
e-mail: yuzo@decom.fee.unicamp.br

R. Arthur
School of Technology (FT), University of Campinas (UNICAMP), Paschoal Marmo Street, 1888-Garden Nova Italia, Limeira—SP, Brazil
e-mail: rangel@ft.unicamp.br

A. K. Tyagi et al. (eds.), *Intelligent Interactive Multimedia Systems for e-Healthcare Applications*, https://doi.org/10.1007/978-981-16-6542-4_18

Another main advantage is the time of diagnosis since the technology includes computer visualization, this results in faster than the diagnoses that use the microscope by human professionals, meaning that it increases capacity and efficiency. Considering that in a traditional laboratory, a glass slide (containing a blood sample) is taken several times from the file to the pathologist's workstation and vice versa; using this slide's digital image, this unnecessary logistics is eliminated, representing in a job becoming faster and more convenient and the specialized team can be allocated to other more productive and technical jobs [4].

In this sense, through artificial intelligence (AI) referring to a set of techniques such as deep learning (Fig. 1), it is possible to emulate human intelligence, giving machines the ability to learn from experiences and perceptions, make decisions and make decisions based on data because it provides information and insights to support professionals in their activities. It also makes predictive analysis possible, by identifying and analyzing different possible scenarios and events, assisting in strategic decision making; however, to learn and continue to develop, just like human beings, AI needs to be powered by data. Emphasizing that the difference between human professionals and AI is that, to ensure assertiveness, AI requires a large amount of data, structured or not, to learn [5].

An artificial neural network is composed of several processing units; associating these units connected by communication channels that are linked to a certain weight, having some training rule, where the weights of their connections are adjusted according to the standards presented (learn through examples), making operations only on your local data, which are inputs received by your connections, typically organized in layers, with units that can be connected to the units in the back layer. Also, relating that convolutional neural networks has the main idea of filtering lines,

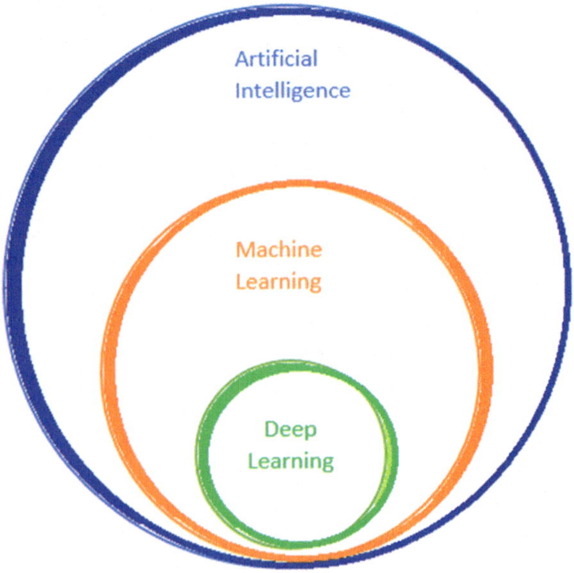

Fig. 1 Artificial intelligence concept illustration

curves, and edges and in each added layer transforming this filtering (convolutions) into a more complex image. Emphasizing that the deeper the layers of the convolutions, the more detailed the traces identified, relating that the depth of the exit of a convolution is equal to the number of filters applied [6].

In summary, the blood test is used to ensure that the patient can undergo surgery, especially because it is an easy test to perform and measure result. It is a blood test much requested by doctors, as it is part of the analysis necessary for any routine exam or annual check-up. Or even applied to check the body's reaction to certain treatments by assessing the quantity and quality of the three main groups of blood cells relating red blood cells (red blood cells, which carry oxygen and nutrients to the body), leukocytes (white blood cells, which act in the immune system), and platelets (which modulate coagulation). This exam assesses health in general, and when there are symptoms such as fever, fatigue, and weakness, among others, in general, it identifies diseases that mess up the blood composition, such as leukemia, anemia, and bacterial or viral infections, or even allergies and hemorrhages can also be detected with this [7, 8].

The data from this examination are interpreted according to standard reference values, which vary according to the patient's age, indicating that changes in red blood cells indicate excessive blood viscosity, if present in large quantities, or even indicate anemia if the number of red blood cells is low. Relating the exaggerated presence of leukocytes indicates bacterial infections, or even the high concentration of other defense cells, such as eosinophils, suggests allergies or the presence of parasites in the intestine. Platelets are important for assessing blood clotting ability, indicating a risk of thrombosis and clogging of blood vessels or, on the other hand, the presence of bleeding. Or summarizing problems in the formation of new cells, problems in containing bleeding and malfunctioning of the bone marrow [7, 9].

It is important to highlight the importance of this examination due to the counting and analysis of these components (main groups of blood cells) allow to assess the clinical condition of the patient, i.e., assess the health and identify diseases, monitor the progression of any adverse medical condition and assess if the treatment is having the desired effect, and not only for the diagnosis of diseases. This is a simple exam, but necessary and essential since it allows several clinical suggestions and helps to detect characteristics of one of our main tissue, the hematopoietic, associating the process of formation, development, and maturation of blood elements (erythrocytes, leukocytes, and platelets) from a common and undifferentiated cell precursor (hematopoietic cell or stem cell), which is inside the bones, allowing an appropriate, safe, and quick treatment when reading its result [10, 11].

In this context, employing Python using Jupyter notebook software, a cognitive approach oriented towards deep learning achieving accuracy at 84.19%, employed at dataset comprising 12,500 medical digital images of human blood smear fields of non-pathological leukocytes, as well as demonstrating the high reliability of the framework. Also, relating the biggest contribution of AI in medicine is the aid in diagnosing pathologies, allowing medical professionals to reinforce the diagnosis encompassing the interpretation and recognition of medical reports for imaging examinations of a certain disease, in this context, is the proposed framework improving diagnostic processes. The continuity of this research is related to techniques based on generative adverse networks (GANs) optimizing cell qualification and identification, classification, and recognition of WBCs, refining the level of segmentation detail related differentiation of T-lymphocyte and B-lymphocyte.

Therefore, the AI-oriented cognitive approach is pointed as a reliable and inexpensive method that can be implemented as a third procedure for blood tests; for that portion of the world population associated with the inaccessible reality of public health derived from underdeveloped and developing nations, facilitating the obtaining of medical diagnostics with low cost and reliability in often underprivileged countries. The structure of this work is Sect. 2 argues Cognitive Computing Concept. Section 3 conceptualizes Neural Networks. Section 4 discusses and presents Metaheuristic Algorithm. Section 5 demonstrates the results of the framework and discusses it. Section 6 displays the Future Research Directions for research, and, finally, in Sect. 7, the findings are explained.

2 Cognitive Computing Concept

The word "cognitive" comes from "cognition", referring to the ability of machines to perceive, interpret and absorb knowledge, i.e., it is a high-level understanding, this is applied to technologies with the capacity to process and distribute information in a way smart. In this sense, cognitive computing creates hypotheses and rationalizes, emulating an artificial brain; it is responsible for obtaining data and giving it a correct destination, with a great difference is that it goes beyond the analysis of pure data, being a technology that analyzes conceptual information, which is helpful in the most complex decision-making processes. Thus, cognitive computational systems are no longer programmed, but learn, adapting to realities [12, 13].

The goal of cognitive computing is to make a computer/machine behave, "think," and interact in the same way that human beings do, simplifying and defining a cognitive system evolves through learning (Fig. 2). Considering that the key to distinguish "traditional" computing from cognitive computing, and intelligent digital learning, this is what is achieved through artificial neural networks (ANN), used in the AI technique known as deep learning, which is a high-capacity technique computational processing, in turn, depends on a lot of information (dataset) to be able to calibrate its artificial neurons and, thus, to respond accurately to each request [12, 14].

A neural network is algorithms and models created from the understanding of the animal brain, emulating the connections between neurons, consisting of architecture with a simple processing model (artificial neuron) composed of multiple highly connected layers (neural network), i.e., processing units that aim to acquire knowledge through experience, and an optimization algorithm that identifies the particular characteristics of patterns presented to the neural network, with the training being categorized into supervised and unsupervised. It is through an interactive training

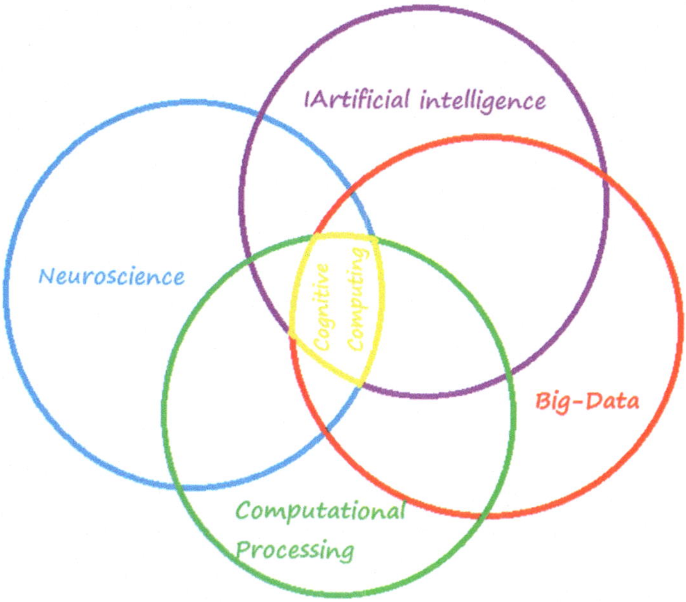

Fig. 2 Cognitive computing illustration

process that the neural network learns to identify the patterns, demonstrating excellent results in applications aimed at the recognition of voice and image patterns, considering the processing capacity is directly linked to the training time of the neural network and the application complexity [15].

It is precisely through these learning techniques, such as deep learning combined with the computational power of data processing and storage that it is possible to consider cognitive computing as a new paradigm, not only in terms related to an "artificial brain," but a system capable to extract information from a huge volume of data sources [1, 16].

Stressing that a digital cognitive system is an extremely powerful helper, and not a substitute for the current paradigm, used in the field of medical research helping doctors in treatments for some types of cancer. This is a valuable aid to be added to the professional's experience physician to make a decision, considering that it is humanly impossible to match this capacity, since, with the evolution of cognitive models, it is possible to guide the development of applications aimed at processing unstructured data [17].

Also, considering that a cognitive system learns given the more access to data it has over time, the more it learns, becoming a continuous process, this can analyze thousands of articles published in scientific journals and correlate them with data obtained in clinical treatments and electronic medical records of patients to suggest new treatments [18].

Like any technological revolution, and with the advancement of digital transformation in health, three technologies cognitive computing, wearable devices, and deep learning, resulting in that this new computational paradigm is to a greater or lesser extent we are already immersed in this technology, pondering over disruptive tools giving traction to the changes promoted by digital transformation, transforming the way management works and helping with medical assistance. Health technology has a widespread impact on the sector since the strategy of a health operator related to the definition of offers to beneficiaries to the clinical area of a hospital, assisting the doctor in the diagnosis and choice of treatment [19, 20].

Thus, cognitive computing is a revolution in the way health strategies are built and impacts all departments of the sector organizations, specifically in the clinical area, it is more assertive diagnoses and treatments, or it can even point out the probability of a patient developing a disease based on your family history, the demographic group you belong to and your personal habits, this is because these cognitive solutions process data from the most varied sources such as patient record, data warehousing, medical knowledge portals (structured data) extremely quickly), and even social media and other digital sources (unstructured data). Besides, solutions based on cognitive computing have properties and characteristics to suggest the treatment of diseases based on clinical protocols and best practices that have proven to be effective, considering that the rapid computational processing of this volume of information provides the physician with elements to decide on what is the best care to be taken with the patient [15, 21].

Cognitive computing has come to facilitate and provide innumerable variables of information about the patient himself, constantly supplied with information from treatment histories, scientific research, among others, allowing greater proficiency in diagnoses and treatments, helping medical professionals both when identifying diseases and in the indication of treatment protocols. Despite this, patients will understand this change through practical knowledge, generating more quality, speed, and the medical safety that technology can generate [22].

Deep learning (Fig. 3) looks for patterns in the data; this allows to generate conclusions without being explicitly programmed to reach them. It is the characteristic that gives AI the ability to improve "its artificial knowledge" and propose more assertive diagnostic treatments, employing attempt, success, and error, cognitive computing learns over time. Based on these conclusions and the feedback obtained, the artificial

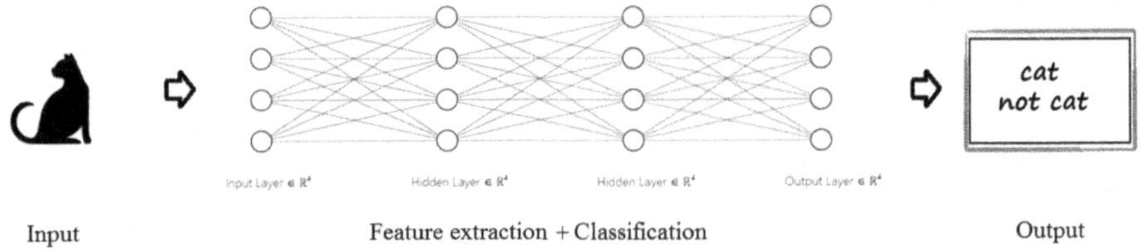

Fig. 3 Deep learning

knowledge generated in a new data set can be used, creating a learning circle that improves the algorithm and its accuracy [23].

Thus, AI is the broadest definition in this source of technology. It can solve problems through methods, algorithms, and techniques are used to create intelligence in the machines, dealing with the technology responsible for the creation of devices that simulate human capacity to think and make decisions. In short, AI aims to bring the machine closer to the man, teaching them to act in a specific way in the most varied situations, allowing these machines to learn to identify the situations and respond accordingly, thus, the intelligence of the machines is born from the teaching given to them [5, 6].

Considering that AI is not just a term but a set of different technologies and methods that seek to train machines with the objectivity of simulating human tasks, within this disruptive technology, there are several subsets of relevant studies, such as cognitive computing, computer vision, data processing, natural language, machine learning, and deep learning among many others. Broadly speaking, AI is the science of machines that simulate human tasks, while deep learning is a method of how machines learn from data (Fig. 4) [5, 6].

But this is not the same definition of cognitive intelligence, differentiating that that AI alone works based on a good database, in large quantities and, with that, it crosses information to find an answer or a vision of something specific. In contrast, cognitive intelligence uses its hits and misses on top of this information base to learn and improve, unlike isolated AI; in this sense, it is worth describing that cognitive intelligence uses AI resources, always aiming to solve existing problems efficiently and effectively [6, 12, 16].

Therefore, cognitive computing is nothing more than the set of all the technologies previously mentioned; based on this technology, it is possible to restructure medical work, with the evolution and increasing use of AI there will be a paradigm break that will cause data are used to treat patients according to what would be ideal for

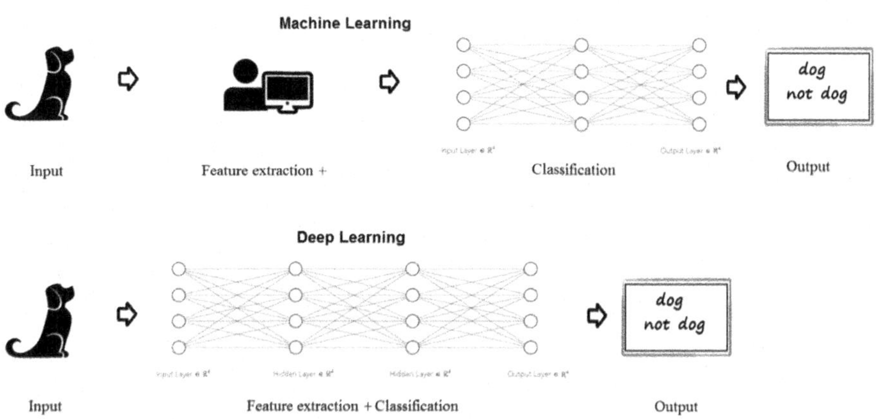

Fig. 4 Machine learning x Deep learning

each one, and no longer what works for the "majority," as it happened in the past and still occurs in some cases. Stressing that in the same way that the telephone did not replace the human voice, but expanded its reach, cognitive computing will increase people's brain potential [6, 12, 16].

Thus, technology in health is already part of the reality of institutions and the trend is that this evolution is increasingly faster and more intense in line with the search for value in the sector through the concept of preventive, predictive, personalized, and participatory health, reaching this level by the continuous investment in tools that allow greater de-hospitalization, more efficient treatments, and disease prediction, increasing the quality of medical care [24, 25].

3 Neural Networks Concepts

In artificial neural networks (ANN) (Fig. 5), several neurons are used in parallel, forming a hidden layer of the neural network, considering that in each neuron signals are received from the input variables and passing on a weighted and treated version of that signal. This is divided into several layers composed of neurons, which are connected by connections to simulate a synaptic connection, relating input layer, hidden layers (intermediate), and output layer. Thus, it is possible to treat the output of each neuron as a variable of the input of another hidden layer, making it possible to stack hidden layers and produce a deep neural network [26].

Artificial neural networks can also be defined as successive nests of several linear transformations followed by some differentiable function, which is applied element by an element of the input matrix. An ANN goes through a process called training, that is, a set of data is provided to the ANN that "learns" the patterns behind the data set and from there can make predictions about that data through an algorithm called backpropagation [26].

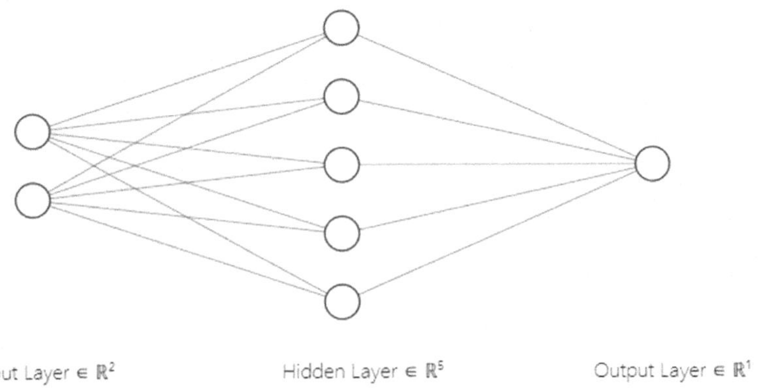

Fig. 5 Neural networks

Concerning nonlinearity, ANN can represent any function, even considering that the cost function optimizes and becomes non-convex and extremely complicated to optimize, considerably hampering the training process, given a sufficient number of neurons, i.e., the greater the number of neurons, the greater the capacity of the learning model. However, ANN's is the most interesting class of machine learning models since they are extremely simple; intuitive, as they allow the interpretation of learning levels of hierarchical abstractions; flexible, which makes them ideal for solving the most diverse types of problems as well as being effective in the quality of the results [27, 28].

In this sense, in machine learning, it is worth noting that the most difficult task is not to train the machine but to engineer variables that assist in learning, considering image recognition, the need for preprocessing relating noise filters, segmentation, contrast enhancement, contour detection, among many others, that the digital image passes before being fed to a machine fastening algorithm. In this context, ANNs appear to solve this, instead of needing to create representative variables manually, ANNs can learn them alone, especially the deep learning neural networks, in addition to learning a mapping between representative characteristics and the desired output, the machine can learn the representative characteristics themselves automatically [29].

A neural network can be interpreted as a processing scheme capable of storing knowledge based on learning (experience), capable of learning and making decisions based on it and making this knowledge available to the application in a specific focus. Considering that there are several ways to develop a neural network, which must be assembled according to the problem to be solved, emphasizing that its architecture must be determined according to the number of layers used, still considering that the amount of neurons in each layer, the type of synapse used, is derived from the problem to be solved [30].

As there are also three types of learning in artificial neural networks; supervised, considering that the ANN receives a set of standardized inputs and their corresponding output patterns, where adjustments in synaptic weights occur until the error between the output patterns generated by the network has the desired value; unsupervised, emphasizing that in this type, the ANN works the data to determine some properties of the data sets, and from these properties is that the learning is constituted; and semi-supervised, considering the "mix" of supervised and unsupervised types since one layer can work with one type of learning while another layer works with the other type of learning [30–32].

Deep learning techniques are mainly based on the use of several hidden layers of a deep neural network as learning levels of hierarchical abstractions, oriented to image recognition, these lower layers (close to the inputs) learn to detect traces and variation of luminosity, while the upper layers learn to join these features in parts of objects, then this is used by a linear model to discriminate between one or the other object [1, 33].

3.1 Convolutional Neural Network

The general applicability of neural networks is an advantage that becomes a liability when it comes to digital images, considering convolutional neural networks (CNN) make a conscious compensation since if a neural network was designed to specifically manipulate images, some generalization should be sacrificed for a much more viable solution [33].

Considering that when considering a digital image, the proximity of the pixels has a strong relationship with the similarity represented in the digital image. This implies that, in a given image, two pixels that are closer to each other are more likely to be related than the two pixels that are separated from each other. Comparatively, in an ANN, each pixel is connected to each neuron, representing an added computational load making the network less accurate [33, 34].

Thus, CNN eliminates many of these connections that are less technically significant, making image processing computationally manageable by filtering connections by proximity. Whereas in a given layer, instead of linking each input to each neuron, CNNs intentionally restrict connections so that any neuron accepts input only from a small subsection of the previous layer, meaning that each neuron is responsible for processing only a certain portion of an image [33, 35–38].

CNN (Fig. 6) is composed of two major stages: extraction of characteristics by the convolutional layers and performing classification, comprising convolutional layers associating filters (Learning/BackPropagation), activation associating neurons (Relu/Sigmoid/TangH), pooling which reduces the scales (Max, Median, among other characteristics) and even fully connected representing the layer that determines the classes (classifier) [33, 37, 38].

In the extraction of characteristics, a digital image is transformed into a vector of characteristics based on a sequence of convolutions, changing the data representation and learning through the filters, activation and pooling's, reducing the scale to the next layer; this is necessary to reduce the quantity filter characteristics (scaling down). Considering that the weights of the filters are calculated automatically (BackPropagation) and considering that each filter learned is an extractor of characteristics since from that point on, this neural network structure is effective for blood cell biology (Fig. 7), meaning that each image resulting from a filter is a map of characteristics [33, 37, 38].

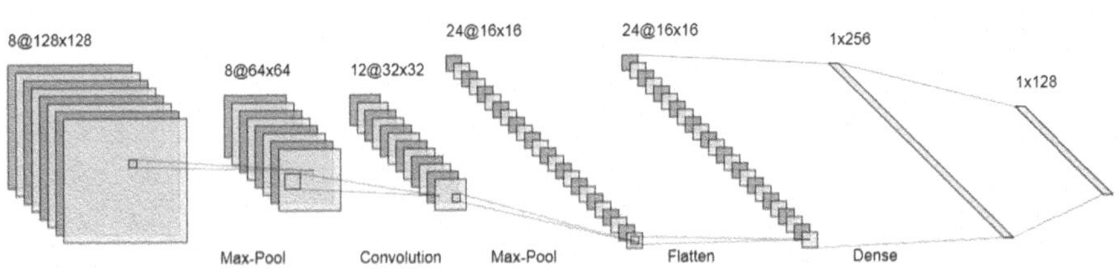

Fig. 6 Convolutional neural networks

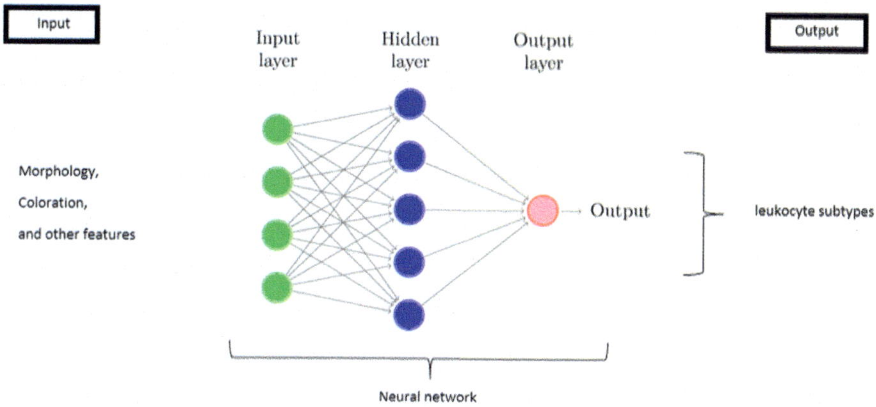

Fig. 7 CNN

In the training of a CNN, the filters and the fully connected layer (Random/Const/Gaussian/Xavier) are initialized, and from the learning phase (depending on the neural network configuration), validation and Backpropagation take place, considering that the of the weights and filters is done throughout the process, and when testing the CNN, these filters and defined weights are used [39, 40].

Thus, CNN is different from dense neural networks or ANN or even fully connected. CNN's are not fully connected, not having the complete connection of all neurons as with dense neural networks, since they are useful for general purpose problems, and can be used for almost any situation. The purpose of CNN is to solve a specific task related to the recognition of digital images, associated with computer vision [39, 40].

4 Metaheuristic Algorithm Proposal

A dataset [41] of microscopic normal peripheral blood cell digital images, related to the objective of microscopy in obtaining enlarged images of an object (blood cell), in the specific case of the research consisting of augmented white blood corpuscles (WBCs), allowing to distinguish details not revealed to the human naked eye. This data set covers 12,500 digital images that were employed on CNN, characterized concerning four morphological subtypes of WBC, i.e., monocytes, neutrophils, eosinophils, lymphocytes, still including a denial logic-oriented basophil (Fig. 8). This dataset also considers a class 2400 augmented WBC images supported at CNN training (Figs. 9 and 10), still considering four more classes of 600 augmented WBC images testing the CNN.

Thus, describing the dataset for the design of CNN, WBC digital images were reduced to a ratio of 60 × 80 × 3, to avoid dimensionality problems in neural

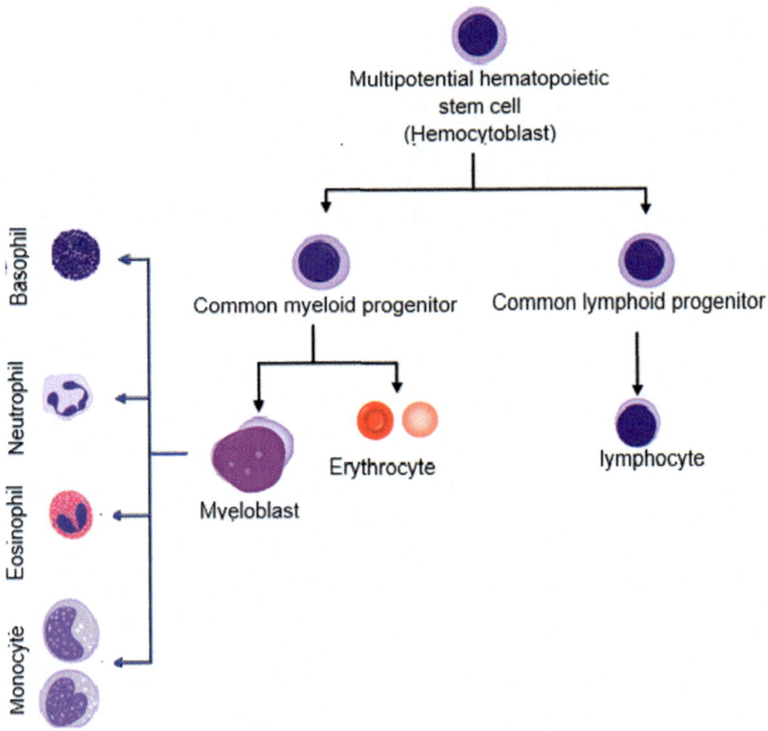

Fig. 8 Blood cell morphological types

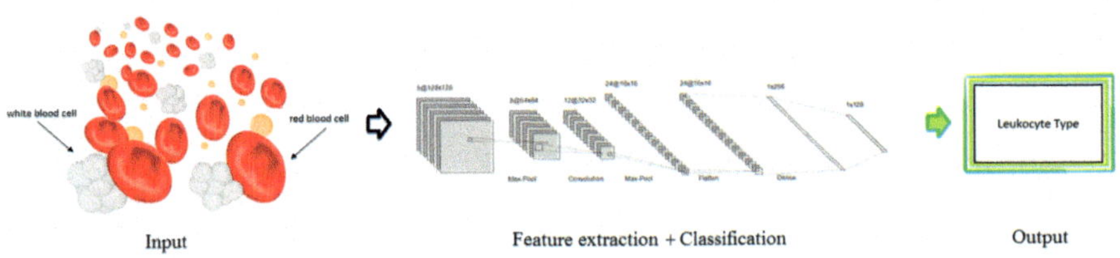

Fig. 9 Proposal modeling

networks, providing dimensionality reduction is a very interesting tool to visualize high-dimension data, optimizing to keep points close to its neighbors allowing to observe some interesting geometric properties of these representations (WBC digital images). After loading it as numerical arrays, due to the computational favor related to training of the neural network. This was possible using Intel Core i3 machine with 4 GB RAM (hardware used for CNN test) com a Kera's open-source library (Python 3.7) directed at training the neural network, also associating Jupyter notebook software (version 0.35.4) for the codification of the CNN source code.

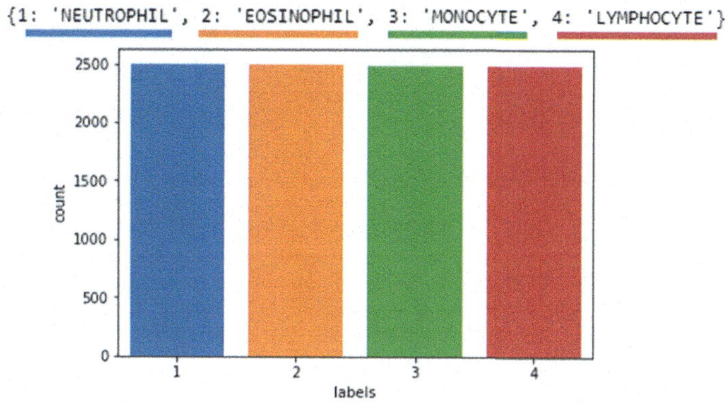

Fig. 10 Leukocyte classes

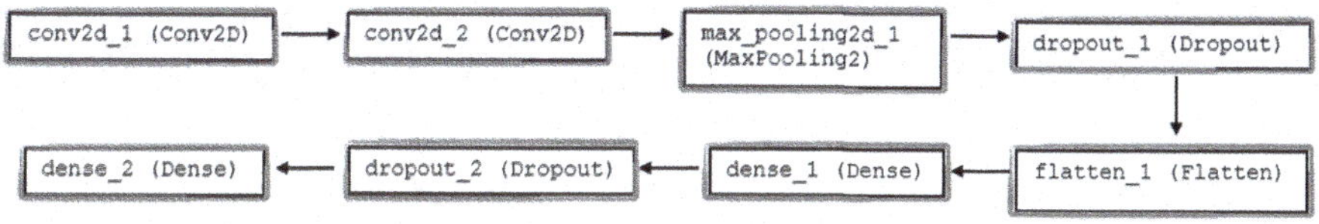

Fig. 11 Leukocyte classes

Considering the structure of the CNN containing methods and objects for dataset processing from Kera's libraries aiming at digital preprocessing images. Relating the characteristics of CNN, consisting of colorful digital images by a 3D matrix, i.e., by tones RGB colors (red, green, and blue), this employs the set of convolution layers, from that is possible to extract resources (from edges) from WBC digital images molding the convolution operation, also relating feed-forward layers combined for WBC augmented digital image for cell classification and qualification.

Also associating that CNN contains operations laborious, compared to those types of a simple neural network, which are unable to obtain learning, or even classify or even identify from features present in a WBC cell digital image relating and associating cell subtypes. So, CNN's logical structure is illustrated in Fig. 11 (flowchart).

5 Results and Discussion

It was achieved an accuracy of 84.19% from 44 simulated epochs with the CNN developed in this study (Fig. 12), emphasizing that accuracy indicates an overall performance of the model, among all classifications, how many the model correctly classified, i.e., the proportion of cases that were correctly predicted, this symbolizes a significant result because of the heterogeneity corresponding to the different WBC

```
A: 34s - loss: 0.2863 - acc: 0.89 - ETA: 33s - loss: 0.2865 - acc: 0.89 - ETA: 32s - loss: 0.2863 - acc: 0.89 - ETA: 32s
- loss: 0.2864 - acc: 0.89 - ETA: 31s - loss: 0.2867 - acc: 0.89 - ETA: 30s - loss: 0.2867 - acc: 0.89 - ETA: 29s - loss:
0.2866 - acc: 0.89 - ETA: 29s - loss: 0.2864 - acc: 0.89 - ETA: 28s - loss: 0.2861 - acc: 0.89 - ETA: 27s - loss: 0.2866
- acc: 0.89 - ETA: 26s - loss: 0.2862 - acc: 0.89 - ETA: 26s - loss: 0.2869 - acc: 0.89 - ETA: 25s - loss: 0.2875 - acc:
0.89 - ETA: 24s - loss: 0.2873 - acc: 0.89 - ETA: 23s - loss: 0.2877 - acc: 0.89 - ETA: 22s - loss: 0.2878 - acc: 0.89 -
ETA: 22s - loss: 0.2873 - acc: 0.89 - ETA: 21s - loss: 0.2870 - acc: 0.89 - ETA: 20s - loss: 0.2869 - acc: 0.89 - ETA: 19
s - loss: 0.2864 - acc: 0.89 - ETA: 19s - loss: 0.2859 - acc: 0.89 - ETA: 18s - loss: 0.2852 - acc: 0.89 - ETA: 17s - los
s: 0.2848 - acc: 0.89 - ETA: 16s - loss: 0.2846 - acc: 0.89 - ETA: 16s - loss: 0.2851 - acc: 0.89 - ETA: 15s - loss: 0.28
47 - acc: 0.89 - ETA: 14s - loss: 0.2850 - acc: 0.89 - ETA: 13s - loss: 0.2851 - acc: 0.89 - ETA: 13s - loss: 0.2854 - ac
c: 0.89 - ETA: 12s - loss: 0.2849 - acc: 0.89 - ETA: 11s - loss: 0.2848 - acc: 0.89 - ETA: 10s - loss: 0.2857 - acc: 0.89
- ETA: 9s - loss: 0.2860 - acc: 0.8930 - ETA: 9s - loss: 0.2856 - acc: 0.893 - ETA: 8s - loss: 0.2861 - acc: 0.893 - ETA:
7s - loss: 0.2861 - acc: 0.892 - ETA: 6s - loss: 0.2858 - acc: 0.893 - ETA: 6s - loss: 0.2858 - acc: 0.892 - ETA: 5s - lo
ss: 0.2860 - acc: 0.892 - ETA: 4s - loss: 0.2859 - acc: 0.892 - ETA: 3s - loss: 0.2854 - acc: 0.892 - ETA: 3s - loss: 0.2
853 - acc: 0.892 - ETA: 2s - loss: 0.2852 - acc: 0.892 - ETA: 1s - loss: 0.2846 - acc: 0.892 - ETA: 0s - loss: 0.2846 - a
cc: 0.892 - ETA: 0s - loss: 0.2847 - acc: 0.892 - 318s 1s/step - loss: 0.2844 - acc: 0.8929 - val_loss: 0.4900 - val_acc:
0.8420

Keras CNN #1C - accuracy: 0.8419782871887489
```

Fig. 12 CNN accuracy result

subtypes morphologies, whether are true-positive, relative when the model correctly predicts a WBC cell subtype, or true-negative, relative to CNN pointing to the WBC cell subtype, and that's right, this also symbolizes the complexity of this type of neural network implemented, capable of processing a large volume of information in minimum time.

Concerning Figs. 13 and 14, it is notable that the CNN training was satisfactory, respective its accuracy achieved, associated the identification, recognition, and classification of the monocyte (Fig. 14), affirming the validity of the CNN algorithm respective to technique deep learning concerning cell biology digital learning.

The digital transformation in the health segment, mainly in the field of diagnostic medicine, is pioneering, driven by digital techniques and devices that are increasingly modern, accurate, high definition, and with lower risks for the patient, meaning the adoption of digital tools can in the search for early and assertive diagnoses and treatments. This presents a universe of possibilities, which impact the way health

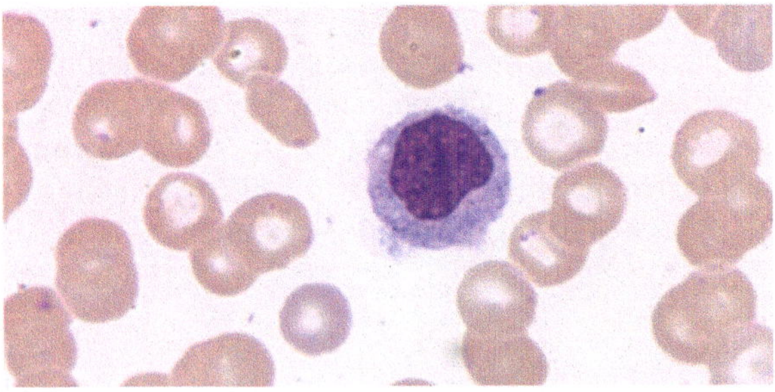

Fig. 13 Monocyte

```
In [42]: preds = model.predict_classes(xi)
         print(preds)

         [3]
```

Fig. 14 CNN monocyte classification

professionals see the ability to provide increasingly better treatments. The use of digital tools would open up the possibility for millions of people to have access to quality health care in both developed and underdeveloped countries, saying that receiving quality health care today is very expensive for patients, in addition to the limitations imposed by healthcare service providers. Cheers. As diagnostic conditions improve, it is inevitable that patients will also feel the difference positively in the performance of examinations and surgeries in much less time, especially when mentioning high-risk diseases such as cancer, for example. Since access to reliable diagnostics plus care and prevention also increases patient safety, noting that from the patient's point of view, digital transformation can mean access to appropriate treatments that were previously impossible, and everyone involved in the healthcare chain is impacted positively by adopting health strategies.

Artificial intelligence is a powerful technology that has been revolutionizing existing healthcare systems to perform more accurate diagnoses and even help to identify major problems, considering the use of artificial intelligence as a diagnostic validator for mammography exams, which controls and audits the quality of diagnostics, providing redundancy, reliability, and security to professional medical radiologists. This results in a better audit of the medical diagnosis, with a reduction in the number of tests recalled, less stress and exposure to radiation to patients, as well as greater refinement of the diagnosis and training of specialist doctors, generating greater assertiveness in the diagnosis and treatment of medication as well as cost savings. In this same panorama, the importance of digital identification, recognition, and classification of human blood cell biology is also reflected. This research is contributing to the early diagnosis of several important diseases, providing a better understanding of the functioning of the human organism and even interaction and functioning between the cells, allowing to deduce from the study of the cellular structure, i.e., this research represents an integrated way with other branches of knowledge and science symbolizing an advance in the most diverse areas related to medicine such as genetics, molecular biology, and even biochemistry.

Through the digital optical microscopy images technology, it allows the visualization of microscopic structures such as cells and cell nuclei; it is possible to contribute to the identification of structures not identified, associating the objective of microscopy oriented in obtaining enlarged images of an object, overcoming the limitation of the capacity of the eyes of human specialists. In this context, the importance of diagnostic imaging comes from this helps in the early diagnosis of several diseases; in addition to further increase human capacity in the field of medical microscopy, allowing healthcare professionals to anticipate or prevent disease progression considering the genetic and environmental factors that can increase a patient's predisposition to the disease. It allows adequate treatment at the right time, which results in a reduction in health costs, still relating that this type of digital imaging diagnosis leads to the best possible treatment for the patient.

The blood count is one of the most important exams for the assessment of the patient's general health, primarily aimed at quantitative and qualitative assessments of the cellular elements of the blood, considering reference value indices that were established in the 1960s. Based on criteria for assessing the health of the world population and factors that occur in the majority of people considered healthy, in this bias, the blood count is not only applied for the diagnosis of diseases but also as a "health assessor" in periodic examinations and check-ups up. Just as this exam has the potential to identify certain complications for human health, evaluating the functioning of organs and glands in a specific way. In this sense, the hemogram test serves to assess the three main cells of our blood, platelets, red blood cells, and leukocytes, noting that blood cell counts have been modernized in recent decades with laboratory technological sophistication, given the respective capacity the differential leukocyte count in five types such as neutrophils, lymphocytes, monocytes, eosinophils, and basophils, given its breadth as a starting point for most medical investigations.

This type of exam is intended to assess overall health; diagnose or monitor a medical condition, such as the patient's fevers, inflammations, and hemorrhages; and to monitor the medical treatment being carried out through the use of medications, helping to diagnose the cause of these prognostic. From the results of this test, abnormal aspects are shown that tend to signal the presence of a variety of conditions related to the number and types of white cells. If it is high, it may constitute inflammation or infection; a number of red cells, and if low, can signal anemia or another type of disease. Change in the size of red cells, if this happens, it can also be a sign of anemia; or even through a laboratory parameter that indicates the percentage of red cells (total blood volume) may signal anemia or excessive bleeding or even show anemia and lung diseases. Or even low platelet counts can mean problems due to excessive bleeding; the size of red cells, if it is larger, can denote that the body is low on vitamin B12 or folic acid, if smaller, can be a sign of types of anemia, for example, iron deficiency; and even more serious aspects like leukemia, among many other conditions.

Through the subtypes eosinophils, basophils, neutrophils, lymphocytes, and monocytes, each performing a different role in the immune system can mean the presence of inflammatory or infectious processes in the body, it is possible to measure the quantity and types of leukocytes (WBC), reflecting that a high number of this can signal leukemia (white blood cell disease), a type of malignant tumor, which causes the accumulation of diseased cells in the bone marrow, replacing healthy ones, and often, its origin is unknown, which represents the need for a bone marrow biopsy or the response to treatment with chemotherapy, radiotherapy, or other forms of therapy.

Seen all this context, associating this scenario among the main AI applications, is deep learning since this learns from the data and improves automatically, without necessarily being programmed. This technology applied in medicine allows faster and more accurate diagnoses, such as the digital classification of these cell leukocyte subtypes through CNN, through digital medical imaging allows to evaluate a patient's clinical condition concerning the initial diagnosis and monitoring of infectious, inflammatory, allergic, toxic, and neoplastic processes, increasing accuracy granting the early diagnosis of various diseases or even following the progression of any adverse medical condition evaluating whether the medical treatment is reaching the expected effect. Deep learning in medicine offers greater precision in the analysis and faster both in the performance of the exams and in the availability of the results, through an extensive database (dataset) of symptoms of patients, in the case of this particular research related to the dataset [41] of microscopic normal peripheral blood cell digital images, making it possible to find patterns in digital images, using this to learn for yourself, performing the task automatically, without human intervention or with few instructions, improving the certainty of diagnosis compared previously conventionally without AI technology, i.e., by human experts.

Thus, this study has the potential to reflect the constant technological and digital evolution related to the identification and classification of cell biology, given the diversity of technology-assisted exams enabling the need techniques for medical human specialists, as deep learning technology implicating equivalently for medical practice standardizing diagnoses of serious and frequent diseases such as bacterial infectious processes that can be analyzed by digital imaging, pointing to chronic myeloid leukemia or even intense reactive leukocytosis, favoring the medical assistance assisting in the decision making and consequently increasing the possibilities of a promising treatment.

Reflecting on the framework developed in this research since the tool can process a high volume of data automatically in a matter of seconds as well as learning to interpret them and identify patterns in that information, and observing the results achieved, it proves how this study is promising for medical areas. From this panorama, it is still possible to reflect on the reality present in medical institutions dependent on high-cost hematological equipment or even specific reagents with restricted purchase options from resellers. This context can be changed from blood tests via a computational device (with the framework presented) reducing the time of the exam result and even producing higher quality.

Or even associating the aspect of employment of AI technology to a large portion of the world which is not indifferent to developing blood disorders, living in situations of extreme poverty, or even a portion of the world with little or no government assistance, and from this type of study is one more step in the possibility of being cured of diseases when discovered in the early stages and even providing personalized medicine and treatment designed according to a patient's specific physiological characteristics, at the same step as it provides more information about his condition, since, in contrast, the practice of medicine in its current model, medical care is quite reactionary, which does not allow a type of personalized medicine with scope.

6 Future Research Directions

This research is aligned with the constant requirement and demand for advancement in the medical field associated with optimizing cell qualification and identification, classification, and recognition of WBCs, refining the level of segmentation detail related differentiation of T-lymphocyte, related to immune system cells of the group of leukocytes responsible for the defense of the organism against unknown agents (antigens), and B-lymphocyte, having an important role in humoral immunity, with the main one being the production of antibodies against antigens, also being an essential component of the adaptive immune system, thus it stands out for the immunological response performed by the production of antibodies capable of neutralizing or even destroying antigens acting as immune memory cells [9, 10, 42].

This research may employ techniques based on generative adverse networks (GANs), which consist of neural networks that generate digital images that look real, consisting of two neural networks, based on two competing neural networks, one of which produces artificial images and the other com the role of deciding whether an image is true or false. That is, there are discriminator neural networks, having the task of judging whether the image is true or if it was artificially generated, and neural networks generating new artificial images, to deceive the discriminating network. However, GANs goes beyond that, it creates new content, so it is considered an important milestone in AI, given their potential to generate 3D models of cars and buildings based on the study of 2D photos [42–44].

Exemplifying the technological use of GANs, it is possible to collect all Picasso's paintings and train a GAN to identify the colors, characteristics, and individual brushstrokes representative of the artist's works. In this sense, the neural network tries to copy Picasso's works, while another analyzes every attempt. GANs imitating by applying their knowledge to produce thousands of new images in the style of Picasso, using characteristics of existing works of art (generator), while another network assesses the similarity between the creations and the style of Picasso and generates a classification (discriminator). The unconvincing results are returned to the imitation neural network (generator) to be improved, so after processing data millions of times, the imitation (generator) network gets better and better at creating Picasso-style paintings (Fig. 15) [42–44].

GAN starts from the premise of the possibility of a neural network being able to go beyond learning what characterizes each of the digits, learning the relationship that the data has and, with this, it can understand what looks like a digit 0 and what looks like a digit 1. This can create a digit 1 or a digit 0, which is very similar to a handwritten digit. This is exactly what GANs can do, instead of simply classifying, GANs create images, or even GANs can serve to reconstruct what has been lost, and this is very useful for society. For example, if the image of a tiger was cut off and there is a neural network that knows how to draw tigers, we can use this GAN

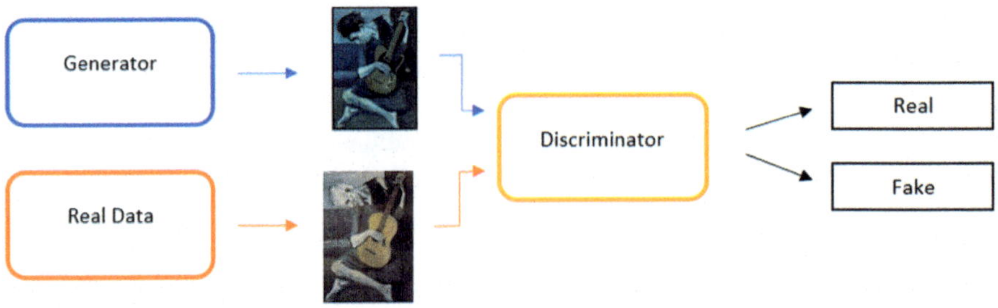

Fig. 15 GANs

to reconstruct that part that was cut off. This is very useful in order not to lose the entire image because of that damage that was caused by the image cut, associating this applicability to the old, historical images, which have some noise or smudges, can be totally reconstructed with the help of GAN's [42–44].

Emphasizing that in computer vision techniques that use dense or convolutional neural networks, when it is intended to increase the size of a digital image, this is done via interpolation or even repetition of the pixels; however, this does not increase the image quality. The digital quality is dependent on how many pixels were collected at the time that image was taken (like a cell microscopy image), and from that, it is no longer possible to manipulate to recreate an image with more quality. GANs increases the quality of the image, creating pixels that did not exist, created not based on an average of the surrounding pixels, nor using any technique based on the image that is already there; GANs create these new pixels based on knowledge from training and digital learning from other images. Also relating that deep learning models are generally used to perform classification tasks; however, it is limited by the number of images available in the training dataset, increasing this volume of data and synthetically generating a larger amount of data, which resembles the original, GANs, on the other hand, it can be applied to generate synthetic and realistic images [45, 46].

Another trend of this research is in the detection and classification of morphologies of healthy and pathological red blood cells, which can vary concerning their normal state associated with the shape of a biconcave disk and anucleated when mature, to assist in the diagnosis of leukemia and anemia. Or even relating the perspective of the development of this research concerning the detection of morphological alterations of platelets (micro-platelets and macro-platelets) to assist in the diagnosis of blood coagulation disorders, since this results in the organism being unable to produce sufficient amounts of proteins that are needed to help the blood to clot. Stressing that normal blood clotting is a complex process, where blood cells heal damaged blood vessels and control bleeding, as coagulopathies occur when clotting factors are lost or damaged, or when the number or function of platelets is debilitated [7, 9, 10, 46].

7 Conclusions

Deep learning (DL) is an area of AI that gives computing devices the ability to learn automatically, emphasizing that this digital learning is acquired through the processing of a large amount of data, which is used by the algorithm to obtain experience and constant improvement, using results from old experiences to make better decisions in the future. This technology used in healthcare takes on those repetitive, tiring, and error-prone tasks (since countless factors must be taken into account in this process) by healthcare professionals, having the potential to make patients' diagnoses and treatments more accurate.

The blood count is the blood test most commonly requested by doctors, being part of the routine of periodic examinations, consisting of the analysis of cells present in the blood and aiming to detect disorders such as anemia, infections, and bone marrow malfunction. The examination is a simple procedure that does not require much preparation, given the possibility of bringing valuable information about the patient's health. There are no contraindications for this test, nor are there any impediments for that more sensitive part of the population, such as pregnant women, children, diabetics, and the elderly; however, some conditions may temporarily alter the result. Therefore, it is important to warn about the use of medications and avoid consuming alcoholic beverages within 48 hours before the exam.

Thus, through the CNNN dataset training applied in the medical context primarily concerned with the construction of solutions that perform diagnostics, it was noted that the classification-oriented model of white blood cells achieved significant results related to 84.19% of accuracy. This represents an excellent score due to the complexity of the studied problem, i.e., a satisfactory distinctiveness in the classification between different blood subtypes. It also can be concluded that the structure modeling parameters allowed the positive exploration of CNN's advantage regarding maintaining the spatial characteristics of a digital image, such as height, width, and even colors, enabling computational processing favored, provided that it receives the digital images as input, interpreting it as values stored in an array by the computational device.

The biggest advantage of AI in medicine is, without a doubt, the aid in diagnosing pathologies, or even performing laboratory tests using technology deep learning, enabling results, suggestive or not, allowing medical professionals to reinforce the diagnosis encompassing the interpretation and recognition of medical reports for imaging examinations of a certain disease, or even serious pathologies, reflecting that health is a vast area suitable related to medical diagnostics by images.

Also reflecting on the proposed framework of this research is highly feasible for the distinct realities (socio-economic) and laboratory models, able to contribute rightly to the access to health of economically disadvantaged populations, still considering the perspective that these exams may be archived in digital files for later consultations, related to the patient's history, confirming the identification of pathologies or even the symptoms can be associated, also eliminating the generation of physical space (use of data storage) for it.

Thereby, the creation of new methodologies, as the one shown in this chapter, aims to reduce the pressure on medical professionals, simplifying the workflow, improving diagnostic processes, associating the vision of the job, and implementation of AI on the individuality of each patient's health. Also associating that the presented framework has immediate implications for the care of the patient, being able to eliminate problems with the handling of biological materials and could detect anomalies as it occurs, as well as meaning in a lesser concern with the risk of loss or damage of biological specimens (blood sample collected).

At the same time, it is worth noting that AI technology, as well as deep learning in the area of health, brings innumerable innovations, but that in no way is it intended to replace the performance of medical professionals. On the contrary, the purpose of this technology is to facilitate the human medical work, comprising machines and computational devices that can interpret information for which it was taught, given the knowledge and human experience of healthcare professionals, feeding these algorithms with specific and technical instructions. Thus, intelligent digital technology and innovation are capable of transforming the experience of patients, facilitating the prevention of diseases, providing clearer and faster diagnoses, in addition to allowing more quality of life.

References

1. França, R. P., et al. (2020). An overview of deep learning in big data, image, and signal processing in the modern digital age. *Trends in Deep Learning Methodologies: Algorithms, Applications, and Systems, 4*, 63.
2. Monteiro, A. C. B., et al. (2018). Toxoplasmosis Gondii: From discovery to advances in image processing. In *Brazilian Technology Symposium*. Springer.
3. Estrela, Vania V., et al. "DICOM's Standardization in Histo-Pathology." Medical Technologies Journal 4.3 (2020): 578–579.
4. Khelassi, A., et al. (2019). Health 4.0: Applications, management, technologies and review. *Medical Technologies Journal.*
5. Matheny, M., Israni, S. T., Ahmed, M., & Whicher, D. (2019). *Artificial intelligence in health care: The hope, the hype, the promise, the peril* (Vol. 154). NAM Special Publication. National Academy of Medicine.
6. Walczak, S. (2019). Artificial neural networks. In *Advanced methodologies and technologies in artificial intelligence, computer simulation, and human-computer interaction* (pp. 40–53). IGI Global.
7. Monteiro, A. C. B. (2019). Proposta de uma metodologia de segmentação de imagens para detecção e contagem de hemácias e leucócitos através do algoritmo WT-MO.
8. Monteiro, A. C. B., et al. (2019). Medical-laboratory algorithm WTH-MO for segmentation of digital images of blood cells: A new methodology for making hemograms. *International Journal of Simulation: Systems, Science and Technology, 20*(Suppl 1), 19–1.
9. Silberstein, L. E., & Anastasi, J. (2017). *Hematology: Basic principles and practice E-book.* Elsevier Health Sciences.
10. Lazarus, H. M., & Schmaier, A. H. (Eds.) (2018). *Concise guide to hematology*. Springer.
11. Monteiro, A. C. B., et al. Hematology: A review of the main methodologies of clinical analyses. In *Proceedings of the 5th Brazilian Technology Symposium*. Springer.
12. Modha, D. S., et al. (2011). Cognitive computing. *Communications of the ACM, 54*(8), 62–71.
13. Gutierrez-Garcia, J. O., & López-Neri, E. (2015). Cognitive computing: a brief survey and open research challenges. In *2015 3rd International Conference on Applied Computing and Information Technology/2nd International Conference on Computational Science and Intelligence*. IEEE.
14. Chen, M., Herrera, F., & Hwang, K. (2018). Cognitive computing: Architecture, technologies and intelligent applications. *Ieee Access, 6*, 19774–19783.
15. Mehta, N., & Devarakonda, M. V. (2018). Machine learning, natural language programming, and electronic health records: The next step in the artificial intelligence journey? *Journal of Allergy and Clinical Immunology, 141*(6), 2019–2021.
16. Judith, et al. (2015). *Cognitive computing and big data analytics.* Wiley; Wang, Y., et al. (2016). Cognitive intelligence: Deep learning, thinking, and reasoning by brain-inspired systems. *International Journal of Cognitive Informatics and Natural Intelligence (IJCINI), 10*(4), 1–20.
17. Skansi, S. (2018). *Introduction to deep learning: From logical calculus to artificial intelligence.* Springer.
18. Meng, W. *Cognitive computing: theory and applications.*

19. Bini, S. A. (2018). Artificial intelligence, machine learning, deep learning, and cognitive computing: What do these terms mean and how will they impact health care? *The Journal of Arthroplasty, 33*(8), 2358–2361.
20. Monteiro, A. C. B., et al. (2018). Health 4.0 as an application of Industry 4.0 in healthcare services and management. *Medical Technologies Journa,l 2*(4), 262–276.
21. Estrela, V. V., et al. (2020). Content-based image retrieval (CBIR) in big histological image databases. *Medical Technologies Journal, 4*(3), 581–582.
22. Behera, R. K., Bala, P. K., & Dhir, A. (2019). The emerging role of cognitive computing in healthcare: A systematic literature review. *International Journal of Medical Informatics, 129*, 154–166.
23. Kelleher, J. D. (2019). *Deep learning.*
24. Monteiro, A. C. B., et al. (2020). Deep learning methodology proposal for the classification of erythrocytes and leukocytes. In *Trends in deep learning methodologies: Algorithms, applications, and systems* (Vol. 129).
25. Monteiro, A. C. B., et al. (2018). Methodology of high accuracy, sensitivity and specificity in the counts of erythrocytes and leukocytes in blood smear images. In *Brazilian technology symposium.* Springer.
26. Flasiński, M. (2016). *Introduction to artificial intelligence.* Springer.
27. Jackson, P. C. (2019). *Introduction to artificial intelligence.* Courier Dover Publications.
28. Gambus, P., & Shafer, S. L. (2018). Artificial intelligence for everyone. *Anesthesiology: The Journal of the American Society of Anesthesiologists, 128*(3), 431–433.
29. França, R. P., et al. (2021). an overview of the machine learning applied in smart cities. In *Smart cities: A data analytics perspective* (pp. 91–111).
30. Stengel, R. (2017). *Introduction to neural networks!.*
31. Wilamowski, B. M. (2018). Neural networks learning. In *Intelligent systems* (pp. 11–11). CRC Press.
32. Levine, D. S. (2018). *Introduction to neural and cognitive modeling.* Routledge.
33. Monteiro, A. C. B., et al. Deep learning methodology proposal for the classification of erythrocytes and leukocytes. *Trends in Deep Learning Methodologies: Algorithms, Applications, and Systems, 129.*
34. Neagoe, V.-E., Ciotec, A.-D., Cucu, G.-S. (2018). Deep convolutional neural networks versus multilayer perceptron for financial prediction. In *2018 International Conference on Communications (COMM).* IEEE.
35. Wu, J. (2017). Introduction to convolutional neural networks. *National Key Lab for Novel Software Technology. Nanjing University. China, 5*(23).
36. Yao, G., Lei, T., & Zhong, J. (2019). A review of Convolutional-Neural-Network-based action recognition. *Pattern Recognition Letters, 118*, 14–22.
37. Negrete, P. D. M., et al. Classification of dermoscopy skin images with the application of deep learning techniques. In *Proceedings of the 5th Brazilian Technology Symposium.* Springer, Cham.
38. Kim, K. G. (2016). Book review: Deep learning. *Healthcare informatics research, 22*(4), 351–354.
39. Véstias, M. P. (2021). Convolutional neural network. In *Encyclopedia of information science and technology* (5th ed., pp. 12–26). IGI Global.
40. Mohapatra, S., Swarnkar, T., & Das, J. (2021). Deep convolutional neural network in medical image processing. In *Handbook of deep learning in biomedical engineering* (pp. 25–60). Academic Press.
41. GitHub—Shenggan/BCCD_Dataset: BCCD Dataset is a small-scale dataset for blood cells detection. BCCD Dataset is under MIT license. [Online]. Available: https://github.com/Shenggan/BCCD_Dataset
42. Yi, X., Walia, E., & Babyn, P. (2019). Generative adversarial network in medical imaging: A review. *Medical Image Analysis, 58*, 101552.
43. Tavakkoli, A., et al. (2020). A novel deep learning conditional generative adversarial network for producing angiography images from retinal fundus photographs. *Scientific Reports, 10*(1), 1–15.

44. Kazeminia, S., et al. (2020). GANs for medical image analysis. *Artificial Intelligence in Medicine*, 101938.
45. Armanious, K., et al. (2020). MedGAN: Medical image translation using GANs. *Computerized Medical Imaging and Graphics*, *79*, 101684.
46. Singh, N. K., & Raza, K. (2020). Medical image generation using generative adversarial networks. arXiv preprint arXiv:2005.10687.

Extreme Learning-Based Intellectual Lung Cancer Classification Using Artificial Intelligence

Prasannavenkatesan Theerthagiri and C. Gopala Krishnan

1 Introduction

Lung carcinoma, also referred as lung cancer, is a high-risk condition that affects lung cells and causes tumors. It affects all peoples of the world. It also affects one's ability to breathe. It is caused by the development of malignant tumors in the lungs as a result of uncontrollably developing cells. It is popular among all chain smokers and those who are frequently exposed to second-hand smoke. In rare circumstances, it is also genetically transferable based on family background. The presence of carcinogens, or cancer-causing agents, in smoke raises the disease's risk factor [1–3].

Abnormal chest pain, coughing, coughing up blood, loss of appetite, shortness of breath, weight loss, shortness of breath, and weakness are some of the vital common symptoms of the lung cancer dangerous disease. The final stage leads to metastasis, or the spread of cancer to other areas of the body. Small cell lung cancer (SCLC) and non-small cell lung cancer (NSCLC) are the two main types of lung cancer (NSCLC). The SCLC is most common in chain smokers, and the NSCLC is the most common form [2].

Cancer-causing cells called adenocarcinomas develop in outer layer of the lungs and squamous cell carcinoma forms in the respiratory tract in NSCLC. SCLC allows tumors to mutate more rapidly than NSCLC. Roughly publics develop both NSCLC and SCLC and cells in exceptional cases. To one side from these two groups, asbestos exposure can contribute to the development of mesothelioma, a form of lung cancer. SCLC cancer stages are divided into two categories: small stages and comprehensive stages. Just one lung can affect by cancer cells in the restricted stage [1].

The cancer cells have been spread in and sections around both lungs throughout the advanced stage. The phases of NSCLC cancer are divided into many classes.

P. Theerthagiri (✉) · C. Gopala Krishnan
Department of Computer Science and Engineering, GITAM School of Technology, GITAM University, Bengaluru, India
e-mail: vprasann@gitam.edu

A. K. Tyagi et al. (eds.), *Intelligent Interactive Multimedia Systems for e-Healthcare Applications*, https://doi.org/10.1007/978-981-16-6542-4_19

Cancer cells are located within one lung in stage one. The Stage 2 cancer cells are present in one lung as well as surrounding lymph nodes. The Stage 3 cancer cells are found within one lung, as well as in the middle of the chest on lymph nodes. Cancer cells are located in lymph nodes on the same side of the chest where they first begin to develop in stage 3A. Cancer cells migrate to lymph nodes on the other lung and lymph nodes above the collarbone in stage 3B. The fourth stage is metastasis.

The rest of the chapter is set out as follows. The Section-II discusses the recent literature works on the lung cancer detection technique. The proposed methodology of the work is given in Section-III. The results analysis and performance evaluation of the proposed works are presented in Section-IV. Section-V concludes the presented chapter with future work.

2 Literature Works

To reduce human error, Kalaivani et al. [1] suggested an automatic early detection of lung cancer through image recognition models and ANN. To add an RGB image as input, the preprocessing, thresholding, histogram equalization, and feature extractions are used. It is translated into a grayscale image in binary form for better lung cancer detection accuracy [2]. Furthermore, with 78% overall performance, a back-propagation algorithm (feed-forward) network has been used for the minimization of the error at each point at each epoch.

Gawade Prathamesh et al. [4] suggested using a CT scan from the patient to detect lung cancer cells. The filtering algorithms like high pass filtering and median pass filtering are applied to the image after it is converted to grayscale [5, 6]. The output resultant image with the cancer depicted region is found after passing the median filtered image through various segmentations such as p-tile thresholding, binary morphology, and watershed segmentation. This research can also be used to detect cancers such as skin cancer.

To detect lung cancer, Ritika Agarwal et al. [7] suggested content-based medical image retrieval. It employs a computer-aided diagnostic (CAD) method to detect lung nodules on chest CT images early. The techniques used include lung area extraction with preprocessing technique and a region-based segmentation method. Following that, features are extracted from an unsegmented area using feature extraction algorithms such as 2D wavelet transformation, gray level co-occurrence matrix, and categorization of the existence of lung cancer to achieve an effectiveness of 80% in lung cancer detection by learning diagnosis.

Kurkure et al. [8] suggested using a genomic approach with CT images, X-ray images, and PET diagnostic images to diagnose lung cancer. Presence of nodules in the lungs is detected early on using an optimization algorithm. To distinguish between cancerous and non-cancerous cells, the classifier called Naive Bayes algorithm is used. Via classification, a significant accuracy of around 80% is achieved.

Pooja et al. [9] presented a study that used image processing and data classification techniques to detect lung cancer. It employs image processing techniques such as a median filter for noise removal, a high boost operator for image enhancement, and a balanced watershed algorithm for image segmentation. The support vector machine (SVM) algorithm is used to categorize images based on their image pattern. The patient's cancer is determined by the nodule's development at various levels.

Prajwal Rao et al. [10] suggested a CanNet architecture that consists of two convolution layers of CNN that is used to distinguish malignant images and benign images from CT scans. This architecture is often related to conventional architectures such as the ANN and the LeNet architecture. The results show that ANN is more accurate than LeNet architecture, with 72.5% and 56% accuracy, respectively.

The entropy degradation method (EDM) was presented by Qing Wu et al. [11] based on a machine learning technique for detecting small cell lung cancer from CT scan for detecting lung cancer earlier, and this algorithm is also used to achieve an accuracy of around 77.8% with a limited dataset. However, by using it in a wider training set and a broader network for different applications, the algorithm can be strengthened.

Wafaa et al. [12] suggested the use of 3D convolutional neural networks in computer-aided diagnosis (CAD) (3D-CNN). The input comes from CNN architecture, which detects nodules in lung cancer patients and detects the interest point using U-Net architecture. This algorithm outperforms current CAD systems with an accuracy of 86.6%.

With the aid of feature extraction, Siddharth et al. [13] proposed a deep residual network for lung cancer detection. Preprocessing is used to highlight the cancerous lung area, and Unet and Resnet models are used to remove the function. Unet and the random forest have a cumulative accuracy result of 74%. Resnet algorithms and XG boost classifier model have a 76% of accuracy; although, if we consider the ensemble of Unet algorithm, Resnet, and XG boost classifiers, the images of CT scan display lung cancer has an 84 percent accuracy.

3 The ELM Methodology

The proposed lung cancer detection algorithm includes an ELM classifier for classification. The successful part of the lung image is obtained by preprocessing. Using the PSO algorithm in the function extraction, the optimized features were accessed to boost the precision of lung cancer detection. The proposed strategy's well-organized system has been examined in the subsections that follow. The workflow of the proposed approach is depicted in Fig. 1.

The Kaggle repository [14] provided the dataset of DICOM photographs of lung cancer. For evaluating lung cancer diagnosis, about 100 photographs of different ages are used.

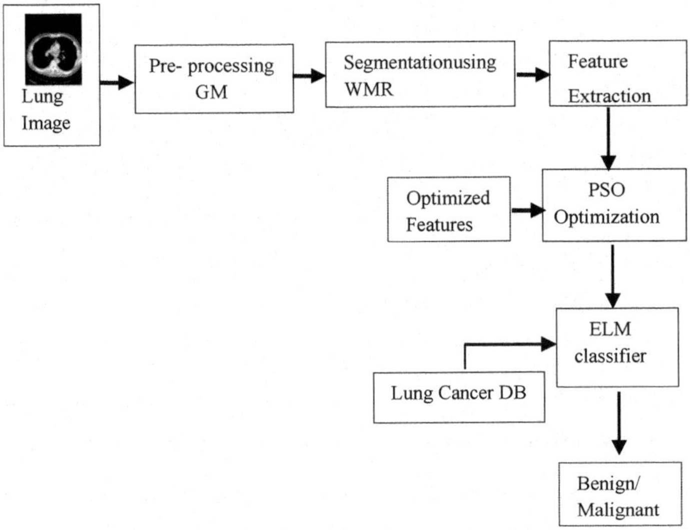

Fig. 1 Block diagram of proposed system

3.1 Preprocessing of Data

In preprocessing, the lung CT image has been processed as the input using a median filter. Median filtering is a common nonlinear method for noise suppression. The median value of the neighborhood (mask) is used to change the noisy value of the digital image or series [15]. The mask's pixels are ranked according to their gray levels, and the group's median value is saved to replace the noisy value [15].

Then, the gradient magnitude has been utilized to get the accurate threshold result. The gradient is usually high at the borders of the objects and low inside the objects. Image gradients can also be used for robust feature and texture matching. Gradient computation of a non-segmented image is a kind of edge detection; it enhances the areas in an image where the rate of change is high [16]. Usually done by subtracting each pixel in a row from the previous pixel (i.e., horizontal gradient) and each pixel in a column from the previous one (i.e., vertical gradient). The preprocessing result of the gray level value of an image is obtained using the gradient magnitude is as

$$\nabla F = \begin{bmatrix} g_x \\ g_y \end{bmatrix} = \begin{bmatrix} \frac{\partial f}{\partial x} \end{bmatrix} \begin{bmatrix} \frac{\partial f}{\partial y} \end{bmatrix} \tag{1}$$

$$\|\nabla F\| = \sqrt{\left[\frac{\delta F}{\delta x}\right]^2 + \left[\frac{\delta F}{\delta y}\right]^2} \tag{2}$$

ΔF is the image gradient; $|\Delta F|$ is the gradient magnitude of an image.

3.2 Lung Cancer Segmentation Using Marker Controlled Watershed Algorithm

The main aim of the CT tumor image segmentation is to acquire a better-segmented image by using marker-controlled watershed segmentation. This segmentation is a reliable and adaptable method for partitioning objects with closed contours and ridges as boundaries [17]. The watershed segmentation marker image is a binary image of the source with either a larger marker or a single marker region [17]. Each linked marker is placed within a target item.

Each initial marker corresponds to a single watershed area, so the total number of markers would be the same as the total number of watershed regions [18]. Following segmentation, the borders of the watershed regions are placed on the desired ridges, dividing each entity from its neighbors. The morphological image reconstruction has been processed as follows:

Let A and B be two images that are defined on the same domain, with $B \leq A$ [18]. The reconstruction of A from B denoted as $\gamma_A^{(\text{recn})}(B)$ is obtained by iterating elementary dilations of B under A until stability is reached,

$$\gamma_A^{(\text{recn})}(B) = \cup\delta_{n\geq 1}^{(n)}(B) \tag{3}$$

where $\delta^{(n)}(B)$ is attained by iterating from an elementary dilation, and the dilation of the relation is defined as

$$\delta^{(\text{I})}(B) = (B \oplus b) \cap A \tag{4}$$

(b stands for flat structuring part of the size I and $\bigcap$ stands for point-wise minimum). Let A and B be two images that are defined on the same domain, with $B \leq A$. The rebuilding of A from B denoted as $\varphi_A^{(\text{recn})}(B)$, is obtained by iterating basic erosions of B under A until stability is reached.

$$\varphi_A^{(\text{recn})}(B) = \cap\varepsilon_{n\geq 1}^{(n)}(B) \tag{5}$$

where $\varepsilon^{(n)}(B)$ can be obtained by iterating an elementary erosion [16], and the erosion is defined as

$$\varepsilon^{(I)}(B) = (B \ominus b) \cup A \tag{6}$$

(b stands for the flat structuring element of the size I and $\cup$ stands for point-wise maximum).

Algorithm 1: Marker-controlled watershed segmentation

i. Read an image.

ii. Use an effective edge detection feature to extend the gradient images.
iii. Use morphological reconstruction to locate foreground objects (i.e., opening and closing by reconstruction).
iv. Calculate regional maxima and minima to obtain strong foreground markers.
v. Overlay the foreground marker picture on top of the initial.
vi. Exclude any dark pixels that are near to the object's edges.
vii. Calculate the markers for the history.
viii. Calculate the segmentation function's watershed transform.

3.3 Feature Extraction

A function is a significant piece of information derived from an image that helps to explain the image more thoroughly. Geometric and intensity-based statistical characteristics, for example, are extracted [19, 20]. Shape measurements are physical dimensional measurements that describe an object's appearance. These characteristics are given as input to the classification. Scale, form, entropy, convexity, homogeneity, eccentricity, concavity, irregularity, location, and perimeter have all been extracted from the texture. The extracted features are optimized using the PSO algorithm, and optimized features are using the ELM classifier for further classification.

3.4 Optimized Feature Selection Using PSO

The method of choosing the redundant function for the classifier is known as feature selection [21]. It will be extremely helpful in reducing the dimensionality of the data to be processed as well as the execution time. The feature selection is primarily used in the data analysis process because it represents a feature that is critical for predicting the rigorousness and relationships between features. Russell Eberhart and James Kennedy proposed particle swarm optimization (PSO) as a bio-inspired meta-heuristic algorithm in 1995. The PSO was used to classify the most significant features among those extracted from the segmented lung area [22, 23].

The group-based search algorithm is the particle swarm optimization (PSO). It is the genetic algorithm (GA) based on the population, and it is similar to the PSO algorithm. The self-adaptive global search method is the PSO [7] that works as manner as to the optimization algorithm. To begin, this algorithm chose a solution at random through the search space that contains every possible solution. Every unit keeps track of its fitness score, location, and velocity. The optimal fitness value is achieved for all particles, called gbest fitness. Also, the finest location of the value is achieved using a unit called P_{best}. There are three stages to it, as follows:

1. Determine the fitness value of each particle.
2. Re-evaluate each person's best health and its roles.
3. Reset the velocity and location of each particle.

Each particle's velocity is restructured by

$$vi(t+1) = wv + c1\,\text{rand1}[x(t) - xi(t)] + c2\,\text{rand2}\,[\text{gbest}(t) - xi(t)] \quad (7)$$

The particle's key is indicated by the letter '*I*' The velocity of the particle '*I*' at time '*t*' is vi(t), and the location of the particle '*i*' at time '*t*' is $xi(t)$. The variables w, $c1$, and $c2$ are user-defined. The values rand1 and rand2, which range from 0 to 1, are generated at random on every update of velocity. The meaning $xi(t)$ represents the unique best optimal candidate solution for unit '*i*' at the time '*t*,' while $g_{\text{best}}(t)$ represents the swarm's global optimal candidate solution at the time '*t*.' Applying the new velocity to the particle's previous location to update the positions:

$$xi(t+1) = xi(t) + vi(t+1) \quad (8)$$

The features are computed for the training lung cancer datasets and provided as an initial solution to the PSO optimization algorithm to obtain the best features for classification. The fitness function is used to choose the features that are suitable for classification using PSO. The random selection of features and assessment of the fitness function was carried out first. This process of calculating the best fitness function and its location is repeated until the highest precision with the fewest possible features is achieved. As a result, the range of features for classification is improved even further.

3.5 Feature Classification Using ELM

The feed-forward neural network with a single hidden layer (1-LFN) is the extreme learning machine (ELM) [24]. For higher learning, the output of the l-LFN should be sufficient for the system to be modeled for data such as weight, threshold value, and activation functions. All of these parameters are iteratively modified for the desired value in gradient-based learning approaches. As a consequence of the probability of being attached to the slow and local minimum, the performance may be bad.

In contrast to FNN, which is renewed based on the gradient in the ELM Learning process, the output weights are determined analytically while the input weights are chosen at random [25]. Since the resolution time and error value will seriously reduce the probability of being fitted to a local minimum in an analytic learning method, the performance rate increases. ELM can be used for activating the hidden layer cells based on a linear function, and also using the nonlinear (sinusoidal and sigmoid), non-derivative activation functions, or periodic activation functions.

The mathematical statement for a network with M neurons in the hidden layer is as follows, with $X = (X1, X2, X3... XN)$ denoting input attributes and $Y = (Y1, Y2, Y3... YN)$ denoting output attributes.

$$y = f(x) = \sum_{i=1}^{P} \beta_i g(w_i, x_j, b_i)$$

$$\sum_{i=1}^{P} \beta_i g(W_i.X_j + b_i) = o_j, j = 1, 2, \ldots., N \tag{9}$$

where $wi = (W_{i1}, W_{i2}, W_{i3} \ldots, W_{in})$ is the output weight in the input layer, $\beta i = (\beta i1, \beta i2, \beta i3 \ldots \beta in)$ is the weight vector that unites the output neurons and the 'i'th hidden neuron, bi is the threshold values and o_j is the output values of the network. g(.) is the activation function. In order to reduce the relative error o_j and Y_k in ELM, rewrite Eq. (9)

$$\sum_{i=1}^{P} \beta_i g(W_i.X_j + b_i) = y_j, j = 1, 2, \ldots., N \tag{10}$$

And the above N equations can be provided as

$$H\beta = T \tag{11}$$

where $H(w1, \ldots, wL, x1, \ldots, xN, b1, \ldots, bP) = \begin{bmatrix} g(wi.xi + bi \ldots & g(wp.xi + bp \\ \vdots \quad \ldots & \vdots \\ g(wi.xi + bi \ldots & g(wP.xi + bP)_{N\times P} \end{bmatrix}$.

where 'H' is the hidden layer output matrix. By solving the linear Eq. (11). The optimal weight of the output matrix as a target attribute,

$$\hat{\beta} = H^{\dagger} T \tag{12}$$

4 The Outcomes and Discussions

In this segment, classifiers such as ENNPSO, RBFN, SVM, and ANFIS have been used to evaluate and test the presented method for detecting lung cancer using ELM [26, 27]. CT scan images are sorted first, and then attempts are made. MATLAB is used to monitor the activities. All of the images are 512 × 512 pixels in size. For the test, approximately 100 sample images are obtained. There are 75 images which are trained from the dataset, and about 25 images are checked using the ELM classification method. Figure 2 illustrates the proposed watershed with morphological reconstruction segmentation results. Figure 3 depicts the performance metrics of

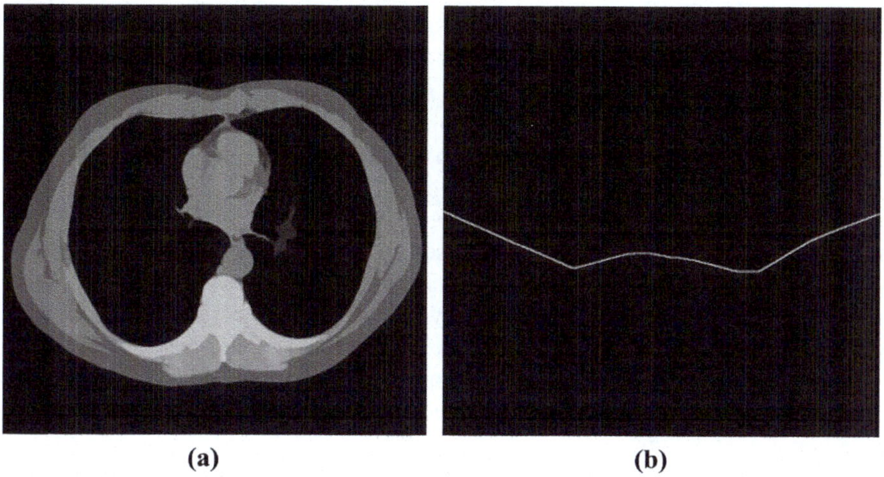

Fig. 2 Proposed watershed with morphological reconstruction segmentation results

Fig. 3 Performance metrics of Proposed ELM

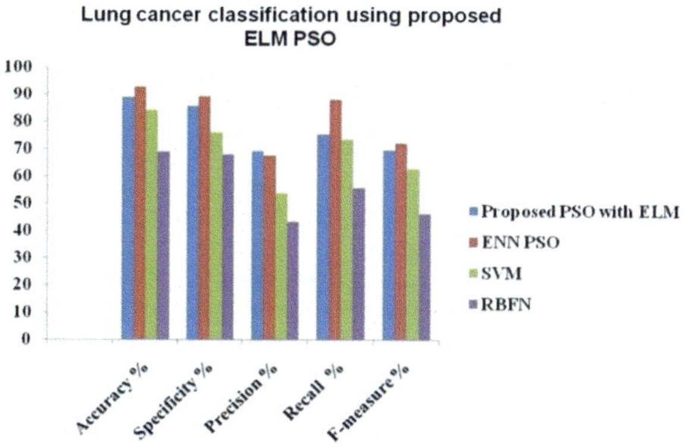

proposed ELM. Table 1 summarizes the performance matrices of proposed model for lung cancer detection method.

Table 1 Performance matrices of proposed model for lung cancer detection method

Performance matrices	Proposed PSO with ELM	ENN PSO	SVM	RBFN
Accuracy (%)	89	93	84	69
Specificity (%)	85.76	89.31	76.14	67.88
Precision (%)	69.25	67.49	53.78	43.50
Recall (%)	75.36	88	73.33	55.68
F-measure (%)	69.61	72.14	62.65	46.42

5 Conclusion

The diagnosis of lung cancer using ELM has been suggested in this paper. The noise in the input DICOM image is eliminated, and the image smoothing is enhanced. The original lung image is segmented through the preprocessed image using a marker operated watershed algorithm with morphological reconstruction to improve precision. Significant features are driven from segmented lung images. Hence, the features are extracted and optimized using PSO. Based on the optimized features, ELM is used to classify the tumor part with higher accuracy. The experimental results show that the proposed ELM attained a less accuracy rate of 89% compared with the existing algorithm as ENNPSO. Based on the above results, predict that ENNPSO has a high accuracy rate when compared with the proposed method. In the future, the sample size will be increased to develop a naval deep algorithm that will make a lung tumor detection more intelligible.

References

1. Karthikeyan, V., & Vijayalakshmi, V. J. (2013, November 13) An efficient method for recognizing the low quality fingerprint verification by means of cross correlation. arXiv:1311.3076
2. Kalaivani, S., Chatterjee, P., Juyal, S., & Gupta, R. (2017). Lung cancer detection using digital image processing and artificial neural networks. In *International Conference on Electronics, Communication and Aerospace Technology (ICECA)* (pp. 100–103).
3. Usha Ruby, A., Theerthagiri, P., Jeena Jacob, I., & Vamsidhar, Y. (2020). Binary cross entropy with deep learning technique for image classification. *International Journal of Advanced Trends in Computer Science and Engineering, 9*(4), 5393–5397.
4. Pratap, G. P., & Chauhan, R. P. (2016). Detection of lung cancer cells using image processing techniques. In *1st IEEE International Conference on Power Electronics. Intelligent Control and Energy Systems (ICPEICES)* (pp. 1–6).
5. Pham, T. P., Durillo, J. J., & Fahringer, T. (2020, January). Programmer sought. *IEEE Transactions On Cloud Computing, 8*(1).
6. Attolini, C. S., Cheng, Y. K., Beroukhim, R., Getz, G., Abdel-Wahab, O., Levine, R. L., Mellinghoff, I. K., & Michor, F. (2010). A mathematical framework to determine the temporal sequence of somatic genetic events in cancer. *Proceedings of the National Academy of Sciences, 107*(41), 17604–17609.
7. Agarwal, R., Shankhadhar, A., & Sagar, R. K. (2015). Detection of lung cancer using content based medical image retrieval. In *Fifth International Conference on Advanced Computing & Communication Technologies* (pp. 48–52).
8. Kurkure, M., & Thakare, A. (2016). Lung cancer detection using genetic approach. In *International Conference on Computing Communication Control and automation (ICCUBEA)* (pp. 1–5).
9. Katre, P. R., & Thakare, A. (2017). Detection of lung cancer stages using image processing and data classification techniques. In *2nd International Conference for Convergence in Technology (I2CT)* (pp. 402–404).
10. Rao, P., Pereira, N. A., & Srinivasan, R. (2016). Convolutional neural networks for lung cancer screening in computed tomography (CT) scans. In *2nd International Conference on Contemporary Computing and Informatics (ic3i)* (pp. 489–493).

11. Wu, Q., & Zhao, W. (2017). Small-cell lung cancer detection using a supervised machine learning algorithm. In *International Symposium on Computer Science and Intelligent Controls* (pp. 88–91).
12. Alakwaa, W., Nassef, M., & Badr, A. (2017). Lung cancer detection and classification with 3D convolutional neural network (3D-CNN). *International Journal of Advanced Computer Science and Applications (IJACSA)*, 409–417.
13. Bhatia, S., Sinha, Y., & Goel, L. (2019). Lung cancer detection: A deep learning approach. *Advances in Intelligent Systems and Computing* (pp. 699–705).
14. Kaggle repository retrieved from: https://www.kaggle.com/kmader/siim-medical-images
15. Kaur, L. (2014, January 1). Removal of high density salt and pepper noise through hybrid of negative selection algorithm and median filter. *International Journal of Computer Applications, 107*(15).
16. Noguchi, M., Fujifilm Corp, assignee. (2014, July 31). Ultrasound diagnostic apparatus and method of producing ultrasound image. United States patent application US 14/166,260.
17. Parvati, K., Rao, P., & Mariya Das, M. (2008, November). Image segmentation using gray-scale morphology and marker-controlled watershed transformation. *Discrete Dynamics in Nature and Society*.
18. Súkeník, J. (2011). Solving of image similarity puzzle–singular value decomposition. *Information Sciences and Technologies Bulletin of the ACM Slovakia., 3*, 109–112.
19. Athira, P. K., & Mathew, L. S. (2015). Fetal anomaly detection in ultrasound image. *International Journal of Computer Applications, 975*, 8887.
20. Tun, K. M., & Khaing, A. S. (2014). Feature extraction and classification of lung cancer nodule using image processing techniques. *International Journal of Engineering Research and Technology (IJERT), 3*(3), 2278–3181.
21. Vryniotis, V. (2013). Machine learning blog & software development news.
22. Benes, R., & Riha, K. (2012). Medical image denoising by improved Kuan filter. *Advances in Electrical and Electronic Engineering, 10*.
23. Wang, D., Tan, D., & Liu, L. (2018). Particle swarm optimization algorithm: An overview. *Soft Computing, 22*, 387–408
24. Prasannavenkatesan, T. (2021). Forecasting hyponatremia in hospitalized patients using multilayer perceptron and multivariate linear regression techniques. *Concurrency and Computation: Practice and Experience*, e6248.
25. Theerthagiri, P. (2020). FUCEM: Futuristic cooperation evaluation model using Markov process for evaluating node reliability and link stability in mobile ad hoc network. *Wireless Networks*.
26. Kim, Y., & Seok, J. (2020, October). Network estimation for censored time-to-event data for multiple events based on multivariate survival analysis. *PLoS One, 15*(10), Public Library of Science (p. e0239760).
27. Krishnan, C. G., Nishan, A. H., Prasannavenkatesan, T., Jacob, I. J., & Komarasamy, G. (2021). Two dimensional and gesture based medical visualization interface and image processing methodologies to aid and diagnose of lung cancer. In J. Nayak, M. N. Favorskaya, S. Jain, B. Naik, & M. Mishra (Eds.), *Advanced Machine Learning Approaches in Cancer Prognosis. Intelligent Systems Reference Library*, Vol. 204. Springer.

Cancer Patient Healthcare Analysis by Genomic Prediction

V. Kakulapati, Subhani Shaik, and S. Mahender Reddy

1 Introduction

One of the most dangerous increases in fatalities throughout the world is due to cancer, and according to the WHO, cancer is second in death rate. Above 8–9 million individuals have died per year due to the disease's prevalence, and a predicting that the number of the fatality rate increases by 50% concluded the approaching in the 21st century. Cancer is characterised by a set of ailments of independent development and transmission of a somatic replica. The characteristic of this type of cancer clone must designate several cell developments that empowers it to ignore the ordinary limitations on cell development, change the neighbourhood microenvironment to support its multiplication, attack through tissue boundaries, spread to different organs and dodge safe surveillance. It cannot be achieved by single-cell development alone. Moderately, there is a vast number of probable pathogenic irregularities from which specific cancers lure its peculiar features: the shared characteristics of obvious highlights across tumours give a false representation of an inconceivably heterogeneous scene of cell anomalies.

Throughout the world, cancer is a significant public health problem, and in the USA, out of four fatalities, one casualty is due to cancer [1]. The primary health issue is cancer in many countries. According to recent health reports from Iran, health care providers stated that cancer is in third place in the fatality rate after cardiac failure and accidents [2]. The fatality rate of cancer has been continuously reducing in the

V. Kakulapati (✉) · S. Shaik
Sreenidhi Institute of Science and Technology Yamnampet, Ghatkesar, Hyderabad, Telangana 501301, India

S. Shaik
e-mail: shaiksubhani@sreendhi.edu.in

S. Mahender Reddy
Otto-Friedrich University of Bamberg, IsoSySc, Germany
e-mail: mahender-reddy.sheri@stud.uni-bamberg

A. K. Tyagi et al. (eds.), *Intelligent Interactive Multimedia Systems for e-Healthcare Applications*, https://doi.org/10.1007/978-981-16-6542-4_20

last two decades. The percentage of cancer fatality rate is reduced by 20% between 1990 and 2010, and this happened mainly because of middle-aged persons whose fatality frequency has weakening by 50%. The disease of cancer occurs based on various symptoms, some profound and some are not profound [3]. Presently, one of the chronic illnesses is cancer, increasingly deliberated as a long-lasting condition [4], and this may affect diverse provinces of cancer patient's quality of life [5] and leads to more economic issues, sadness, and loneliness in the persistent [6].

In human body cells, most of the work is done by genes that transmit the instructions to develop proteins, and the changes occur in these genes are caused by cells to avoid usual development regulators and leads to cancer. One type of cancer caused by gene changes, for example, is one in which protein intensification leads to cell nurturing and, as a result, non-functional protein development usually restores cellular impairment.

Cancer occurrence due to genetic variations can be inherited from parents if the variations exist in origin cells, which are the propagative cells of the form. These variations are known as germline variations that originate in every single cell of the progenies.

Cancer disease-causing genetic changes damage DNA, such as procured during one's lifetime, smoking, and radiation. For instance, a bright stream of lights from the sun initiating genetic variations can also attain. As a result, these can happen as cells split or form acquaintance with toxic elements that harm DNA, for instance, some chemicals in tobacco, and contamination, such as ultraviolet rays. These genetic variations may occur after conception, known as somatic variations. Several types of DNA variations exist, and some are affected by one segment of DNA known as a nucleotide. A nucleotide can get replaced by another nucleotide or misplaced. Some other variations encompass a more significant part of DNA [7], consisting of redisposition, omissions, or replications of a large portion of DNA.

The significance of variation in the human genome [8] sequencing genetic basis may lead to various chronic diseases related to health issues such as diabetes mellitus, coronary artery diseases, hypercholesterolemia, hypertension, osteoporosis, and other cancer types [9]. Because of this variation, predicting the onset of an illness will be improved, investigations will be developed and improved, and effective disease prevention, regulation, and diagnosis methods will most likely result [10] in screening the genes that are responsible for causing cancer to assist in the purpose of risks later in life [11].

Malignancy is multifaceted, and it is hereditary and extremely assorted [12]. The accumulation of and selection for mutations in genes are known as carcinogenesis, which can then drive, among different procedures, cell expansion, invulnerable avoidance, genomic precariousness and intrusiveness. The perception of a malignancy gene apprehensions the machine-like prerequisite for a cell to affect ordinary cellular and skin homeostasis and endorse neoplasia and cancer. The gene mutations are frequently retreating loss-of-function abrasions, illustrated by lump gene suppressors, but they can act predominantly as oncogenes. Defining which alterations or genes turn as blockages in the cohort of cancer is nervous with issues, as cells resonant one or more alterations will also transmit a vast set of co-selected changes which establish most of the ordinary somatic modification of the developed malignant growth cell yet which do not legitimately produce the neoplastic phenotype [13].

Evaluate the effect of malignancy diagnosis with various measurements. This work is mainly focused and taken to understand, categorize, and document analysis of cancer patients—their common symptoms, genes analysis and genetic variations in the process of malignancy diagnosis.

2 Related Work

Malignancy is a polygenic ailment where numerous hereditary variables look as if they play significant roles in ailment expansion in its diverse subtypes of malignancy [14]. A functional interaction network [15] is developed to recognize analytical biomarkers for cancers like breast and ovarian. This network integrates gene system [16] explanations and province–province communications and protein-protein communications and gene appearance. Markov clustering is utilized to predict diagnosis to recognize gene appearance segments from this. Then recognized linear amalgamations of segments that are extremely associated with persistent existence.

A neural network-based method for diagnosis prediction [17, 18] is developed by combinatorically dysregulated subnetworks, and this network identified the dysregulation in the lump and metastatic models. This approach of subnetworks can be utilized as precise prognosticators of projecting consequence for colorectal malignancy and glioblastoma multiformat. Researchers envisaged that the cost of sequencing a specific genome generally denotes the initiation of new DNA sequencing stages [19]. The significant expense of customized genomic medication and medical procedure stays an obstruction to its far-reaching clinical application for the general public, though, as novel sequencing methodologies, named "next-gen" stages, remain to expand. It is not behind the prospect that an individual genome succession will turn into a future standard segment of each patient's clinical records. The genetic variations can affect personal health in many ways. The mutations in genes warn the menace of convinced illness before medical signs and symptoms appear. Therefore, approaches to anticipation and early intervention can develop. For instance, two genes (BRCA1 and 2) are life-threatening to essential cell procedures [20, 21], and changes of these genes subsidize to tumorigenesis in breast cancer and ovarian cancer tissues. Another investigation demonstrated that life-threatening risk for women who have breast cancer ranges below 14% in Europe and the USA [22], although women with germline BRCA alterations between 36 and 85% of life are at threatening risk of emerging breast cancer [23–25].

Moreover, abnormalities of these genes' intensification of a woman's coincidence of emerging ovarian cancer between 25 and 60%, and in contrast, a stark report demonstrates a 1.7% chance among women who do not convey these gene alterations [26, 27]. Many investigations of genomic menace analysis directed the CDS (clinical decision systems) about destructive observation drivers, such as improved incidence of mammography or even prophylactic surgery, as well as mastectomy and amputation of the ovaries. In [28], they developed a recommendation system that ill people undertake for premature and consistent screening colonoscopy in the determination to intensify the coincidence for early recognition of cancer [28]. Even if ongoing GWASs have connected numerous interminable illnesses and pervasive malignant growths to hereditary pointers, further investigations are required to control the scope in which the information acquired will convert into applied clinical involvements for persistent.

A few computational strategies have been useful for diagnosing tumour growth alterations, depending on the non-arbitrary spreading of variations within proteins [29]. Predictive analytical tools such as PolyPhen and SIFT are broadly utilized to support manual curing; in any case, they have not recognized themselves as the prominent features in clinical decision making [30]. Many researchers developed machine learning models on feature training, secondary structures, fundamental ailments, DNA-obligatory, phosphorylation, maintenance, foreseen structure, and homolog amount to advance the accuracy of abnormality classification, to integrate high-dimensional data sets, and to combine the abnormal construal among test centers. For example, DNN (deep neural networks) [31], DT (decision tree), RF (random forest) and SVM (support vector machine).

3 About Genomic Analysis of Cancer

a. Genetic factor controls by what method cells work by the construction of proteins, and these have explicit capacities and performance as a communicator for the cell. Every genetic feature has the proper directions for constructing the proteins, which can allow protein functioning properly. Suppose one or more genetic features are altering, which leads to malignancy, generates an irregular protein and avoids the construction of protein. This type of protein delivers changed information when compared with normal protein, which causes the cell to reproduce irrepressibly and turn out to be a malignancy.
b. Genetic feature mutations

Two types of gene feature mutations are there

Gain mutations. This type of variation is the utmost basis of malignancy, which can occur from impairment to genes in a specific cell in an individual's life. For instance, a chest cell or a colon cell drives on split countless times leads to form a lump, which is nothing but abnormal form. This type of occurrence of cancer as gained mutations is known as sporadic malignancy. These are not initiating in every cell in the human body and not transferred from parent to child.

Reasons that occurs for these mutations:

- Smoking
- Electromagnetic radiation

- Infections
- Age.

Germline mutations. This type of variation is not shared and occurs in a sperm or egg cell, transfers from parental to a kid at the time of commencement. For example, the embryo produces into a baby, and the first sperm or egg cell mutation passes into each cell inside the human body due to the variation moves propagative cells; it can permit from peers to peer group. This type of variation is known as genetic cancer, and it occurs in 5–20% of all other types of cancers.

c. Cancer and mutations

Metamorphosis occurs frequently, and it may be helpful, destructive, or unbiased, which is based on the occurrence of alteration in the gene. Naturally, the human body stimulates the maximum mutations. Cancer will not occur based on a single mutation, and malignancy depends on multiple variations in a person's life. Due to this, a fatality occurs more frequently in aged people, and there are more chances of developing the mutations.

d. Cancer-causing types of genes

Cancer-causing genes can be classified as:

i. **Lump suppressive genome**. This type of genes are known as caring genes [32] and can curb cell development by:
ii. Intensive care on how cells split into new-fangled cells
    - Restoring incompatible DNA
    - Monitoring as soon as a cell decease.

At the time when a lump suppressor inheritable factor metamorphoses, cells expand irrepressibly and may cause forming of a lump.

For example: *BRCA1*, *BRCA2* and *p53* or *TP53*.

BRCA1 or *BRCA2* genetic feature changes intensification risk of emerging inherited breast or ovarian malignancy, and, for males, risk of emerging inherited prostate malignancy. These also cause pancreatic and malignancy in both genders.

p53 or TP53 are more frequent changes in genetic features in humans with malignancy. Lost or abnormalities of this gene cause 50% malignancy out of all cancers, which is an acquired type of mutation. There are infrequent, but persistent, who transmit this type of genetic factors are at danger of emerging several kinds of malignancy.

iii. Understanding cancer genetics

Most of the investigations analyse that the genes play a vital role in the occurrence of cancer, but most of the tumours are not related to any specific genetic factor. Furthermore, the DNA segment cooperates with their location, which more obscures empathetic of the protagonist genetic factors' performance in malignancy.

Many researchers are continuing their investigations to analyse the mutations of genes involved in the development of malignancy. Predicting the enhancement in curing of cancer in terms of early identification of cancer, reducing fatality rate, diagnosis methodologies and persistence.

These investigations of genetic features may assist physicians for better diagnosis:

- Forecast a patient risk of malignancy.
- Analyse state of cancer.
- Therapy methods of cancer.

The genes which are causing cancer

- **Oncogenes**
  - Gene mutations that give the addition of capacities oncogenes can influence development malignant growth.
  - Gene mutations with development-endorsing consequences on the cell.
  - Frequently heterozygous.
- **Lump suppressive genes**
  - Gene mutations that deliberate damage of function can confer to malignancy.
  - Characteristically homozygous.
- **Chromosome preservation of genes**
  - Secondary consequences on malignancy progress by not restoring DNA or modifying mutations.

Hereditary assessments [33] are presenting for types of malignancy. Those are breast, ovarian, colon, thyroid, prostate, pancreatic, melanoma, sarcoma, kidney and stomach cancer.

This assessment can assist in:

- Analysis of forecast of risk of specific disease.
- Screening for predicting cancer.
- Make available information for better healthcare.

No assessment can give assurance that cancer will develop, and it can provide the evaluation of only the possibility and risk of disease. Sometimes cancer can occur in family members, which is not originated by an inherited mutation. Let's say, lifestyle such as smoking can source malignancy to progress between families. Few people may fall in malignancy due to genetic factor variations.

e. Critical features for hereditary malignancy

A genetic malignancy is cancer instigated by an inherent protein sequence variation, and this protein sequence variation is acquiring from parents to kids in a family. The following aspects are a probably improved chance for genetic cancer:

- Background of family.
- Acquiring malignancy at a younger age.
- Various types of cancer in family members.
- Sporadic cancers.

f. Reasons to study genomic testing for malignancy

This genomic testing is an individual choice based on several aspects, and it may be a multifaceted decision. This testing may contain some constraints and psychological issues. Those are depression, anxiety or guilt, family tension. Sharing results with other family members, insecurity, unclear results and testing cost.

DNAs [34] have a structure like thread in cells that contain genetic factors, and 46 chromosomes are arranging in 2 sets of 23; these sets are acquired from parents.

4 Methodology

4.1 Hybrid Discriminant Analysis (HDA)

Many researchers utilized PCA and LDA in disease analysis, including clinical notes analysis. Some application uses PCA component vectors give more accurateness than LDA, whereas in some other form, LDA is better than PCA. The performance of both techniques relies on the data distribution due to the dimensionality frequently come across in classification methods. Many investigations integrate both methods, and PCA is implementing on lower-dimensional data, then applying the LDA to dimensionality reduction. HDA is a new technique, and it varies significantly from performing PCA and LDA as it merges the optimization in PCA and LDA and limits feature vectors utilizing the formation of new functions.

4.2 PCA

One of the oldest dimensionality reduction techniques is PCA [35, 36], and it pursuits for linear amalgamations of the unique dimensions known as principal components, which can successfully characterize the consequences of the aspects. Principal components are quartic to each other, and computational easiness and efficient statistical analysis make PCA widely utilized in several applications. It can also use in bioinformatics investigations, including genetic analysis and dimensionality reduction [37].

4.3 LDA

It simplifies Fisher's linear discriminant, which utilizes statistical analysis and machine learning approaches [38]. LDA is based on probabilistic topic modelling, which is an analytical technique used to find document topics depicting classes of text. It applied to gene sequences instead of the documents, attains the occurrence of static-length k-measurements, and develops a propagative technique for a training set of genes sequences and model acquired concluded with the LDA algorithm, which is utilized to categorize a massive volume of genomic sequences.

5 Implementation Results

In this chapter, taking data set from Kaggle and after pre-processing of the dataset, then classifying the dataset based on the mutations and apply hybrid discriminant analysis, which is a combination of both principal component analysis (PCA) and linear discriminant analysis (LDA) for analysing the cancer based on the genomic function.

Data pre-processing: Dataset contains feature selection—a primary pre-processing phase in machine learning techniques which is operative in dimensionality reduction, eliminating inappropriate data, enhancing learning accurateness and improving accurate consequence, removing missing values such blank fields and outliers in the data set.

Scores: The data set is split into a training set and test set. A model built on the training set, and then this model is validated by the test set.

- Accurateness
- Prediction error:
- Recall
- Precision
- Sensitivity
- Specificity.

Position of components:

	PC1	PC2	PC3	PC4	PC5	PC6	PC7	PC8
Std	2.3704	1.2177	0.71055	0.44704	0.38619	0.21041	0.005096	0.003407
Pv	0.7024	0.1853	0.06311	0.02498	0.01864	0.00553	0.000000	0.000000
CP	0.7024s	0.8877	0.95084	0.97582	0.99446	1.00000	1.000000	1.000000

where Std: Standard deviation, Pv: Proportion of Variance, CP: Cumulative Proportion (Figs. 1, 2, 3 and 4).

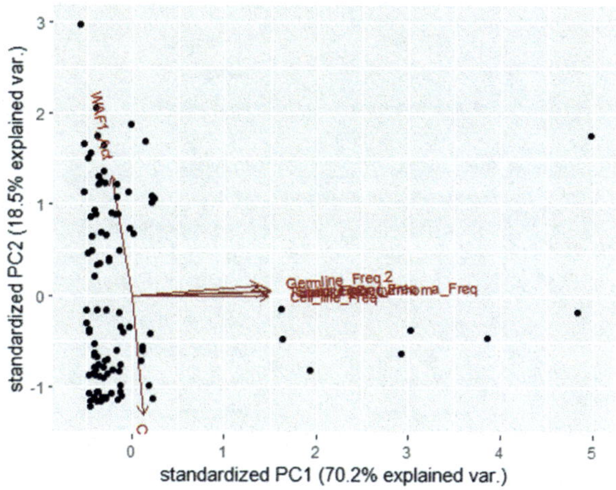

Fig. 1 Importance of principal component analysis with 18.5%

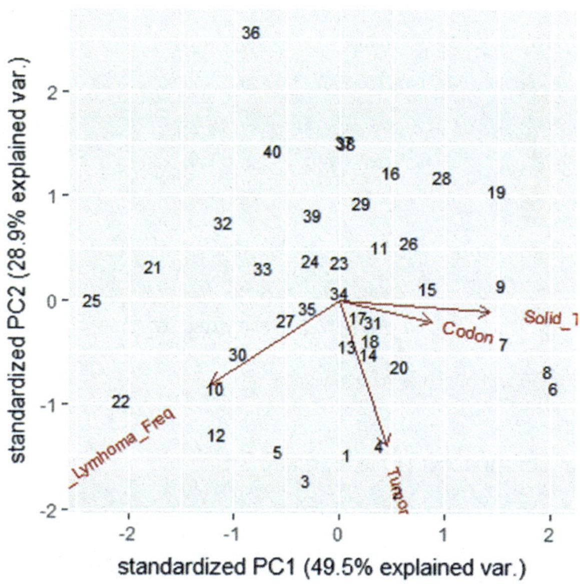

Fig. 2 Importance of principal component analysis with 28.9%

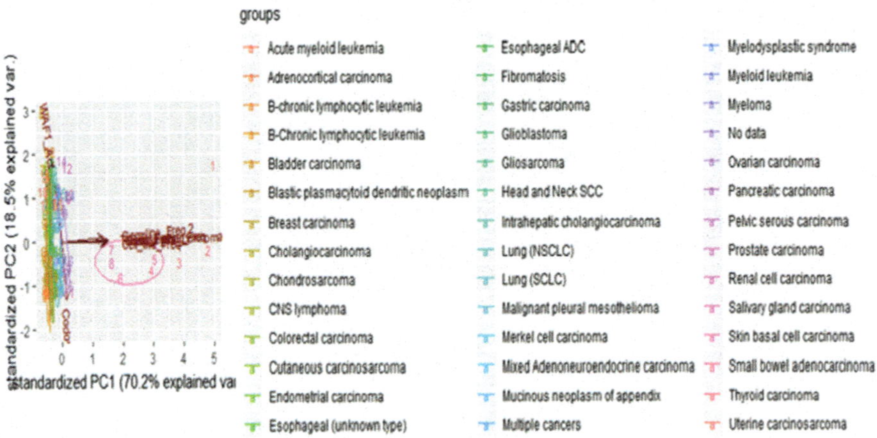

Fig. 3 Principal component analysis with dimensionality reduction

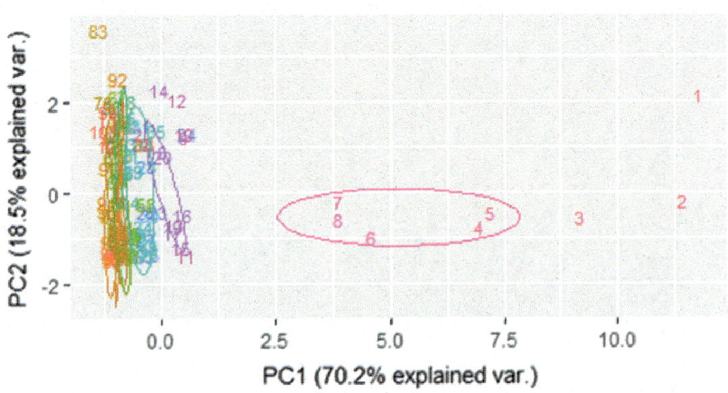

Fig. 4 Principal component analysis with variance

Importance of components (Figs. 5, 6 and 7):

	PC1	PC2	PC3	PC4	PC5
Std	2.3053	1.7328	0.94474	0.78598	0.68976
PV	0.4831	0.2730	0.08114	0.05616	0.04325
CP	0.4831	0.7561	0.83720	0.89337	0.93662

	PC6	PC7	PC8	PC9	PC10	PC11
Std	0.59823	0.40978	0.3541	0.21210	0.02625	0.01756
PV	0.03253	0.01527	0.0114	0.00409	0.00006	0.00003
CP	0.96915	0.98442	0.9958	0.99991	0.99997	1.00000

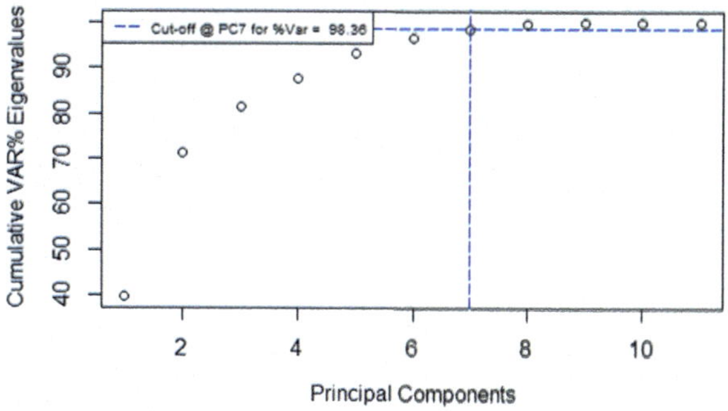

Fig. 5 Cumulative variations Eigen vectors of principal component analysis

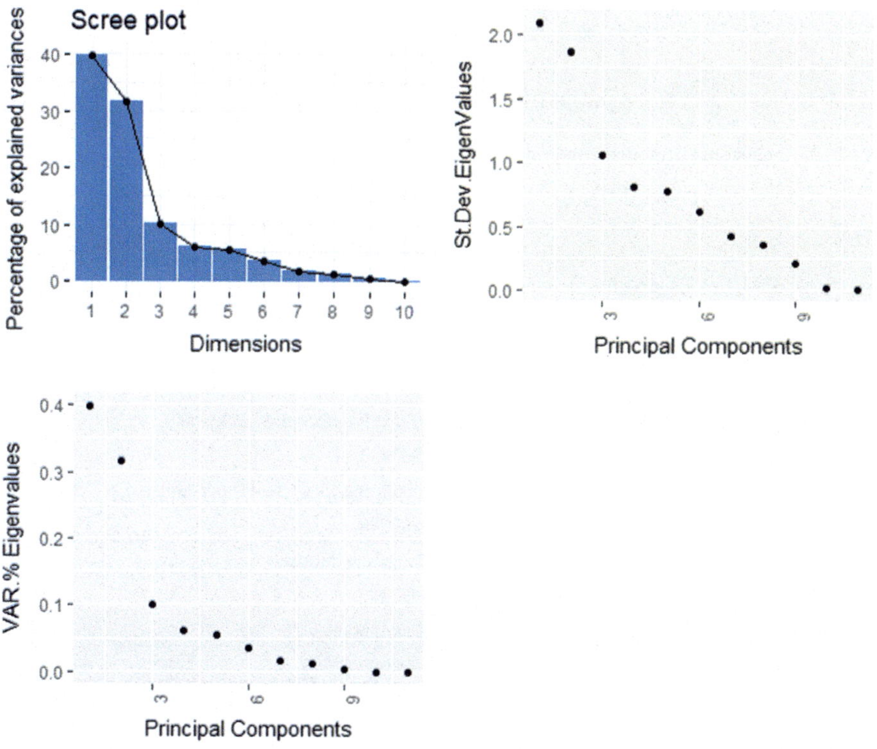

Fig. 6 Percentage and Eigen values and standard deviation of principal component analysis

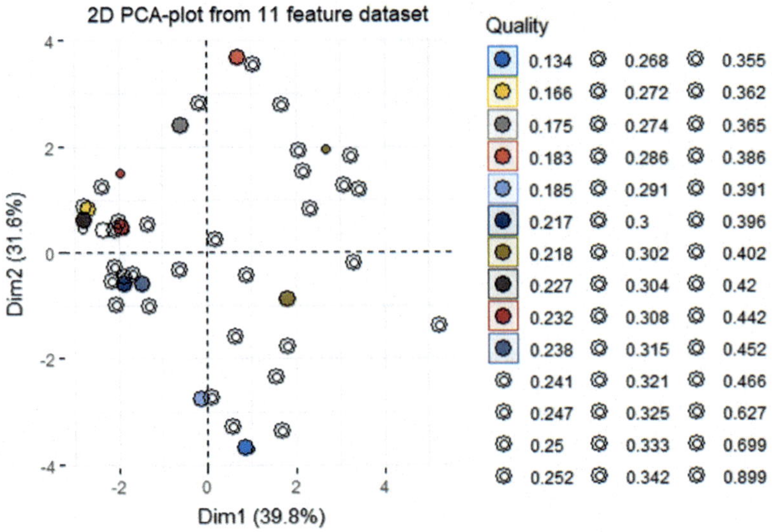

Fig. 7 2-dimensional principal component analysis of 11 features

LDA

Prior probabilities of groups:

Acute myeloid Leukemia	Adrenocortical carcinoma
0.02970297	0.02970297
B-chronic lymphocytic Leukemia	B-chronic lymphocytic Leukemia
0.01980198	0.06930693
Bladder carcinoma	Baltic plasmacytoid dendritic neoplasm
0.02970297	0.00990099
Breast carcinoma	Cholangiocarcinoma
0.07920792	0.01980198
Chondrosarcoma	CNS lymphoma
0.00990099	0.00990099
Colorectal carcinoma	Cutaneous carcinosarcoma
0.09900990	0.00990099
Endometrial carcinoma	Esophageal (unknown type)
0.01980198	0.00990099
Esophageal ADC	Fibromatosis
0.00990099	0.00990099
Gastric carcinoma	Glioblastoma
0.01980198	0.04950495
Gliosarcoma	Head and neck SCC
0.00990099	0.01980198

(continued)

(continued)

Intrahepatic cholangiocarcinoma	Lung (NSCLC)
0.00990099	0.08910891
Lung (SCLC)	Malignant pleural mesothelioma
0.01980198	0.00990099
Merkel cell carcinoma	Mixed Aden neuroendocrine carcinoma
0.00990099	0.00990099
Mucinous neoplasm of appendix	Multiple cancers
0.00990099	0.00990099
Myelodysplastic syndrome	Myeloid leukemia
0.01980198	0.01980198
Myeloma	No data
0.00990099	0.00990099
Ovarian carcinoma	Pancreatic carcinoma
0.05940594	0.01980198
Pelvic serous carcinoma	Prostate carcinoma
0.00990099	0.00990099
Renal cell carcinoma	Salivary gland carcinoma
0.01980198	0.01980198
Skin basal cell carcinoma	Small bowel adenocarcinoma
0.02970297	0.00990099
Thyroid carcinoma	Uterine carcinosarcoma
0.01980198	0.00990099

Group means:

	Codon Leukemia_	Lymhoma_Freq
Acute myeloid leukemia	150.6667	0.19833333
Adrenocortical carcinoma	279.0000	0.09933333
B-chronic lymphocytic leukemia	266.0000	0.33100000
B-Chronic lymphocytic leukemia	249.0000	0.16800000
Bladder carcinoma	218.3333	0.32866667
Blastic plasmacytoid dendritic neoplasm	138.0000	0.23000000
Breast carcinoma	241.1250	0.17062500
Cholangiocarcinoma	276.0000	0.27050000
Chondrosarcoma	274.0000	0.10800000
CNS lymphoma	244.0000	0.10800000
Colorectal carcinoma	230.3000	0.23250000
Cutaneous carcinosarcoma	244.0000	0.20300000
Endometrial carcinoma	231.0000	0.15550000

(continued)

(continued)

	Codon Leukemia_	Lymhoma_Freq
Esophageal (unknown type)	337.0000	0.21600000
Esophageal ADC	127.0000	0.13500000
Fibromatosis	244.0000	0.40500000
Gastric carcinoma	177.0000	0.25000000
Glioblastoma	172.0000	0.19480000
Gliosarcoma	280.0000	0.20300000
Head and neck SCC	188.5000	0.19600000
Intrahepatic cholangiocarcinoma	214.0000	0.29700000
Lung (NSCLC)	208.3333	0.35411111
Lung (SCLC)	258.0000	0.29050000
Malignant pleural mesothelioma	245.0000	0.16200000
Merkel cell carcinoma	176.0000	0.51300000
Mixed Adenoneuroendocrine carcinoma	216.0000	0.75600000
Mucinous neoplasm of appendix	205.0000	0.28400000
Multiple cancers	238.0000	0.68900000
Myelodysplastic syndrome	267.0000	0.20950000
Myeloid leukemia	218.0000	0.37150000
Myeloma	272.0000	0.68900000
No data	158.0000	0.12200000
Ovarian carcinoma	213.1667	0.68216667
Pancreatic carcinoma	224.5000	0.35800000
Pelvic serous carcinoma	245.0000	0.64800000
Prostate carcinoma	163.0000	0.58100000
Renal cell carcinoma	232.0000	0.62800000
Salivary gland carcinoma	201.0000	0.82400000
Skin basal cell carcinoma	250.0000	1.77833333
Small bowel adenocarcinoma	273.0000	2.10700000
Thyroid carcinoma	260.5000	3.99150000
Uterine carcinosarcoma	175.0000	2.91800000

Solid_Tumor_Freq Tumor_Freq

Acute myeloid leukemia	0.1126667	0.1190000
Adrenocortical carcinoma	0.1280000	0.1290000
B-chronic lymphocytic leukemia	0.1135000	0.1250000
B-chronic lymphocytic leukemia	0.1277143	0.1331429
Bladder carcinoma	0.1296667	0.1450000
Blastic plasmacytoid dendritic neoplasm	0.1410000	0.1550000

(continued)

(continued)

Breast carcinoma	0.1612500	0.1625000
Cholangiocarcinoma	0.1635000	0.1820000
Chondrosarcoma	0.1850000	0.1730000
CNS lymphoma	0.1950000	0.1950000
Colorectal carcinoma	0.1906000	0.1957000
Cutaneous carcinosarcoma	0.2110000	0.2100000
Endometrial carcinoma	0.2170000	0.2090000
Esophageal (unknown type)	0.2020000	0.2180000
Esophageal ADC	0.2330000	0.2330000
Fibromatosis	0.2160000	0.2340000
Gastric carcinoma	0.2390000	0.2355000
Glioblastoma	0.2572000	0.2562000
Gliosarcoma	0.2700000	0.2710000
Head and Neck SCC	0.2895000	0.2855000
Intrahepatic cholangiocarcinoma	0.2840000	0.2970000
Lung (NSCLC)	0.2964444	0.3060000
Lung (SCLC)	0.3475000	0.3400000
Malignant pleural mesothelioma	0.3630000	0.3420000
Merkel cell carcinoma	0.3390000	0.3520000
Mixed Adenoneuroendocrine carcinoma	0.3120000	0.3600000
Mucinous neoplasm of appendix	0.3750000	0.3860000
Multiple cancers	0.3450000	0.3840000
Myelodysplastic syndrome	0.4055000	0.3775000
Myeloid leukemia	0.3850000	0.3760000
Myeloma	0.3820000	0.4090000
No data	0.4440000	0.4200000
Ovarian carcinoma	0.4385000	0.4650000
Pancreatic carcinoma	0.5950000	0.5665000
Pelvic serous carcinoma	0.5960000	0.6060000
Prostate carcinoma	0.6330000	0.6430000
Renal cell carcinoma	0.6935000	0.6995000
Salivary gland carcinoma	1.1405000	1.1160000
Skin basal cell carcinoma	2.0513333	2.0383333
Small bowel adenocarcinoma	2.8440000	2.8030000
Thyroid carcinoma	2.9540000	3.0070000
Uterine carcinosarcoma	4.4060000	4.3280000

Cell_line_Freq Somatic_Freq.2

Acute myeloid leukemia	0.18133333	0.1203333
Adrenocortical carcinoma	0.10366667	0.1260000
B-chronic lymphocytic leukemia	0.15550000	0.1295000
B-Chronic lymphocytic leukemia	0.08142857	0.1312857
Bladder carcinoma	0.18966667	0.1490000
Blastic plasmacytoid dendritic neoplasm	0.02600000	0.1520000
Breast carcinoma	0.19737500	0.1628750
Cholangiocarcinoma	0.10350000	0.1750000
Chondrosarcoma	0.31100000	0.1790000
CNS lymphoma	0.15500000	0.1880000
Colorectal carcinoma	0.19670000	0.1959000
Cutaneous carcinosarcoma	0.18100000	0.2080000
Endometrial carcinoma	0.28500000	0.2105000
Esophageal (unknown type)	0.15500000	0.2120000
Esophageal ADC	0.12900000	0.2250000
Fibromatosis	0.15500000	0.2310000
Gastric carcinoma	0.34900000	0.2380000
Glioblastoma	0.21220000	0.2516000
Gliosarcoma	0.20700000	0.2680000
Head and Neck SCC	0.27200000	0.2835000
Intrahepatic cholangiocarcinoma	0.18100000	0.2880000
Lung (NSCLC)	0.28188889	0.3021111
Lung (SCLC)	0.46550000	0.3420000
Malignant pleural mesothelioma	0.51800000	0.3460000
Merkel cell carcinoma	0.46600000	0.3550000
Mixed Adenoneuroendocrine carcinoma	0.28500000	0.3570000
Mucinous neoplasm of appendix	0.15500000	0.3690000
Multiple cancers	0.23300000	0.3740000
Myelodysplastic syndrome	0.54350000	0.3880000
Myeloid leukemia	0.45300000	0.3785000
Myeloma	0.49200000	0.4100000
No data	0.51800000	0.4180000
Ovarian carcinoma	0.53066667	0.4643333
Pancreatic carcinoma	0.90550000	0.5765000
Pelvic serous carcinoma	0.36200000	0.6050000
Prostate carcinoma	0.62100000	0.6340000
Renal cell carcinoma	0.69900000	0.6910000
Salivary gland carcinoma	1.10000000	1.1040000

(continued)

(continued)

Skin basal cell carcinoma	1.94933333	2.0153333
Small bowel adenocarcinoma	2.87300000	2.7740000
Thyroid carcinoma	4.32200000	3.0455000
Uterine carcinosarcoma	3.77800000	4.2600000

Germline_Freq.2 WAF1_Act

Acute myeloid leukemia	0.08633333	−1.186667
Adrenocortical carcinoma	0.00100000	−1.565667
B-chronic lymphocytic leukemia	0.95250000	−1.123000
B-Chronic lymphocytic leukemia	0.15444286	−1.279000
Bladder carcinoma	0.08333333	−1.451667
Blastic plasmacytoid dendritic neoplasm	0.08300000	−0.432000
Breast carcinoma	0.07267500	−1.343625
Cholangiocarcinoma	0.04155000	−1.074000
Chondrosarcoma	0.00100000	−1.552000
CNS lymphoma	0.00100000	−1.592000
Colorectal carcinoma	0.07502000	−1.481000
Cutaneous carcinosarcoma	0.41400000	−1.570000
Endometrial carcinoma	0.49700000	−1.553000
Esophageal (unknown type)	0.66200000	−1.154000
Esophageal ADC	0.00100000	−1.132000
Fibromatosis	0.24800000	−1.564000
Gastric carcinoma	0.08350000	−1.144500
Glioblastoma	0.04984000	−1.241400
Gliosarcoma	0.08300000	−1.566000
Head and Neck SCC	0.10000000	−1.137500
Intrahepatic cholangiocarcinoma	0.08300000	−1.470000
Lung (NSCLC)	0.35166667	−1.414444
Lung (SCLC)	0.09150000	−1.565000
Malignant pleural mesothelioma	0.33100000	−1.588000
Merkel cell carcinoma	0.10000000	−1.047000
Mixed Adenoneuroendocrine carcinoma	0.08300000	−1.577000
Mucinous neoplasm of appendix	0.08300000	−1.260000
Multiple cancers	0.16600000	−1.056000
Myelodysplastic syndrome	0.12450000	−1.389000
Myeloid leukemia	1.24200000	−1.418500
Myeloma	0.16600000	−1.265000
No data	0.08300000	−1.287000

(continued)

(continued)

Ovarian carcinoma	0.28966667	−1.360167
Pancreatic carcinoma	0.12450000	−1.154000
Pelvic serous carcinoma	0.24800000	−1.513000
Prostate carcinoma	0.49700000	−0.922000
Renal cell carcinoma	0.13300000	−1.337000
Salivary gland carcinoma	1.49000000	−1.422500
Skin basal cell carcinoma	2.20733333	−1.566333
Small bowel adenocarcinoma	1.40700000	−1.550000
Thyroid carcinoma	4.09800000	−1.572000
Uterine carcinosarcoma	4.47000000	−1.134000

MutPred_Splice_General_Score

Acute myeloid leukemia	0.3523333
Adrenocortical carcinoma	0.2516667
B-chronic lymphocytic leukemia	0.3670000
B-Chronic lymphocytic leukemia	0.3195714
Bladder carcinoma	0.2690000
Blastic plasmacytoid dendritic neoplasm	0.2000000
Breast carcinoma	0.3612500
Cholangiocarcinoma	0.4020000
Chondrosarcoma	0.2410000
CNS lymphoma	0.2910000
Colorectal carcinoma	0.3756000
Cutaneous carcinosarcoma	0.1770000
Endometrial carcinoma	0.2145000
Esophageal (unknown type)	0.8160000
Esophageal ADC	0.3450000
Fibromatosis	0.1490000
Gastric carcinoma	0.2490000
Glioblastoma	0.2918000
Gliosarcoma	0.2680000
Head and Neck SCC	0.2610000
Intrahepatic cholangiocarcinoma	0.3650000
Lung (NSCLC)	0.2486667
Lung (SCLC)	0.2780000
Malignant pleural mesothelioma	0.1340000
Merkel cell carcinoma	0.1540000
Mixed Adenoneuroendocrine carcinoma	0.6270000

(continued)

(continued)

Mucinous neoplasm of appendix	0.3210000
Multiple cancers	0.3500000
Myelodysplastic syndrome	0.2100000
Myeloid leukemia	0.2330000
Myeloma	0.2680000
No data	0.1120000
Ovarian carcinoma	0.3173333
Pancreatic carcinoma	0.2960000
Pelvic serous carcinoma	0.1460000
Prostate carcinoma	0.1440000
Renal cell carcinoma	0.4410000
Salivary gland carcinoma	0.1790000
Skin basal cell carcinoma	0.2843333
Small bowel adenocarcinoma	0.8080000
Thyroid carcinoma	0.2435000
Uterine carcinosarcoma	0.1390000

Coefficients of linear discriminants

	LD1	LD2	LD3
Codon	−2.194058e−04	9.310438e−03	3.781651e−03
Leukemia_Lymhoma_Freq	−5.726692e+00	−1.072922e+01	−1.365504e+01
Solid_Tumor_Freq	−6.306260e+01	−1.202353e+02	−1.060045e+02
Tumor_Freq	1.762542e+02	1.601819e+02	8.596712e+01
Cell_line_Freq	1.029310e+01	1.273649e+01	7.181842e+00
Somatic_Freq.2	−1.053398e+02	−4.509528e+01	2.590555e+01
Germline_Freq.2	−1.222934e+00	1.328251e+00	−4.029367e−01
WAF1_Act	1.014680e+00	9.093851e−01	3.580351e+00
MutPred_Splice_General_Score	−1.200601e+00	−1.008578e+00	−4.458542e−01
	LD4	LD5	LD6
Codon	0.01970284	−9.263175e−03	−2.035329e−03
Leukemia_Lymhoma_Freq	2.81109680	−2.001418e−01	−1.330230e+01
Solid_Tumor_Freq	19.12204116	−2.677779e+01	−1.188940e+02
Tumor_Freq	−104.56897471	−1.222026e+02	6.509440e+00
Cell_line_Freq	−6.86133491	−7.546731e+00	−8.550405e−01
Somatic_Freq.2	91.15359438	1.593539e+02	1.239199e+02
Germline_Freq.2	−0.28020202	−7.944629e−01	2.733395e+00
WAF1_Act	2.84895278	1.454218e+00	7.381861e−01
MutPred_Splice_General_Score	2.32591414	−9.470634e−01	−4.053792e−01

(continued)

(continued)

	LD1	LD2	LD3
	LD7	LD8	LD9
Codon	−0.01021928	1.647282e−03	5.811873e−03
Leukemia_Lymhoma_Freq	−5.35991277	−1.767700e+01	2.118094e−01
Solid_Tumor_Freq	−57.78668818	−1.715295e+02	−2.040748e+01
Tumor_Freq	50.26202115	−2.236784e+01	1.614160e+02
Cell_line_Freq	1.58913274	−2.004890e+00	5.658735e+00
Somatic_Freq.2	10.24258804	2.138881e+02	−1.478776e+02
Germline_Freq.2	0.76673238	3.868351e−01	−1.643132e−01
WAF1_Act	−1.18932902	−1.333907e+00	3.810576e−01
MutPred_Splice_General_Score	4.99411196	−1.587779e+00	−2.867997e+00

Propotion of trace (Fig. 8)

LD1	LD2	LD3	LD4	LD5	LD6	LD7	LD8	LD9
0.9322	0.0246	0.0115	0.0094	0.0070	0.0061	0.0042	0.0027	0.0023

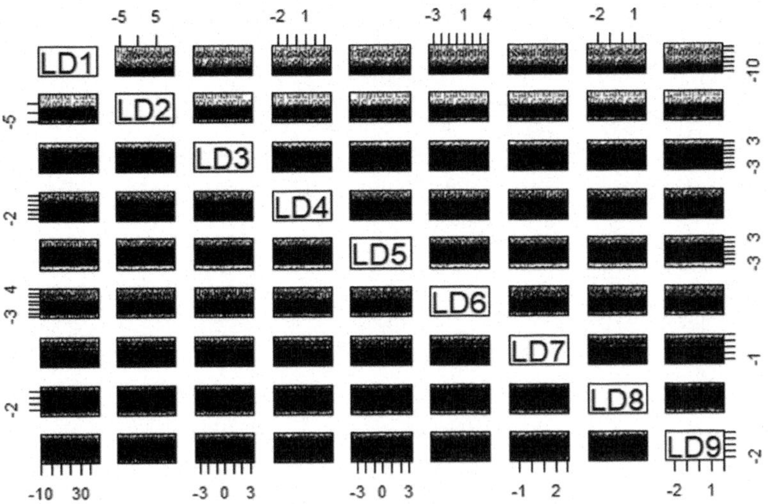

Fig. 8 Linear discriminant analysis components

[1] Uterine carcinosarcoma	Thyroid carcinoma
[3] Thyroid carcinoma	Small bowel adenocarcinoma
[5] Skin basal cell carcinoma	Skin basal cell carcinoma
[7] Skin basal cell carcinoma a	Salivary gland carcinoma
[9] Renal cell carcinoma	Renal cell carcinoma
42 levels: acute myeloid leukemia	Uterine carcinosarcoma

Acute myeloid leukemia Adrenocortical carcinoma B-chronic lymphocytic leukemia (Fig. 9)

1.	0.000000e+00	0.000000e+00	0.000000e+00
2.	0.000000e+00	0.000000e+00	0.000000e+00
3.	5.059047e−303	5.639437e−305	0.000000e+00
4.	3.041306e−280	2.147601e−283	6.023054e−316
5.	5.820236e−148	3.800494e−150	1.047395e−170
6.	1.423080e−116	3.957467e−116	6.443859e−138
7.	4.744755e−81	3.959044e−83	1.955987e−101
8.	1.920607e−41	4.585166e−42	3.039027e−52
9.	6.659249e−19	9.242570e−21	7.022982e−34
10.	5.053036e−18	1.549504e−20	1.206648e−29

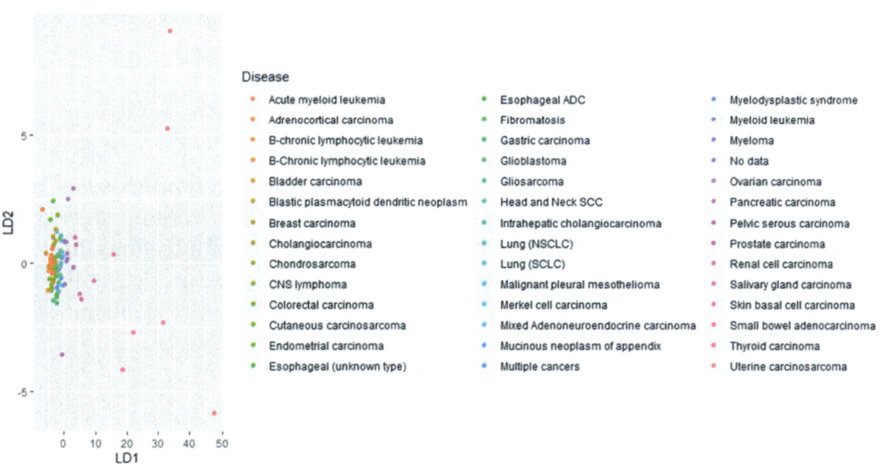

Fig. 9 Genome sequencing

	LD1	LD2	LD3	LD4	LD5	LD6	LD7
1.	47.494344	−5.8334184	1.5910233	0.06045421	−0.1474315	2.802844485	−0.2352143
2.	33.879256	9.0275874	−3.0153115	−0.13703445	2.5431554	0.738714822	−0.9282841
3.	33.086358	5.2228887	0.1980456	−0.27493323	−0.3918145	0.809935972	0.5878109
4.	31.573602	−2.3258452	1.9663069	1.29498852	−1.4821459	−3.144690543	1.5520795
5.	21.888378	−2.7128237	−3.0644510	0.80341874	−0.1459279	−0.001841049	−1.7006616
6.	18.602860	−4.1434948	−0.6866197	0.05746609	−3.2723779	0.682196581	−0.9057033
7.	15.658400	0.3507651	−1.5813215	0.38266117	1.5504461	−1.569360706	1.7061104
8.	9.539552	−0.6762131	−2.1866510	−0.02726318	−11,502,966	3.620470166	0.3070011
9.	5.408362	−1.4211918	1.1334370	−2.13505819	−0.4737918	−2.082459095	−0.9864448

6 Conclusion

In this work, the results reveal that genomic analysis-based on mutations and protein sequencing may be used to anticipate genetic and medical understandings. Utilizing both intra and intertumoral heterogeneity deliberated for apprehending the probable of the omics-type lump. Furthermore, applying a novel method that exhibits transformations in correlation among genetic factors in developing malignancy, by analysing the genetic factor by using protein sequencing, predicting the different types of cancers. The results demonstrated that it recommended the requirements to analyse significantly more genetic tests for early detection of cancer and reduce the cancer fatality rate. In this work, hybrid discriminant analysis was implement, which combines LDA and PCA to optimize the performance analysis.

7 Future Enhancement

In the future, utilizing topic modelling in the analysis of infectious diseases with the help of machine learning techniques. Further, utilize deep learning algorithms based on the neural networks for predicting the consequences of infectious diseases. Also, analyse patient's emotional recognition of infectious disease persistent. Further, analyse the psychological development occupied in the emotional alteration to persistent disease, mainly emotion-extraction.

References

1. Siegel, R., et al. (2014). Cancer statistics, 2014. *CA: A Cancer Journal for Clinicians, 64*, 9–29.
2. Taghavi, A., et al. (2012). Increased trend of breast cancer mortality in Iran. *Asian Pacific Journal of Cancer Prevention, 13*, 367–370.

3. Heydarnejad, M. S., et al. (2011). Factors affecting quality of life in cancer patients undergoing chemotherapy. *Health Science* 266–270.
4. Dehkordi, A., et al. (2009). Quality of life in cancer patients undergoing chemotherapy. *Oman Medical Journal, 24*, 204–207.
5. Roiland, R. A., et al. (2011). Symptom clusters and quality of life in older adult breast cancer survivors. *Oncology Nursing Forum, 38*, 672–680.
6. Pinquart, M., et al. (2010). Depression and cancer mortality: A meta-analysis. *Psychological Medicine, 40*, 1797–1810. https://www.cancer.gov/about-cancer/causes-prevention/genetics
7. Lander, E. S., et al. (2001). Initial sequencing and analysis of the human genome. *Nature, 409*, 860–921.
8. Pang, C. P., et al. (2000). Hunting for disease genes in multi-functional diseases. *Clinical Chemistry and Laboratory Medicine, 38*, 819–825.
9. Gottesman, et al. (1994). The role of the human genome project in disease prevention. *Preventive Medicine, 23*, 591–594.
10. Chung, W. K. (2007). Implementation of genetics to personalize medicine. *Gender Medicine, 4*, 248–265.
11. Hanahan, D., & Weinberg, R. A. (2011). Hallmarks of cancer: The next generation. *Cell, 144*, 646–674.
12. Garraway, L., & Lander, E. (2013). Lessons from the cancer genome. *Cell, 153*, 17–37. http://www.sciencedirect.com/science/article/pii/S0092867413002882
13. Schully, et al. (2011). Cancer GAMAdb: Database of cancer genetic associations from meta-analyses and genome-wide association studies. *European Journal of Human Genetics, 19*, 928–930.
14. Wu, G., Feng, X., & Stein, L. (2010). A human functional protein interaction network and its application to cancer data analysis. *Genome Biology, 11*, R53. [PMC free article] [PubMed] [Google Scholar]
15. Wu, G., et al. (2012). A network module-based method for identifying cancer prognostic signatures. *Genome Biology, 13*, R112.
16. Chowdhury, S. A., et al. (2011). Subnetwork state functions define dysregulated subnetworks in cancer. *Journal of Computational Biology, 18*, 263–281.
17. Patel, V. N., et al. (2013). Network signatures of survival in glioblastoma multiforme. *PLoS Computational Biology, 9*, 1003237.
18. Mardis, E. R. (2006). Anticipating the $1, 000 genome. *Genome Biology, 7*, 112.
19. Farmer, H., et al. (2005). Targeting the DNA repair defect in BRCA mutant cells as a therapeutic strategy. *Nature, 434*, 917–921.
20. Venkitaraman, A. R. (2002). Cancer susceptibility and the functions of BRCA1 and BRCA2. *Cell, 108*, 171–182.
21. Roukos, D. H., et al. (2007). Individualized preventive and therapeutic management of hereditary breast ovarian cancer. *Nature Clinical Practice Oncology, 4*, 578–590.
22. National Cancer Institute. BRCA1 and BRCA2: Cancer risk and genetic testing. http://www.cancer.gov/cancertopics/factsheet/risk/brca
23. Struewing, J. P., et al. (1997). The risk of cancer associated with specific mutations of BRCA1 and BRCA2 among Ashkenazi Jews. *New England Journal of Medicine, 336*, 1401–1408.
24. Ries, L. A. G., et al. (2006). SEER cancer statistics review, 1975–2003. Bethesda: National Cancer Institute.
25. Narod, S. A., et al. (2005). Prevention and management of hereditary breast cancer. *Journal of Clinical Oncology, 23*, 1656–1663.
26. Wiesner, G., et al. (2009). *Genomic it personalized medicine* (pp. 879–897). Elsevier.
27. Manolio, T., et al. (2008). A HapMap harvest of insights into the genetics of common disease. *The Journal of Clinical Investigation, 118*, 1590–1605.
28. Porta-Pardo, E., et al. (2017). Comparison of algorithms for the detection of cancer drivers at subgene resolution. *Natural Methods, 14*(8):782–788.
29. Adzhubei, I. A., et al. (2010). A method and server for predicting damaging missense mutations. *Nature Methods, 7*, 248–249.

30. Bromberg, Y., et al. (2008). SNAP predicts effect of mutations on protein function. *Bioinformatics, 24*:2397–2398.
31. Jolliffe, I. T. (1986). *Principal component analysis*. Springer.
32. Johnson, R. A., et al. (2001). *Applied multivariate statistical analysis*. Prentice Hall. https://www.cancer.net/navigating-cancer-care/cancer-basics/genetics/genetics-cancer
33. Knudsen, S. (2006). *Cancer diagnostics with DNA microarrays*. Wiley. https://www.cancer.net/navigating-cancer-care/cancer-basics/genetics/genetic-testing-cancer-risk
34. Tahmasebi, P., Hezarkhani, A., & Mortazavi, M. (2010). Application of discriminant analysis for alteration separation. *Australian Journal of Basic and Applied Sciences, 6*(4), 564–576. https://www.cancer.net/navigating-cancer-care/cancer-basics/genetics/genetics-cancer
35. Jolliffe, I. T. (1986). *Principal Component Analysis*. New York. Springer.
36. Johnson, R. A., et al. (2001). *Applied multivariate statistical analysis*. Prentice Hall.
37. Knudsen, S. (2006). *Cancer diagnostics with DNA microarrays*. John Wiley and Sons.
38. Tahmasebi, P., Hezarkhani, A., & Mortazavi, M. (2010). Application of discriminant analysis for alteration separation. *Australian Journal of Basic and Applied Sciences, 6*(4), 564–576.

The World with Future Technologies (Post-COVID-19): Open Issues, Challenges, and the Road Ahead

A. V. Shreyas Madhav and Amit Kumar Tyagi

1 Introduction

The COVID-19 crisis has caused a global disruption in the daily lifestyles of the working population while mounting tremendous pressure on the world's healthcare sector. The highly transmissive virus led to increased panic and restricted people to their homes. Immersing people of most countries in a continuous series of lock-downs, the recent pandemic brought the world to a standstill. The resumption and recuperation of abandoned operations by organizations and the government have only been possible with the support of appropriate technology. The technological world has gone through a rapid transformation to adapt to the instant needs of critical industries in order to provide them with the necessary options to resume their operations. Remote communication has become the new normal, and socially distant working environments have become essential to control the spread of the virus. Vital applications in the COVID world have risen from new and upcoming domains like AI, machine learning, blockchain, and the Internet of things. These fields have seen humongous growth due to the impact of COVID, which has resulted in their growing demand to facilitate and support the functioning of critical applications. Insights into the current trends of each field can help analyze and attain an understanding of what technology reserves for a post-COVID world. The field of artificial intelligence has risen as one of the most promising fields in assisting humans and automating repetitive tasks in an intelligent manner. The advent of COVID 19 has positioned AI as the most popular emerging field in technology today. Before discussing the applications

A. V. S. Madhav · A. K. Tyagi (✉)
School of Computer Science and Engineering, Vellore Institute of Technology, Chennai, Tamilnadu 600127, India

A. K. Tyagi
Centre for Advance Data Science, Vellore Institute of Technology, Chennai, Tamilnadu 600127, India

A. K. Tyagi et al. (eds.), *Intelligent Interactive Multimedia Systems for e-Healthcare Applications*, https://doi.org/10.1007/978-981-16-6542-4_22

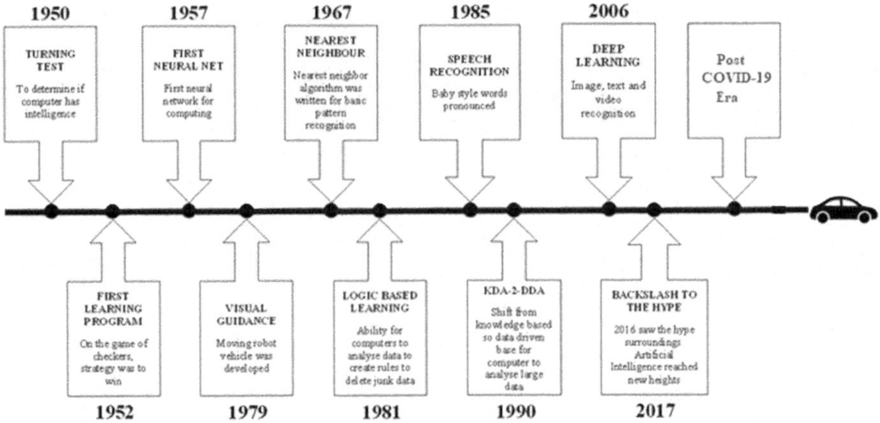

Fig. 1 Milestones of artificial intelligence since 1950

and problems solved by AI, it is essential to understand the answer to one question; what is artificial intelligence?

Artificial intelligence has several definitions and its true meaning cannot be encapsulated into a single statement. Enabling computers to develop human-like intelligence for efficient decision making and computational analysis is a generic expression of what AI aims to accomplish. The roots of AI run deep to the early philosophers who expressed the notion of the non-living things being instilled with human thoughts. The official introduction and advent of AI in the technological world are considered to have taken place in the 1950s. Figure 1 describes the brief timeline that marks important milestones in the field of AI/ML and its development.

AI is now spreading across different domains of technology and integrates as part of other large-scale applications for enabling intelligent computations, analytics, prediction, security, and intensive calculations. Machine learning-based modeling is considered a major subset of AI and is growing at an exponential rate, providing low-cost solutions for highly computational tasks. The COVID-19 pandemic has accelerated the growth and needs for emerging technologies like AI to support the increasing requirement for automation and prediction of uncertain events of the future. The healthcare industry is also under massive pressure to support the huge inflow of patients. This has been made possible only by increasing the pace of operations, making use of technological assistance. Due to the impact of COVID-19, human emotions are influencing decision-making processes indirectly in panic situations. It is essential for AI to step in to assist humans in battling this unfortunate situation through mechanisms for diagnosis, healthcare management systems, and an overall reduction of manual labor. Other Industries and organizations have also turned to emerging technologies like IoT, AI/ ML, and blockchain for facilitating their remote operations in a secure manner.

The Internet of things (IoT) has also gained recent traction in enabling critical applications and essential services to manage their functioning remotely with effective communication. The idea of establishing a network of connected devices that have the ability to share data and interact with each other forms the core idea behind IoT technology. Establishing smart systems that have the ability to record information and take decisions based upon their data or through human control makes IoT imperative for creating a smart and efficient future for both commercial and personal purposes. The mass migration of all companies and organizations to a homebound work environment has resulted in a surge in the need and production of IoT technology. Remote monitoring of COVID-19 patients in hospitals, public places, and in their homes would have been impossible without the intervention of IoT. Apart from this, IoT has also constituted a major role in the critical applications of a country and the government. The development of vehicle-based communication techniques has also enabled the scope for completely autonomous opportunities. Authentication and identity management of IoT devices and personnel accessing the network are also crucial in ensuring secure connections for interactions. The rise of IoT and AI/ML technology has also caused an increase in the security risk and vulnerabilities of a system. Security of an IoT network is of prime importance for critical applications as the consequences of hacking and exploitation of the network are extremely dangerous and highly disadvantageous in nature. Leakage or modification of patient data can lead to identity theft, change in medical records, and potentially death due to prescription of wrong treatment by misinformed doctors. Access to controls of autonomous vehicles can lead to improper navigation, kidnappings, and severe road accidents. Hence, a strong security system should be in place for ensuring proper authentication and mitigation in case of intrusions. Blockchain technology is now seen as the state-of-the-art application for this purpose and has received recognition for its high security while maintaining transparency.

Blockchain can be elucidated as a distributed system of immutable transaction ledgers that are transparent and decentralized in nature. This in turn promotes trust within the internal members and helps keep track of all the intermediate transactions and interactions that have taken place. The scalable nature of the technology and its robust security have made it one of the go-to technologies where members of any organization or a group of organizations can keep count of their past interactions in an open and safe manner. Blockchain has now established a significant position for itself in the healthcare system during this pandemic situation. Tracking disease outbreaks via public health monitoring with blockchain promotes accuracy and efficiency in reporting active cases. Early detection of disease symptoms by fast processing of data can help fasten the rate of treatment and prevent the development of the spread into a pandemic. Blockchain can also aid the government in creating a secure platform for multi-industry interactions involving doctors, healthcare personnel, city officials, media, government officials, and technology experts for drafting solutions toward COVID-19. The use of cryptographic techniques for encoding sensitive data in blockchains has also increased its reliability and provides access only to registered participants. Several essential services and industries are adopting blockchain technology for securing their application and preventing cyber-attacks. The monumental rise of new technological applications modeled for a post-COVID world has shifted the future of the technological era onto a new path. This article aims to provide an overall projection and review of the existing technologies and their future directions due to the impact of COVID-19. This paper explores the most promising emerging technologies including IoT, ML, blockchain applications, and their viable implementation to critical applications. Issues and challenges surrounding future emerging technologies are also discussed to provide comprehensive insights into the respective fields and their hope for the future.

Fog computing and edge computing are decentralized computation paradigms that focus on reducing the complexity of data transfer in large networks by performing the computations near the data source. This computing approach performs the intended calculations near the edge nodes and carries out a significant amount of calculations and storage on a local scale, supported and routed through the backbone of the Internet. Huge volumes of raw data are obtained by the edge devices in the sensory or manual inputs, and the transfer of this unprocessed data to remote cloud-based servers will be cumbersome and pose high bandwidth requirements. The usage of computing units positioned closer to the end node devices helps carry out the initial processing of the data before transmitting only the most relevant information to the cloud centers. The bandwidth required is reduced significantly due to these measures, and the latency of transmission is also greatly reduced. The decrease in transmission and response time plays a major role in critical applications that require immediate actions. Another added benefit arises from previous observations which show that the point at which a data source arises will be the point requiring computations to the done on the data. While fog computing and edge computing are very similar in their working, a slight differentiation can be achieved by analyzing the location of their computing power and intelligence. Embedded automation controllers are utilized to provide processing power for edge computing. Fog environments mostly depend upon LAN to transmit data to the appropriate locations for processing via a gateway. The rapid growth in complexity and size of IoT networks has placed this paradigm in the forefront for battling bandwidth requirements and processing power necessities.

Organisation of the work: Further, Sect. 2 proceeds to draw a comparison between the use of machine learning and other emerging technologies before and after COVID-19. Section 3 summarizes the motivation behind writing this article. Section 4 focuses on the different applications and implementations of artificial intelligence in the healthcare sector. Section 5 discusses strategies aimed toward protecting autonomous and semi-autonomous vehicles and the associated networks. Section 6 provides an overview of security and standardizations for smart and critical applications. Several technologies like blockchain and machine learning have been explored under this section. API Security, authentication, and standardization techniques have also been briefed in this part of the article. Section 7 identifies the prospects of technical security applications for financial institutions and banks. Section 8 investigates privacy issues in different fields of technology. Section 9 throws light upon open issues and challenges faced in emerging technologies. Section 10 looks at some of the possible future directions of research that can be explored moving forward. Note that in this work terms "Internet of things," "smart things," and "Internet connected things" and "smart devices" have been used interchangeably.

2 Comparison of Scope of Machine Learning Techniques Pre-COVID and Post-COVID-19 Era

Machine learning is a subfield of artificial intelligence and helps develop automated systems that can learn on their own. The machine then improves its efficiency by learning from experience without any interference by humans. This lets the machines make decisions which are completely data-driven. Whatever the machines learn from past experience, they use it to make predictions. In fostering global initiatives to solve COVID-19, developments in data science and artificial intelligence/machine learning (AI/ML) play a crucial role. The versatility of AI/ML technology helps scientists and technologists overcome an impressively large range of technological, epidemiological, and socioeconomic challenges. Before the COVID, i.e., pre-COVID-19 era, we have numerous scopes of machine learning, such as:

- Automotive industry: One of the fields where machine learning excels by changing the definition of "healthy" driving is the automotive industry. There are a few big companies like Google, Tesla, Mercedes Benz, Nissan, and so on that have invested heavily in machine learning to come up with new technologies. Yet Tesla's self-driving car is the industry's best. These self-driving cars are constructed using machine learning, IoT sensors, HD cameras, voice recognition systems, etc.
- Robotics: Robotics is one of the areas that often attract both the attention of researchers and the general interest. George Devol invented the first programmable robot in 1954, which was called Unimate. After this, Hanson Robotics developed the first AI-robot, Sophia, in the twenty-first century. With the aid of machine learning and artificial intelligence, such inventions became possible.
- Quantum computing: In the field of machine learning, we are still at an infant level. There are several advances to accomplish in this region. Quantum computing is one of the ones that can push machine learning to the next level. It is a method of computing that uses quantum mechanical phenomena like entanglement and superposition. By using the superposition quantic principle, we can construct systems (quantum systems) that can simultaneously exhibit multiple states. On the other hand, the theory of entanglement is when two distinct states can be related one to another. It helps to explain the connection between a quantum system's properties.
- Computer vision: Computer vision, as the name implies, provides a view of a computer or machine. Here comes to mind what Google's Head of AI, Jeff Dean, once said, "The improvement we made from an error of 26 percent in 2011 to an error of 3 percent in 2016 is incredibly impactful. The way I like to think is now

computers have evolved working eyes." The aim of computer vision is to give a machine the capacity to recognize and analyze images, videos, graphics, etc. Progress in the field of artificial intelligence and machine learning has allowed the faster achievement of the computer vision target.

Now, if we will discuss the scope of Machine Learning Post-COVID-19 in brief.

Officials around the world are using different outbreak prediction models for COVID-19 to make informed decisions and implement appropriate control measures. Among the traditional COVID-19 global pandemic prediction models, simple epidemiological and statistical models have drawn more attention from authorities and are popular in the media [1]. In the face of the global public health crisis, data scientists and AI/ML innovators may be inclined to ask: are we ready for this? Can we find a responsible path to ethically and safely exercising our technological effectiveness? In what follows, I argue that these crossroads do not need to cause confusion as to how we should go, and in fact, to find the right way forward, they give us straightforward signage [1]. In the fields of diagnostics, prognostics, genomics, drug creation, epidemiology, and mobile health monitoring, biomedical AI/ML innovations have also made major strides in assisting physicians and researchers when pressed into action for the public good. And although the great promise of helping healthcare professionals to solve COVID-19 is held by each of these growth areas, they also present substantial ethical hazards. Actionable ways of coping with these are what we need now. In order to advance higher-performance models for long-term prediction, future research should be devoted to comparative studies on various ML models for individual countries. Due to the fundamental differences between the outbreaks in different countries, the creation of global models with generalization potential would not be feasible. Table 1 provides a comparison summary of emerging techniques pre-COVID-19 and post-COVID-19.

To summarize, in the post-COVID-19 era, we have shifted more toward IoT-based cloud applications and prefer things that can work automatically, i.e., we rely on programmed machines. But, as discussed above, these machines or solutions come with several negative impacts, which have been discussed in [2, 3].

3 Motivation

The COVID-19 pandemic has become a significant checkpoint in the technological world as well as the health industry. Controlling the fast growing pandemic has attained utmost importance and the world has been transformed into a socially distant place for this purpose. The healthcare industry has turned to technology for immediate response assistance to prevent, control, diagnose, and treat the COVID-19 virus. The areas of artificial intelligence and machine learning have attained massive attention due to their computational ability in monitoring and predicting future outcomes of the disease. Contact tracing [4] and monitoring of the population to ensure social

Table 1 Comparison of emerging techniques popularity pre-COVID-19 and post-COVID-19

Emerging technologies	
Pre-COVID-19	Post-COVID-19
Artificial intelligence/machine learning	
Advantages: The ability of computers is to recognize patterns and perform computations in minimal time form the basis of this technology. It is highly efficient in mimicking human jobs and performing its tasks with much more accuracy in lesser time	*Advantages*: AI cost has decreased significantly due to the expansion of operations by AI companies to meet the growing demand for autonomous applications. Several popular applications in today's remote world are almost completely powered by machine learning algorithms to accommodate the massive surge in the online population
Disadvantages: Although machine learning has found its way into several organisations and applications, The field of AI is distant from attaining its true potential. The cost for implementation is considerably high, lacks creativity, and poses a threat to human jobs. The risk of unemployment sets an unsettling environment for employees of a company and may lead to a decrease in morale	*Disadvantages*: The inflow of data may lead to bias in the decision-making process of AI and hinder the widespread factors that are to be accounted for before deriving a conclusion. Mainstream application brews a whiff of hostility and emotionless interactions. In critical industries, humans feel far more comfortable dealing with other humans than when compared to dealing with automated models
Fog/cloud computing	
Advantages: Cloud storage can hold humongous amounts of data at very minimal costs compared to traditional servers. Data restoration and backup features of cloud-based servers enable organizations with the ability to retrieve deleted content efficiently. Accessibility of the data stored is also eased from location restrictions	*Advantages*: The wide scale adoption of IoT networks has increased the need for fog computing in all domains. The increase in inflow and outflow of raw data has propelled cloud technology to the next level for assuring remote storage of large data volumes
Disadvantages: Vendor lock-in, lack of Internet connectivity, and limited controls over the data are few of the disadvantageous aspects of the cloud paradigm. Fog computing applications face problems in authentication and maintenance due to their decentralized nature	*Disadvantages*: The increase in cloud platforms and servers also leads to an increase in the points of vulnerability. Data security might be sacrificed if the clouds do not store encrypted versions of the data. In a fog environment, the increase in computational complexity leads to an increase in the processing power requirements that may not be satisfied by intermediate resources
Internet of things	
Advantages: IoT network applications enhance data collection, facilitate remote operations, and reduce the requirement of physical presence. Intercommunication of the devices promotes informed data transfer and analysis to make insightful conclusions	Advantages: The implementations of IoT have expanded past the conventional use cases. From health care to the military, remote monitoring techniques have taken different forms and prove highly efficient when compared to physical observations

(continued)

Table 1 (continued)

Emerging technologies	
Pre-COVID-19	Post-COVID-19
Disadvantages: The heterogeneous nature of the network, arising from the different devices used, poses a problem for compatibility and interoperability for different IoT networks. Node device vulnerabilities also expose the network to major exploitations	*Disadvantages*: Several issues concerning the complexity, privacy, security of the IoT networks have been discovered due to the large-scale application of IoT in such a short period of time
Blockchain	
Advantages: The transparency associated with blockchain builds trust among the concerned parties on any transactions carried out. All blocks are time stamped, and hence, a timeline can be envisioned. The chain is highly secure and follows standard encryption rules for the content within its blocks	*Advantages*: The need for blockchain applications for the healthcare industry increased rapidly during the COVID-19 period. Blockchain today plays an imperative role in managing EHRs and other confidential data due to their transparent, immutable, and decentralized nature
Disadvantages: Although several fields have proposed the use of blockchain to strengthen their applications, the implemented applications of blockchain are limited to transactional data and financial information	*Disadvantages*: The decentralized and block-based architecture of this system makes scalability difficult. High cost of implementation for large-scale organizations builds reluctance incorporates and makes them seek other options that might provide security solutions at a lower cost
Summary: While technologies were being developed at a steady pace, the wide scale and mainstream application of emerging technologies was deemed possible only in the next couple of decades. Traditional and manual processes were preferred for work operations while remote work was offered only in special cases	*Summary*: The urgent and dire need to cope with the rapid changes brought about the pandemic has accelerated the growth. Consumer behavior after the pandemic will not revert back to normal. More jobs will be remote and the purchase of services and goods will remain predominantly online. A major increase in the need for security applications was observed. The adoption of emerging technological applications proved vital for crisis management and recuperation of the world from the impact of the virus

distancing have been facilitated by the use of AI. Predictive modeling for detection and diagnosis of COVID-19 based on images is also a viable application [5]. All the above-mentioned applications have opened up new opportunities and gateways for the development of new applications that suit the purpose. This has given rise to several innovations that have been created and brought to fruition in a considerably short period of time. Companies and organizations have also transformed their working nature to accommodate the restrictions that have been brought about by the pandemic. This has led to the accelerated development of digital applications to deal with remote operations and manage work at home employments for businesses to sustain their professional activities. Although most of these applications were developed as temporary solutions for a problem that was once considered to last for a short period of time, the impact of this rapid expansion of applications and data has led to a complete transformation in the field of technology. Education has undergone a paradigm shift to enable students to pursue their learning from home as a way to maintain proper social distancing. Students are undergoing live online schooling through video communication services in most parts of the world and are graded upon their projects and assignments submitted through learning management systems. This transformation has led to massive data flow, and relevant implementations have been developed to support this rapid expansion. Video communication platforms have seen a massive inflow of users and have been expanding their features at a speedy rate to provide learners with the best educational experience possible.

Existing technology has also gone through heavy modifications to enable contactless and socially distant usage. IoT has now become an imperative asset for connectivity and monitoring of several health systems over the Internet without the need for physical presence. The intercommunicating nature of this domain proved useful particularly in a situation where physical contact has to be minimized. Automation and remote communication have become necessary not only for the healthcare industry but also for normal people to continue their daily tasks in a safe manner. Patient monitoring and personalized care can be achieved while maintaining an appropriate physical distance. The Internet of health things [6] plays an imperative role in many hospitals for providing interconnectivity between the health devices present for doctors to easily access all the data in a holistic manner. Wearable technology that monitors patient vitals like smart thermometers and RFID-based monitoring [7] has all attained importance during this lockdown scenario. The dire need for contactless and remote monitoring technology during this pandemic has given rise to several IoT systems and startups that are now focussing on solving this issue.

With this boom of online data, the risk of breaches and chances of exploitation also increases. Due to the abrupt need for employees to work from home, employers have had to set up new applications and portals to support the working of their employees. This opens up pathways for several potential security threats due to the inexperienced nature and low testing period of the new applications. Communication interfaces such as Zoom are not known to provide end-to-end encryption to enable secure communication of sensitive information. The security of the networks used by the employees and the security of their own computers is also of concern. Hospitals are at the utmost risk of cyber-attacks and ransom attacks that aim to extract ransoms by threatening to compromise confidential patient information. Access to patient records is considered the holy grail to any hacker as this data is highly valuable and can be sold for a significant amount of money. Hence, there is a big need for improvements in cyber-security measures to adapt to the current situation faced by the working population. Being aware of these possibilities of security breaches will help organizations and individuals secure themselves from intruders and protect their data. Blockchain technology has also been instrumental in establishing a decentralized system that maintains data integrity and transparency while maintaining no single point of failure. This feature of blockchain-based security makes it trustful and a viable asset for maintaining security across several platforms. The transfer of everyday affairs is now completely online. Technologies that were once categorized as specific and niche have now become essential for daily mainstream usage. At this point in time, It only seems appropriate to analyze the new direction in which the technological advancements are heading due to the monumental alterations in lifestyle brought about by COVID-19.

4 Artificial Intelligence in Health Care and Other Sectors: Hope or Hype?

There is an increasing demand for healthcare services and medical practitioners, especially in an epidemic situation. While the healthcare industry struggles to keep up with the great advancements in the field of medical technology, patient expectations have also increased with respect to the level of infrastructure and treatment services expected. Although the field of artificial intelligence has been present and developing considerably over the past few decades, the hype created around artificial intelligence in recent times portrays it in a different light altogether. Multimedia applications have also become vital for the smooth functioning of the healthcare space and its integration with artificial intelligence and machine learning ideas are of great interest. Figure 2 describes an overview of the various multimedia applications present in the healthcare space and of high interest for AI-based inclusions. Today, AI is regarded as one of the most instrumental fields for technological and societal development. It is essential to take a step back at this point and weigh the positive and negative aspects of AI to arrive at a solution on whether AI will live up to its expectations.

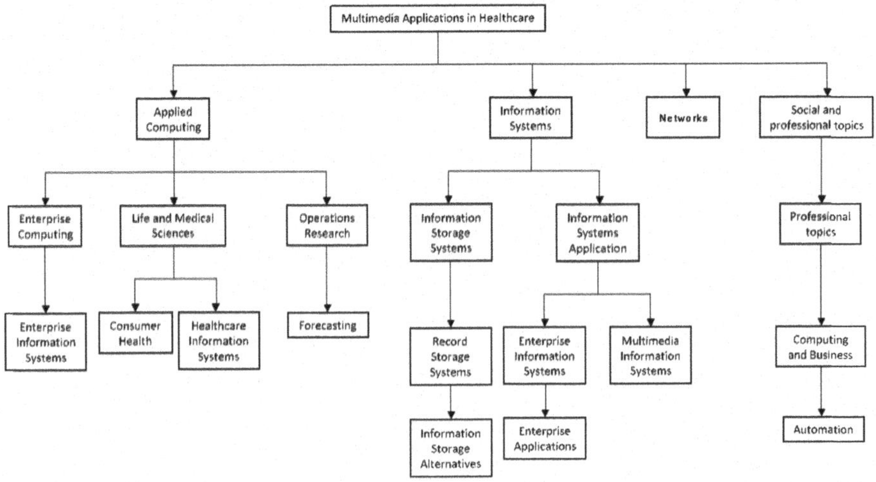

Fig. 2 Multimedia applications in health care

Computer vision and AI go hand in hand, and this is no different in the case of the medical domain. Surgery applications have employed computer vision and AI techniques for skill augmentation in repairing wounds. John Hopkins University demonstrated the ability of their Smart Tissue Autonomous Robot (STAR) in aiding doctors in animal surgeries. Although autonomous robots for complete surgical procedures have not achieved practical application, automating and assisting surgeons by providing valuable insights about their surgical procedures has been made possible. One prime example of this was proven by Alpen-Adria Universität Klagenfurt using surgery videos for identification of the surgical method employed by the surgeon. For example, when an act of dissection or cutting is performed on the patient's tissues or organs, the algorithm recognizes the likelihood of the intervention as well as the specific region in the body [8]. Apart from visual interpretations, AI technology also has reached the realm of development to think and make decisions based upon audio inputs. Force cough-based diagnosis of COVID-19 for both symptomatic and asymptomatic patients has been made possible using CNNs-based architecture, providing a binary prescreening diagnostic [9]. The largest database of COVID-19 coughs was created for this purpose using positive cough audio recordings. This AI speech-based framework enables non-invasive testing based upon acoustic biomarkers with almost zero cost. Integrative approaches for diagnosis of the coronavirus have also proven effective, where lung ailment categorization for both COVID-based and non-COVID-based complications was carried out [10]. X-ray-based diagnosis methods have also enabled AI systems to learn and classify COVID-19 positive cases efficiently. Individual adaptions of medical treatments based upon medical history, gene profile, diagnostic report, and treatment effects have become essential in ensuring maximal benefit for any patient. Individual biology of a person is considered for treatment rather than considering the general biological profile of the relevant population. This direction of approaching treatment, called precision medicine, relies upon advanced modeling and prediction for diagnosis and prescribing treatment based upon an individual's comprehensive biological report. While precision medicine is developing with huge steps forward, it is at the beginning stages of complete implementation and only time can tell how dominant it will be. Apart from diagnostic purposes, artificial intelligence has also found its place in other domains and departments of the healthcare sector. Medical coding and billing industries can further the efficiency of their operations and billing procedures with the help of AI. Natural language processing helps formulate a methodology to match medical codes accurately and reduces the error rate and the cost required to mitigate the errors. Contextualizing unstructured data through analytics and interconnections, computational programs can categorize and sequence data from various mismatched sources to form a timeline of EHRs and medical histories, helping in the reduction of reporting errors and record mismanagement. Bill forecasting and expenditure predictions benefit the patient in attaining a proper understanding of how much and where the money is required to be spent. Ensemble architectures with novel combinations of data mixing and node dropout regularization give hospitals and patients to predict the individual financial costs on hospital rooms and medications.

People have grown hesitant to approach hospitals or health centers due to the fear of contracting a disease or the heavy sum of consultation fees. This leads them to self-diagnose themselves based upon unverified information sources on the Internet. This often proves detrimental effects on the person's mental and physical health if misdiagnosed and improper medicines are consumed. Healthcare chatbots have been purposed to solve this problem and ensure proper diagnosis and advice for people from the comfort of their homes. Based upon the severity of the diagnosis, the chatbot prescribes over the counter treatment or escalates the diagnosis to a verified healthcare professional. Interactive chatbots that have been trained on a large and wide variety of symptoms, risk factors, and treatment can handle user health queries with ease, especially in the case of COVID-19. The World Health Organization (WHO) in collaboration with Viber (messaging app) promotes an informative and interactive chatbot that spread awareness and accurately resolves doubts about COVID-19 in several world languages [11]. The massive size of libraries used in drug screening and selection of drug trial candidates is highly difficult for researchers to review manually. Machine learning and artificial intelligence can step in and accelerate the development and testing of drugs in an exponential manner. The different roles of AI in drug discovery can be briefed into three main segments.

- Characterizing potential compounds based upon their properties for synthesis rather than exploring every ineffective compound in detail. This helps researchers identify the required and most effective compounds in a shorter span of time compared to the manual classification of the compounds based upon their known chemical attributes. Expenditure toward the drug's research is also reduced as many unnecessary chemical tests can now be averted.
- Exploring and coming up with completely different perspectives on entirely new or relatively unknown compounds that have the capability of being modeled into an entirely new drug with different medicinal and chemical properties such AI-based methodologies can rapidly increase the rate of drug discovery and production, enabling drugs to reach patients faster especially for relatively new diseases.
- Analytical processes are now automated with higher accuracy of processing leading to an enormous reduction in the number of laboratory hours required to be put in by researchers for a specific analysis. This also enables the researchers to dedicate their time toward the next steps required and increases the efficiency of the intermediate processes involved in drug development.

All these advantageous aspects of artificial intelligence pose a big question-Why is the technology not in much greater use, considering the vast benefits and efficiency factor associated with it?

First of all, machine-based interpretations of X-rays/medical scans and the research work surrounding it are highly expensive in nature and most often are specific to a particular machine (machine dependant). Several payment models are being tested for the practical implementation of machine learning where the hospital gets paid for a machine interpreted X-ray and refers a radiologist for further reviews whenever an X-ray is classified as not normal. There is also the issue of trusting a non-human entity. Practitioners and patients feel uncertain about the results obtained from what the machine have learned as they cannot perceive how the learning has taken place. Automation of billing and other manual processes are under doubt for errors made by the machine. As machines lack emotional intelligence, patients are not really comfortable communicating their worries and symptoms with the non-human consultant. They also find it difficult to trust AI, which is usually shrouded with mistrust. Therefore, AI implementations are focused on handling essential tasks, while primary patient management and appointments are handled by human doctors. Several trials have been conducted for using AI to calculate the target locations of a person's body to deliver radiotherapy treatments more accurately but an interventional radiologist is primarily responsible for delivering the treatment and ensuring an extra layer of assurance.

There is also the risk of deterioration of human intelligence. If AI takes over most of the tasks done by humans and requires them only for vital reviews, humans will lose their knowledge due to a lack of real-life practice. For example, if doctors are required only to verify abnormal scans occasionally, they are likely to forget other aspects of what makes a normal scan and its anomalies. Another demonstration of this is when people have adapted to completely autonomous self-driving vehicles/cars, their driving skills will be degraded over a long period of time. Although they might still remember how to drive, the ease and skill with which they once drove a vehicle will be reduced. There are also not enough legal, ethical, and moral standards in place by which AI is expected to adhere to. The thought of AI exploiting people gives rise to fear among humans. Taking into account all of these positives and negatives of AI, It is safe to say that even if artificial intelligence does not match the current hype of being regarded as a technological brilliance, there is a strong hope that AI will provide a brighter future for various different industries in the future leading to low cost and effective applications. Note that AI importance/existence in near future can be found in smart storage at cloud computing, cyber-vulnerabilities detection/digital forensics, education, agriculture, health care, transportation, data science, and industry 4.0.

5 Emerging Techniques for Automotive (Connected and Autonomous Cars) Security

The disruption caused by the COVID pandemic in the automotive industry and its sales has pushed automotive manufacturers to reassess their production and security strategies. The introduction of new threat vectors due to the remote nature of functioning has made automotive manufacturers make modifications to their existing technology. Autonomous and connected cars gained a lot of interest as a result of the pandemic and are moving toward becoming mainstream due to the cautious nature of people in avoiding contact and public transport [12]. New and latent production vehicles such as connected and autonomous cars have been subjected to increased security evaluations and new innovative security measures to overcome the hackable nature of the cars. Connected cars are characterized by their ability to connect to the Internet or an external wireless network and establish communication with both internal and external devices in order to exchange data for the purpose of making better decisions and ease passenger control. The connective nature of the car makes it vulnerable to network attacks and security breaches that may gain control of the vehicle or steal protected data for unsolicited purposes. Intruders can gain access to internal passenger systems which lead to unauthorized control over doors, ignition, and airbag systems. Misdirecting the driver toward wrong decisions by displaying false navigation info, installing malware to corrupt the car's user interface, or controlling the brake system of the car are other attacks that could be carried out and result in great physical and cyber-damage.

Most of the communication channels that are currently in use are vehicle-to-vehicle communication channel (V2V) or communication of the vehicle to external/internal devices and infrastructures [13]. V2V communications are the most target part for exploiting a car and its inner controls. Recent research into connected car security strategies in the USA/UK has concluded that gaining illegal access to the network of the car can result in absolute control over the car's functionalities. The exploitations of any possible loopholes in these networks can provide the intruders with authority over the car's controls and in some cases, both the vehicle and the connected devices. This exploitation is similar in view to intruding into an IoT network. This motivates manufacturers and consumers to ensure the presence of proper security infrastructure in these types of automobiles. The primary course of action should be directed toward the protection of the network channels against data stealing and manipulation of the transmitted data. Encryption of the transmitting data and authentication procedures to ensure the integrity of transmission are imperative steps toward solving this problem. Identification of the communicating devices confirms that the two devices are known to each other, and the data transmission has reached the proper location for further processing. Integrity checks on the received data can be conducted based on their digital signatures, which follow public key cryptography and encryption of the data can be done using public key algorithms. These methods are initial strategies that provide a layer of security on otherwise exposed data. A relevant selection of security policies and validation tests for ensuring the proper executions of intended security parameters have to be met. The installation of security into smart cars is multifold, taking place at different stages in the production of the smart car. These methods include:

- Uniform process and standard process policies that define the entire process of car development. This process of planning security from the analysis and planning of the development until the final test phase of the smart communication in the car promotes robustness. This enables automotive producers to plan out all possible vulnerabilities and correct them at the right stages of development.
- State-of-the-art electronic control unit software and constant updation to cater to the changes in nature of the possible vulnerabilities and loopholes of the system propagate safe interactions and provide additional assurance of security. Security

protocols along with cryptographic key employment should also be reliable and ensure long-term security benefits for the consumers.
- Immediate response to intruder alerts from the system or by the owner should be addressed as a priority and minimizes loss of property and data. Consumers should be provided with the ability to lock and secure their data in case of breaches. Companies should have recovery and response systems to mitigate the effects of unauthorized entry and data exploitation attacks.

Recent advanced security for connected cars has taken into account the importance of integrating security of connected cars right from the production stages rather than implementing security software after opening up to consumers. Contemplating the security of a connected car is to be interwoven into the life cycle of a car and should not be regarded as a separate component for later. Intruder detecting cloud services for smart vehicles [14] conducts service-based clustering to provide a secure and quality user experience. This has come into play in the recent past with assigned mediator structure between the providers and requestors. Intrusion detection measures employ a three-layer system of combating cyber-attacks for validation of approved and legal service requests. Reduction and classification of the data are being facilitated by the use of decision trees and deep models in continuous cloud frameworks used for smart connected cars. Secondary challenges for connected car security include the necessity to revoke the public key and decreasing the time taken for authentication to validate communication between vehicles to infrastructure networks. Vehicle-to-infrastructure validation checks and short time management schemes have proven efficient in recent years for service-oriented networks [15].

Autonomous cars comprise the next level of car development technology and possess the ability of self-driving. Sensory inputs of the surrounding environment provide the car system with the necessary information to navigate and localize itself with very minimal human interference. Most attacks are directly targeted at the vehicular ad hoc networks of autonomous cars and are susceptible to DoS attacks. Vehicular ad hoc network (VANET) is responsible for establishing interactions between other vehicles in the same area network and bear influence on the car's decisions [16]. Current protection technology includes intruder detection systems for the autonomous vehicle systems that protect the controller area networks and other external channels. These systems detect general intrusions and fuzzy attacks on the protected networks. More efficient computational IDS systems have come into fruition to facilitate the growing need for low-cost security for the ramp up of autonomous car production [17]. Intruder protection not only assures the security of the concerned vehicle and also adds to the security of the IoT device in contact with the car. Artificial intelligence and neural networks have been instrumental in increasing the robustness of security systems. Trace file data reading to predict attacks on the networks can now be carried out to assess VANET intrusions with the help of ANNs [18]. Anomaly-based detection of malware entries can estimate the state of the system and its integrity. Preservation of safety constraints based on Bayesian Kalman filters can now ensure safety constraints when sensors present in the vehicle have been compromised [19]. False data injection attacks and data manipulation attempts can be detected via the above-mentioned method.

Connecting smartphones to our cars have also proven beneficial for customer comfort of ease of usage. The only drawback faced in such a situation is the additional component of security that is required to ensure intrusion detection to the mobile ad hoc network. A fuzzy-based algorithm for intruder detection was proposed by Chaudhary et al. in [20] that assured detection of malicious attacks and unauthorized interactions with the autonomous system via the mobile ad hoc network (MANET). While artificial intelligence proved efficient in assisting automotive companies in gaining trust and solving their cyber-security challenges, the field of blockchain technology also started gaining traction due to its decentralized and open nature of transacting data. Ledger-based architecture is employed within the car. Recent developments in this direction are making sure that the information provided to adaptive algorithms (e.g., sensory inputs based) is correct and validated [21]. The technological world is now slowly realizing the rise of autonomous cars and formulating standards to ensure uniform application of security standards throughout the world. New developments in cyber-security standards have come to fruition with recent updates in 2020. ISO 21434 is one of the standards developed for the vehicle-to-vehicle interaction security [22]. UNECE WP.29 is another major regulatory and safety framework for ensuring vehicle safety. It provides a collection of threats and risks that automotive manufacturers should keep in mind for creating secure automobiles. Although general automotive sales have gone down due to the impact of COVID-19, the fields of autonomous automobiles have seen exponential developments in their technology and security standards as mentioned above. As the world moves toward a lifestyle of minimal physical contact, IoT devices have also become mainstream in nature. The next section describes the use of blockchain technology for security in a country's critical applications that employ online sharing of data and IoT technology like health care, defence, transportation, waste management, and many more.

6 Security and Standardization for Smart and Critical Applications

Security is an essential component for any trusted system, and the security validation process of any system contains components like authentication, identity management, which depend on standardization actions that have been put in place. Previously, a biometric-based system was considered more secure, while today blockchain has taken the credibility of securing a system with required features. A few of related techniques have been discussed here:

6.1 Blockchain-Based Security in Critical Applications

In the recent decade, several revolutions in blockchain have been seen in previous decade like Blockchain 1.0, Blockchain 2.0, Blockchain 3.0, and Blockchain 4.0. Blockchain 4.0 is the recent and useful revolution with respect to industry point of view, i.e., creation of decentralized applications. Blockchain technology has gained great interest for security over the past decade for security and transparency, which was proven with the operations of bitcoin cryptocurrency/blockchain technology. A generalized description of blockchain is that it provides a decentralized and transparent block-based structure that is linked and acts as a multinode structure. Every block contains information encapsulating the block timestamp and hash address of the previous linked block. Other data in the block is determined based upon the domain of operations [23]. All these beneficial factors of blockchain make it the best possible option for critical applications in a county, which require the most secure due to the confidential nature of data being stored. The healthcare world deals with large amounts of patient and drug data and requires access to this data on a regular basis. Analysis of healthcare data can improve and influence patient outcomes, prevent disease outbreaks and pandemics, reduce patient costs, and ensure the provision of drugs. The healthcare sector is undergoing a complete digitization process as a result of the pandemic and it is imperative to analyze recent developments in blockchain security as a viable option to secure electronic health record databases. Several platforms for blockchain-based patient data management like MedRec [24] have been established which provide patients with the authority to view their data logs and their access information. Permissions for using data for clinical and research purposes can now adhere to a standard and more formal approach when done via a blockchain. Currently, most of the healthcare information remains in the hospital systems while blockchain stores the distinct properties of the data (location, audit logs, etc.). Encryption of patient data also helps maintain anonymity and concerned parties can only access the data after assurance from registration info data [25]. Even if access is attained by an unauthorized party, the data cannot be used easily due to its encrypted form.

Another critical application that transcends countries and acts as an imperative energy production asset is nuclear technology and nuclear power plants. Nuclear energy is essentially energy produced by nuclear fission and produced in nuclear thermal plants. Nuclear plants have been prime targets of criminals who wish to cause mass destruction and damage to a country and its development. The breach into a nuclear power plant can lead to massive explosions and radioactive release into the atmosphere causing severe materialistic and health damages to the surrounding population. Pressurized water nuclear plants are most common and blockchain technology has found its way recently into SG tube inspections for an open process of assuring regulators and surrounding civilians that the plant is robust and cannot be hacked into. Korea Hydro and Nuclear Power (KHNP) and nuclear fuel storage systems in Russia are fine examples of integrating blockchain technology for tamper-free operations for a sensitive government entity [26]. Adherence to international regulations and the possibility of expanding nuclear fuel production can be seen as achievable goals with the use of blockchain technology. Tracking irregularities between the development models and production reality can be essential in confirming the security and can be accomplished using blockchain. Management of event logs and history assures stakeholders and regulators with the assurance of a safe record of events. Considering the paramount importance of the data and the need for secure access makes blockchain technology the perfect deployment option for building trust and confidentiality in the government.

Communication between army troops yields coordination and proper planning to defeat their targets and accomplish the intended final points is paramount. Battlefield management and communication is a matter of high security where interception by the enemy could lead to catastrophic physical and human losses. IoT technologies have been proposed in this field for formulating attack and defence plans, sensing data about a target location and monitoring crucial locations of interest. Sensor-based inputs are received from drones and UAVs used in the aerospace defence for monitoring and attacking target vectors. Combat engineering vehicles also have GPS and all the components mentioned above are connected to a centralized IoT-based network. This network approach opens up possibilities of intrusion through any node to gain access and collapse the entire system during critical times. Misdirection and manipulation of army transmission data can also lead to severe consequences for the troops and the country. Hence, systematic and standard security deployments are essential for ensuring the integrity of the army and government plans. Isolating the harmed points of intrusion is the first step of mitigation in tackling enemy attempts to exploit the system. The NATO has proposed standards for all types of organizations to safeguard cooperative application establishments.

Proper registration parameters help distinguish known military entities and IoT devices and validate their relations. Current registration processes employ individual and unique ID assignments to each device that are categorized as part of the network. During the course of operations and procedure in the army, the devices are validated and integrity checks are carried out using asymmetric key cryptography [27]. Hence, any manipulative measures on the data can be detected. The system components transmit the army activities and operations, enabling authorities to monitor action plans and their execution by the troop members. The non-modifiable nature of data storage makes certain that a uniform standard is maintained across different bases and domains of the army. Procurement of missiles and other associated machinery in the aerospace industry require confidential transactions between countries. All transactional data is recorded and exchanged between concerned parties through e-mails or fax. Eavesdropping into such information exchanges can help enemies assess the preparedness and available firepower of the opposition. This leads to a disadvantage in combat situations since the enemies are aware of what the army has up its sleeve. Blockchain technology provides a vital structure for transparency among the buyer and seller, avoiding disputes at a later stage.

Drone swarms are an autonomous collection of drones that operate synchronously for the assessment of potential targets tracking enemy movements, recognize victims in need of emergency evacuations or for the protection of aircraft and combat helicopters. This is a relatively new technology that is deemed as the future of AI solutions in the defence industry. The drone swarms follow a global voting-based procedure to complete their objectives. The head drone collects votes from the swarm members on its own decisions and assigns probability factors to each observation. The conclusion is reached when all the opinions of all the drones are combined to attain the most probable observation. Blockchain technology comes into this process for secure recording of the observations of each drone. False voting by an unregistered drone can change the original decision process and should be detected and disregarded. The probabilities of each member drone's decision are recorded into the blockchain. The final result can be derived from this structure while ensuring that the retrieved data is not manipulated.

Waste management is one of the defining factors for a sustainable and environmentally friendly country. Although the requirements of security are high when compared to other critical applications, blockchain plays a key part in facilitating social currency allocation for the social and financial inclusion of social volunteers [28]. Applications use crypto coins as a replacement for printed cards that are now in usage among citizens and social volunteers. This acts as a proof of concept for the integration of blockchain technology in similar applications for the sake of managing the production of physical currency and cards. Other domains of interest in assuring security in critical applications include machine learning and AI-based solutions. In the next section, deep learning and model-based solving of security challenges in critical applications are discussed.

6.2 Machine and Deep Learning-Based Security Techniques for Critical Applications

The implementation and inclusion of network-based operations for communicative interactions in various critical applications have opened up possibilities for machine learning-based security options that can adapt and predict the security measures and their effectiveness. In the field of global health care, the ubiquitous emergence of the Internet of things in medical devices had developed a smart network-based healthcare system. The pandemic has fast tracked this integration due to the urgent need for remote healthcare and monitoring practices. The implantation of monitoring devices in a patient to get constant feedback on their vital signs and possible diseases has become pretty common and comprises a major part of the smart healthcare network. The increase in devices and functionalities also introduces vulnerabilities into the system which can become entry points for attackers. Manipulation of patient data, infusing false readings, and the overall collapse of the medical device are major breaches and require a proper security component in place to detect and prevent such events from happening. Detecting intrusions in a smart healthcare system is facilitated by using machine learning-based secure frameworks. One such example is HealthGuard [29], which aims to understand the relative changes and correlations and identifies discrepancies in vital signs of the connected devices of a patient to categorize readings as malicious or non-malicious activities using four model-based techniques (e.g., K-nearest neighbor, ANN, random forest, and decision trees) and proved efficient in detecting three main malware attacks with an accuracy of greater than 90%. Another approach which is following the principle of prevention is better than cure. Instead of detecting and mitigating after an intrusion, preventing unauthorized access to the healthcare system and its nodes can reduce the effort of mitigation. Data processing in a cloud-based environment for health scans with image processing is present and done with the help of SVM and fuzzy C-means clustering [30] for efficient classification of image pixels. Protection of data and image segmentation in a parallel manner was performed most efficiently by support vector machines. A cloud-based module is also fed as an extra layer of security to prevent unauthorized disclosure. These observations not only validate machine learning and also open up pathways for cloud services integration in the healthcare industry.

The introduction of autonomous and wireless communication-based technologies in the transportation industry has revolutionized the pace of technological advancements. The communication technologies present in the vehicles provide connections with external and internal IoT devices for customer experience enhancement while connections are established with the locality's traffic management centers to analyze and predict congestions and breakdowns by the city authorities. Connections are also made between two vehicles for collision avoidance and getting information of their directional changes. Quality of service in such applications sees a decrease with an increase in robust security parameters. Balancing both QoS and security constraints helps attain an even composition. Machine learning models have been instrumental in providing insights on enhancing QoS through adaptive verification methodologies [30]. Driving of autonomous cars also requires significant computer vision and machine learning technology for detection and avoidance of obstacles and for escaping hazardous situations. Hence, the field of autonomous driving is highly dependent on AI and machine learning for its base functioning and for its secure processing.

Aeronautical systems are also developing from traditional technology to smart intelligent communications based on sensory inputs/outputs. Aerospace cyber-physical systems have reached a certain point of development in wireless and analytical tools where the infusion of proper security into the system has become highly essential. Frameworks for hybrid intrusion detection [31] use machine learning models to predict and identify the type of attack on the system using data from the 6LoWPAN compression header. Three-layer processing for preprocessing and filtering the data helps classify malicious data. Hence, machine learning models can be employed in cyber-security for predictive and classification-based decision-making problems. The difficulty of destruction analysis in advanced nuclear facilities requires an alternate solution for authorities to carry out nuclear material balance analysis, process monitoring, and ensure real-time accountability. Data analytical models in machine learning are employed in such sectors for accurate and safe predictive processes in nuclear safeguards. Surveillance and radiation detection processes are carried out through predictive modeling using data attained from sensors and imaging. The decision making of machine learning models is accurate to a major extent and can alert the operators to check on the faulty points detected. Hence, predictive models are of great assistance in the visualization of data, maintaining security, and preventing mishaps in nuclear facilities.

6.3 Application Programming Interface (API) Security for Critical Applications

Application programming interfaces are predominantly used by businesses and organizations to connect their application services and transmit data. Intercommunication helps establish improved services to the consumers while providing automation strategies. The nature of data transmitted is a major factor in the type of API security required. Before the mainstream usage of Web APIs, SOAP Web services were considered to be popular. XML was highly used during the period of service-oriented architecture Web services. To ensure API security, awareness about how connected third-party applications funnel data back onto the Internet is highly essential. With the recent growth of cloud environments and services, big organizations and companies now possess several API stacks due to past acquisitions and mergers. The healthcare industry has gained interest in APIs for facilitating the data exchange between dissimilar systems to achieve interoperability between their backend applications and electronic health records. This allows electronic health records to be accessed by authorized users without compromising the systems to malware attacks. Government entities have also raised support for the implementation of APIs in healthcare's system infrastructure. The Centers for Medicare and Medicaid Services (CMS) believe that providing patients with the necessary tools for electronic access to their healthcare records can be achieved feasible by introducing APIs. The office of the National Coordinator for Health Information Technology has also voiced its support for APIs in the healthcare sector.

Banks and financial institutions have to abide by strict regulatory compliance rules and have unique attributes to their APIs. The high confidentiality and security requirements push this sector to use high grade security APIs to ensure strong protection and control. Access control of financial data is of utmost importance as this data will be accessed by authorized banking staff, auditors, and law enforcement agencies in addition to the actual account holders in addition to controlled access, data integrity must be maintained and any alterations in the data must be accounted for. Backing up the ledgers and detecting wrong or unauthorized write procedures are required to be made possible. The Equifax breach of 2017 [32] was an important point in time that pushed banks to ensure that their system and API security are working at their utmost potential. The Equifax Attack released highly confidential personal and financial information of half the population of the USA, leading to widespread occurrences of identity theft, insurance claims, and credit card frauds.

This decapitated the market share of Equifax, leading to a cost of close to $4 billion. This attack proved to be an eye-opener, which was followed by highly stringent regulations for institutions handling financial data. Banks have now started working toward opening their customer's accounts to third parties through Web-based APIs known as Open banking APIs. Third parties can now handle user bank accounts, get need information, and initiate transactions. Standards to protect customer data and meet the high grade security requirements like the OpenID Financial-grade API (FAPI) are now being backed up by major industry players. FAPI [33] employs code and Token Binding (including mTLS and OAUTB), JWS Client Assertions, and Proof Key for Code Exchange to provide maximum resistance and prevent attacks even from the strongest of intruders.

There is still a lingering fear, however, about the possibility of APIs opening up new security loopholes and vulnerabilities where a hack will cause a continuous flow of confidential data rather than one at a time like Web site hacks. Authorized users may also gain access to excess data rather than the exact data requested by them. Hence, different levels of confidentiality and exposure must be done to ensure that the total vulnerabilities are minimal. The development rate of APIs is also worrisome. Deployment of APIs without the presence of proper monitoring and testing of the access controls has increased significantly due to the evolution of continuous integration and deployment practices. Commercial software products that are mass produced usually have planned APIs ready to go. An administrator can open up APIs to unauthorized access during software installation, if not installed carefully. API security should not be supplied as an add-on after implementation but must be an integral part of the entire life cycle of the integration. Continuous and constant monitoring of API behavior will expose relatively more loopholes required to be corrected than checking for harmful code and modify access controls. A rigorous analysis of risks and vulnerabilities can help address problems that could open up gaps for a potential cyber breach. Recent approaches that provide protection against message alteration attacks (for SOAP messages) and XML injection attacks [34]. API service mesh creations must be reliable and secure in order to ensure increased performance and security. Security frameworks for this purpose have been established using Kubernetes and Istio along with novel association models to coordinate new APIS to extant categories of the mesh framework [35].

There are some generalized steps that can be followed to provide a basic layer of API security. Token-based authentication to confirm the identities of established and trusted users before relinquishing access controls and encryption methodologies can enable initial resistance to external attacks. Signature-based analysis of the accessed accounts can verify the integrity of data modifications and decryptions. Sniffers can be used to detect and track data leakages. Complete knowledge about the OS, drivers, networks, API components, and their overall working is a necessity to identify vulnerabilities that can be used to infiltrate the API. API call patterns that present as aberration most often indicate abuse or programming errors. Throttling rules can help prevent denial-of-service attacks. API gateway usages can help monitor traffic and derive a deeper analysis on the usage of APIs. Also, API security often boils down to proper API management.

6.4 Authentication and Identity Management in Smart Applications

Identity management deals with administration and standardization for the creation, maintenance, and de-provisioning of user accounts. Online services require proper identity management to ease the process of user provisioning. Smart identity management systems can work based upon internal agreements between the providers to adapt the data privacy rules and ownership. Blockchain applications are usually incorporated to facilitate this functionality in an open manner. Smart contracts are used to verify legitimate access and verification [36]. Third-party authentication services can be eliminated with the use of the smart contract generator to provide authentication for concerned parties and provide autonomous functions for a defined set of actions. Credential replication has been discouraged and the required information based on demand. These methods require proper reliability and trust between the online services and concerned parties. So, similar identity management procedures can conduct authentication of a user who accesses applications via the Internet. However, in IoT networks authentication methods have now increased concentration on the ability to single sign on users without exposing any weak points of the system. This approach can access an IoT edge device that is not connected to the Internet in addition to enabling context adaptation using a two key scheme. The above implementation was rendered feasible with negligible overhead for messages in close to 50 appliances [37].

Authentication decisions can also be made by studying user behavior to detect anomalous patterns in the observations. This emerges particularly helpful in the case of mobile applications as they act as a rich source for acquiring user location, nature of usage, and communication patterns to profile every individual. In most IoT environments and smart grids, securing intermediate interactions is pivotal for the success of the network. Apart from the mainstream authentication methods of one way, two ways, three-way, distributed and centralized methodologies, authentication protocols to mitigate the drop in security performance balance [38] based upon elliptic-curve cryptography have been regarded highly for their capability to identity protection and mutual key agreement. However, there is still a dire need for a highly robust mechanism of authentication like cancellable biometric systems and mutual authentication systems that exchange a collection of mutual collection of equal sized keys. These algorithms proved efficient in managing the computational restrictions of IoT networks while providing maximal security.

6.5 Standardization Activities for Securing Smart and Critical Applications

With the rise in complexity of technological products and software, several diverse standards have risen for applications associated with a single industry. Standards

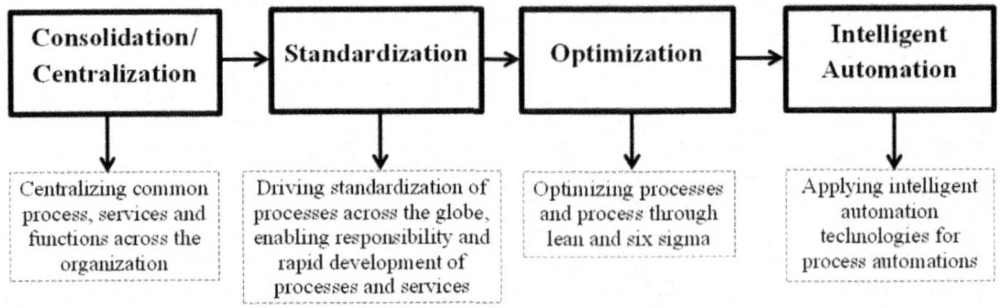

Fig. 3 Standardization chart of automation process

play a vital role in ensuring a secure and unbiased experience for the users. Enforcement of common standards also promotes integration opportunities as it reduces the degree of heterogeneity among systems built for different purposes. Standards have a huge effect on the entire life cycle of development. Standardization can be based upon the product or independent of the nature of the product. IEEE recognizes the imperative need for standards in all emerging technologies. Efforts toward standardization of blockchain have been undertaken by IEEE Standards Association, by recognizing and conducting activities like the virtual workshops on blockchain namely "Advancing HealthTech for Humanity" which was conducted recently. A separate initiative has also been put in place by IEEE to progress blockchain standards. Other workshops relating to the use of blockchain in health care and pharmaceuticals have been pioneered by IEEE. Figure 3 illustrates the critical role of standardization in a product's life cycle.

Artificial intelligence, on the other hand, has several challenges in modeling policies with the requirement of coordinated global responses. International standards that are in place can assist and support AI standardization on a global scale. ISO and IEEE are currently at the forefront of ongoing standardization activities in the field of artificial intelligence. Once strict guidelines have been set for general AI, specific and voluntary protocols enforced by domain-specific institutions can also be adopted if necessary. However, several AI leaders have expressed their concerns about the absence of policy objectives from ongoing standardization work.

Another technological domain in the spotlight for standardization is the field of IoT. Standardization of IoT communication protocols and description of standard models can accelerate the rate of integration and complexity of IoT networks. Several major corporations have made efforts to define M2M protocols and detect the need and market presence of IoT standardization but complete incorporation of standards is yet to take place. There are multiple hurdles present in the path of IoT in achieving global standardization, for example, platform compatibility, connectivity extensions, business models, and many more. However, no universal body has been formed yet. While organizations like IEEE, Internet Engineering Task Force (IETF), ITU-T, OneM2M, 3GPP, etc., are active at the international level, Telecommunication Standards Development Society, India (TSDSI), Global ICT Standardization Forum for India (GISFI), Bureau of Indian Standards (BIS), Korean Agency for

Technology and Standards (KATS), and so on, are active at the national level and European Telecommunications Standards Institute (ETSI) in the regional level for standardization. The authorities behind formulating regulations should provide some instructions and guidance to the industry experts, companies, and protect consumer rights. The private sector companies can also undertake the responsibility to ensure compliance with the existing regulatory guidelines.

7 Security Issues in Finance and Banking and Solutions in Many Other Applications Through Emerging Techniques

To establish a successful financial institution or banking system, the essential requirement is safeguarding the assets, money, and resources from theft or exploitation for personal benefit. Arriving at a critical juncture due to the impact of COVID-19, the financial sector is focused on closing down on any vulnerabilities and loopholes to promote trust among customers. Banks have started experimenting and proving the effectiveness of AI/ ML and blockchain-based security in the financial world. Even though these technologies prove superior in promoting security in most cases, they do have their pitfalls in certain scenarios. With blockchain security receiving praise for its transparent and robust nature, it is also imperative to analyze the possible downsides of this emerging technology. Some perceived risks of blockchain technology are mentioned here:

- The distributed ledger-based architecture of blockchain applications has given rise to new domains related to blockchain development that has been capitalized by many third-party companies. Usage of third-party blockchain applications can open up spots of vulnerabilities as the security of the system is only as strong as the system and data security of the vendor company. If the vendor company has flawed security in place with loopholes in their systems, intruders have the ability to exploit the weaknesses and attain access to the company's information. If the smart contract of a company is attained by an unauthorized member due to insecure systems of the vendor, the exploitation will be catastrophic for both the company and the vendor, leading to a lot of financial wastage in the form of resources and legal pursuits.
- Vulnerabilities at user endpoints where the blockchain and human operators coincide are critical. Although this problem might not fall under risk in a blockchain, we consider the entire system as a single entity and characterize this risk as part of blockchain security. The devices used to input, access, or modify the information in the blockchain serve as a medium of exploitation for intruders. Gaining control of the user end system due to weak credentials and poor authorization can let hackers access the confidential information present in the blockchain. Even when a blockchain system is equipped with cryptographic public and private

keys, access to a user end system can expose the keys without any need to hack the blockchain structure in the first place.

- Lesser period of complete testing makes blockchain a highly experimental field of technology. Although the stability of blockchain has been proven with crypto-currencies in the past, implementations of blockchain for security in other industries are a relatively new concept. Hence, it is essential to increase the testing period of these applications and train them for various scenarios to ensure a proper and well-round security system. High peer review of the application's source code and making followed by smart contract testing by different testing facilities can help strengthen the security features by rectifying loopholes.
- Considering that the implementation of blockchain security is a relatively new concept, it is understandable that the standards and regulations by which blockchain-based applications should abide by are very limited. Non-standard technology of any domain poses several vulnerabilities due to the difference in rules and regulations set by each individual companies and concerned parties. At any point of integration, the difference in characteristics and properties of the two systems, due to differences in standards, will result in a coalition where the security system to cope with both systems will not suffice.

Apart from blockchain, banks have also turned toward machine learning and artificial intelligence to formulate the "perfect" security plan to protect their technology and financial resources. However, the machine learning-based applications also exhibit a few downfalls in certain areas, discussed below. Machine-based decision-making processes promote high rates of accuracy in very little execution times but the process of arriving at a particular decision is not transparent to the users. The inability to perceive the way in which a machine learning application makes a decision based upon factors provided in a situation leads to discontent and unwillingness to accept the decision. Unknown biases in the decision-making processes could be catastrophic for the customers as well as the organization. Hence, the training schemes and the way in which a machine learning application are constructed to operate, play a huge role in its trustability and ensuring customer satisfaction. Another complaint put forth by consumers is the fact that machine-based interactions reduce the warmth and touch of interacting with a human being. Socially backward communities which are not digitally well-equipped feel the need for communicating their concerns and queries with a human before proceeding with a major financial decision. The approachability of an automated bank is drastically reduced when compared with a normal bank operating with human employees. Financial institutions have also received a lot of backlash for a reduction in employment and job opportunities due to the automation of several daily computational tasks. Employees face severe competition and feel the need to compete with AI, which proves far more efficient in executing repetitive calculations. Hence, they are fired from their jobs or moved to other jobs that they are unfamiliar with, to give way for automation. Although AI accelerates the competitive advantage and level of a bank to greater heights, it is instrumental for them to analyze the potential disadvantages and find possible ways of minimizing them.

8 Privacy Issues in e-Healthcare, Telecommunication, and Other Applications Through Emerging Techniques

With the introduction of any new technological domain integration into daily life applications, one important question that is fixated upon the mind of its users is whether their data and identity are safe. The satisfaction and trust it attains from a customer play a major role in determining the success of any technology. Security and ensuring privacy lead the list of factors that influence customer trust. When diving into possible privacy concerns, we contemplate the amount of data required to train a machine learning application. Algorithmic bias is highly undesirable. To prevent wrongful decisions from being taken, proper information and sufficient data content should be fed for training the application. Increasing the quantity of data and sources of obtaining data also increases the probability of infringing upon a person's private information. Catering to a very diverse group of consumers hikes the need for systems to address the problem of data deficiency and the ethical stopping point for means of attaining this data. Device heterogeneity is a cause of major concern that arises during the process of integration or scaling of applications. IoT devices and networks are often ruled by different standards according to rules and regulations set by concerned parties. This gives rise to different properties and characteristics of different networks. Managing several devices or combining two or more networks becomes particularly difficult due to their heterogeneity and compatibility issues. Authentication inefficiencies and the inability to deploy a universal security solution make the management of heterogeneous networks hard. These system vulnerabilities open up opportunities for intruders to breach the system and hence have to be prevented.

Recording of personal data for commercial purposes and duration of storing private data are both surrounded by legal implications if violated. General Data Protection Regulations by the European Union ensure that data obtained from consumers should not be held by the organization in perpetuity. Most data protection laws provide individuals with the right to request deletion of their personal info from company databases. The implementation of this law becomes tricky when a blockchain has been used to store the data. In the healthcare world, blockchain architectures are dominant and help store patient information in a transparent manner. Another concern about the use of blockchain for storing patient data is the diverse formats in which healthcare data is available. The ability of blockchain to traverse through extensive treatment plans and imaging data is highly unclear. This questions the ability of blockchain to adapt to order industries where the nature of data stored is not transactional. The best approach to try and solve this existing problem is to maintain storage of certain data off-chain in regular databases while their corresponding hashes are present in the blockchain for reference. This enables the editing and deletion of the data records while keeping all the concerned parties aware of the changes that have been made via the blockchain. Blockchain security is praised for its robustness but an integral part of maintaining the integrity of the blockchain system lies in the safety of the user credentials.

Concerned users are a part of the system import their own private key and no third-party companies are involved in this process. Hackers can exploit the lack in randomness of the signature process in ECDSA [39] to gain entry into the blockchain system, masking under the identities of legitimate users. It is close to impossible to retrieve a lost account due to the absence of monitoring and account retrieval systems administered by trusted third-party affiliations. Hence, these possible circumstances assert the fact that while several emerging techniques are qualified to provide protection of data, it is important to analyze the vulnerabilities of each technology to understand the most suitable security implementation for a given application.

9 Open Issues and Critical Challenges with Future Technology/Toward Post-COVID-19 Era

Technologies like AI and machine learning do not necessarily adhere to traditional safety methods that are supported by strong and expensive infrastructure. As most of the applications rely on computers and their networks, developers can create AI applications with just strong knowledge and basic hardware. AI programs are also not very transparent in their functioning and analysis. This in combination with the lack of proper regulatory controls can lead to catastrophic failure of the AI application. Hence, to ensure AI safety and equality, existing regulations are not sufficient and rule makers must study the ethical issues revolving around AI in a much deeper manner. The public should accept the principle of ethical requirements for the technology of AI and the principles must adhere to the broad consensus of the society. Human ethical values should be included during the stage of development itself. The final goal of AI is the understanding of human psychology. This gets imbibed so as to deliver the highest benefits for humanity and the natural atmosphere, taking into consideration the rights of the human, reduction of technological risks, and have a positive effect on society. The outside society and its environmental nature should be the goal of the policies and laws that go toward developing AI rules. Knowledge about safety procedures should be imparted to the public so that nobody can abuse the public using AI technology. The decisions of the AI systems should be unbiased ethically. For example, if historical data used for training the algorithms has some trait like gender discrimination or biased method of selection, then the algorithms, while executing the repetitive loop of the selection process in mass data, will reflect the same trait. If unaudited properly, this will become a pattern in the admission process itself, leaving undesirable effects on society. Some diseases statistically affect a particular demographic of a society more than others. Models that have been trained incorrectly may use this information to exhibit extremely racist or sexist behavior if left to complete automation. Conformation of AI to basic ethical standards must be made a top priority in terms of regulation.

IoT systems, on the other hand, encounter a different set of problems. Most IoT implementations are completely mission-oriented and cannot be interrupted unless absolutely necessary. The wide range of systems and heterogenous devices make IoT network security highly volatile. The integrative compatibility of IoT systems depends on several factors and subjective to every IoT network and the type of nodes on the network. Apart from the difficulty in interoperability, IoT system security is also weakened by the mismatch of protocols and node properties. All these issues in IoT are yet to be solved with a proven and regulated solution. A centralized IoT network architecture possessing proper configuration can override the processing throughput of most existing blockchain solutions. The increased cost of consensus functionalities in blockchain exacerbates the problem. The process of splitting the blockchain into shards to increase the overall performance of the nodes involved is also being reviewed by the Ethereum community.

9.1 Internet of Things and Cloud Computing in Post-COVID-19 Era: Applications and Challenges

In the past decade, we have seen major developments in technology and the price fall of smart gadgets. Smart devices are generally called as Internet of things, i.e., the things which run through Internet or access services through Internet. These smart objects are also called Internet-connected things. Similarly, cloud uses have been emerged in the past decade and at a very high rate, its demand has also increased. Storage or energy is two major problems of computing. Storage problem is solved by cloud computing, by storing data at edge or at cloud's edge and this data is accessible from anywhere, at any-time. Hence, these two important technologies have been used at a rapid rate in post-COVID-19 era. Thus, section will discuss various challenges faced during implementation of IoT and IoT-based cloud applications in solving real-world problems.

9.1.1 Challenges in Internet of Things (IoTs)-Based Cloud Applications

As of late, Internet of things (IoT) and distributed computing have been generally contemplated and applied in numerous fields, as they can give another strategy to savvy observation and association from M2M (counting man-to-man, man-to-machine, and machine-to-machine), and on-request use and proficient sharing of assets, individually. Specifically, the accessibility of information at up to this point unheard of scales and worldly longitudes combined with another age of wise preparing calculations is posing as a challenge for the Internet of things-based cloud applications. Information put away in the cloud is similarly delicate as different pieces of the IoT biological system. The foundation ought to have the option to secure information put away in the cloud. Insurance measures incorporate proper encryption, get to control, etc. Security vulnerabilities consistently exist regardless of how much endeavors we pay to upgrade your item code and equipment. For this situation, we should initially have the arrangement to fix mistakes and rapidly discharge patches, rather than leaving the blunders unfixed for an extensive stretch. Next, we need the necessity of furnishing clients with an immediate and secure technique to fix blunders. Right now, it is well known to refresh online gadgets over the air, yet we should guarantee that the above strategy itself would not become security vulnerability. IoT gadgets are frequently situated in open fields and are unattended and not genuinely ensured. We should guarantee that they would not be malevolently messed with by horrible association, penetrated by programmers, or worked utilizing a level head screwdriver. Likewise, we should ensure information that gets put away on the gadgets in any structure. Despite the fact that it is expensive to insert a security assurance part on each IoT gadget, it is as yet critical to scramble information on these gadgets.

(a) **Privacy**: In light of the previously mentioned security defects, numerous other security and protection issues present themselves in Internet of things. IoT utilizes Internet as a major framework used in interconnecting various topographically expanded IoT hubs and hence cloud is utilized as a key backend supporting foundation. In the writing, the assortment of the IoT hubs and the cloud is all in all called as an IoT cloud. Tragically, the IoT cloud experiences different disadvantages, for example, colossal system inactivity as the volume of information which is being prepared inside the framework increments. To lighten this issue, the idea of haze registering is presented, in which fog computing is situated between the IoT hubs and the cloud framework to locally process a lot of local information. Contrasted with the first IoT cloud, the correspondence inertness just as the overhead at the backend cloud foundation could be essentially decreased in the haze figuring upheld IoT cloud, which we will allude as IoT mist. Hence, a few significant administrations which were hard to be conveyed by the conventional IoT-based cloud. A couple of them are listed below as:

   - Burglary of delicate data like bank secret phrase.
   - Simple openness to individual subtleties likes contact address, contact number, and so on.
   - It might prompt open access to classified data like money-related status of an establishment
   - An assault on any one gadget may bargain the respectability of the various associated gadgets. In this manner, the interconnectivity has an immense disadvantage as a solitary security disappointment can disturb a whole system of gadgets.
   - The dependence on the Internet makes the whole IoT engineering powerless to infection assault.

A noteworthy forward jump in beating any boundary among virtual and physical universes began from the vision of the Web of Things (WoT), which uses open Web quantifies in achieving information sharing and articles interoperability. Social Web of Things (SWoT) further loosens up WoT to join sharp articles with casual associations and supposedly connects among physical and virtual universes just as support continued with participation between physical devices and human.

(b) **Security**: The security issues of the Internet of things (IoT) are straightforwardly identified with the wide utilization of its framework. Starting with presenting the engineering and highlights of IoT security, among these well-being estimates concerned, the ones about recognition layer are especially expounded, including key administration and calculation, security steering convention, information combination innovation, just as validation and access control, and so forth. A huge segment of the executed information between IoT gadgets is private data, which must not at all be listened stealthily on or altered. Security in IoT gadgets is in this manner of principal significance for additional advancement of the innovation. Such gadgets ordinarily have constrained region and vitality assets, which utilizes great cryptography restrictively costly. Physically Unclonable Functions (PUFs) are a class of novel equipment security natives that guarantee a change in outlook in numerous security applications; their generally straightforward engineering can answer a large number of the security difficulties of vitality compelled IoT gadgets. RFID is one of the empowering innovations of the Internet of things. RFID can possibly empower machines to recognize objects, comprehend their status, and convey and make a move if vital, to make "ongoing mindfulness." The inescapability of RFID innovation has offered to ascend to various significant issues including security and protection concerns.

(c) **Trust**: Trust the executives assume a significant job in IoT for dependable information combination and mining, qualified administrations with setting mindfulness, and upgraded client protection and data security. It assists individuals with conquering the impression of vulnerability and chance and participates in client acknowledgment and utilization on IoT administrations and applications. In any case, not many explore about trust system for Internet of things (IoT) could be found in the writing, however we contend that impressive need is held for applying trust component to IoT. We decay the IoT into three layers, which are sensor layer, focus layer, and application layer, from parts of framework synthesis of IoT. Each layer is obliged by trust the board for specific explanation: self-created, loaded with feeling coordinating and multiorganization independently. Likewise, an official decision creation is performed by organization requester as showed by the assembled trust information similarly as requester' system. Finally, we use an ordinary semantics-based and fluffy set speculation to see all above trust part, the result of which gives a general framework to the headway of trust models of IoT. The assets ought to be doled out to gadgets as per the framework strategy, which relies upon the data gave by industrial Internet of things (IIoT) gadgets. In the event that there are any asset requesting gadgets, they can report controlled vindictive data for their own enthusiasm to get more assets. That is, the brilliant assembling framework might be defenseless because of narrow minded shrewd assembling gadgets' practices. This lessens the effectiveness of the whole framework and besides stops the plant-wide procedure, while many exploration commitments identified with the trust processing target distinguishing vindictive hubs.

Hence, we can say that privacy, security, and trust are major issues in IoT-based cloud environments/applications. Industries are investing billions of dollars for providing users a hassle-free/secure environment to access their service. In other words, industries are spending a lot of money in avoiding any kind of cyber-attacks on their databases or businesses, any breaching on data reflect trust of consumer directly.

9.2 *Internet of Things Challenges and Solutions*

Protection of IoTs in the post-COVID-19 era: In the fight against COVID-19, technological advancements are continuously making a difference to healthcare systems. The speed of progress in the Internet of things (IoT) systems, in particular disease tracking, human movement, the identification of potential carriers and the remote monitoring of health conditions, is now being used and developed worldwide. According to Forrester Research analyst Chris Sherman [40], two US hospitals have already been targeted via virtual care systems, after a hacker exploited a loophole in a medical IoT device (specifically, a remote patient monitoring sensor) and obtained access to hospital patient databases. And in another type of attack, the Fresenius Group, a maker of medical devices and the largest private hospital operator in Europe, has been hit by ransomware.

(a) IoTs Privacy in the post-COVID-19 era: Most workers worked from offices in the pre-COVID-19 era, where the local area network (LAN) as well as the desktops/laptops were adequately protected. Sophisticated technologies could defend against cyber-attacks that mainly originated from the Internet and targeted the network of enterprises. Only support staff or those who need direct system/hardware access, e.g., testing laboratories, direct consoles, unique printing machines in the banking environment, etc., operate from the office in the post-COVID-19 period. In contrast to those at the workplace, the majority of the workforce is working from home and exposed to more insecure networks.

(b) Performance of IoT applications: Elasticity, which refers to the ability to add or subtract resources according to the needs of the application or service, is one of the most essential cloud computing services. The use of this facility is especially applicable to the Internet of things (IoTs) scope, as IoT requires a middleware that should be capable of handling high data volumes in real time.

(c) Ethical issues in IoT applications: The underlying information security issue in IoT is that there are many communicator-coupled sensors in IoT devices, for example, a camera, microphone, microchip or other sensors that collect environmental/communicated data. In this security issue, there is a connected communicator that transmits the communicated data to a remote located server like a cloud or other proprietary (authorized) server. Although many of the components have some security features, such as passwords that limit user access, a large part of the IoT security problem is that those passwords are typically set to a factory default and have never been changed [41]. However, the default passwords are widely accessible online [42]. The responsibility of the consumer is another problem. For starters, if changing passwords was simple enough, we might think that this is a core user duty [43]. It would be similar to seat belts in vehicles in this regard; it is the obligation of the driver to put them on. But that assumes that the modifications are simple; in other words, that users have the time and cyber-literacy needed to handle safe passwords.

(d) Sustainability of IoT infrastructure: The Internet of things is regarded by business and organizations as an opportunity for the present and the future that will digitize many operations and offer enormous benefits. Yet it also has the potential to help battle and protect the world from climate change. This is how the Internet of things in various fields, such as water use and energy efficiency, will affect the planet's sustainability. There is a long way to go for IoT technology compatible with the SDGs. The World Economic Forum is currently estimating that 75% of IoT ventures are small- and medium-sized, focusing on business, urban energy conservation, renewable energy, health, and responsible consumption. Public–private investments are crucial for projects to expand, Guerrero says. This will generalize IoT use, minimize costs, and extend its use. "Training, raising awareness in society of the importance of sustainability and demystifying technology are important for the large-scale implementation of IoT sustainable development projects," he says.

(e) Scalability in IoT: The fundamental property of an IoT system is that it will provide exclusive recognition for the advancement and creation of usefulness and applications of each "thing" and its virtual personification. Scalability is a very critical component of the modern and revolutionary developments in technology that occur every day [44]. As more and more devices or "things" are linked to the Internet, the various problems that occur as a result of this are a matter of utmost concern. For scalability in the IoT, there are countless things that need to be held in mind.

(f) IoT applications maintenance: In the coming years, the IoT will be instrumental in improving productivity and performance everywhere. This can lead to more efficient power management at plants and factories by automatically adjusting environmental control systems to reduce energy use when it is not necessary. The IoT will then change the way assets are handled in seven respects, but there are certainly several more:

- Greater adoption of predictive maintenance
- Real-time data analysis
- Accurate performance metrics
- Automatic software upgrades
- Recommended repair actions
- Tighter parts and inventory control

- Remote assets.

9.3 Cloud Computing Challenges and Solutions

Cloud reflects the concept of a distributed infrastructure consisting of a series of virtual machines that can be dynamically provisioned to meet the varying resource requirements of a client [45], and the entire basis of this cloud–customer relationship is governed by the service-level agreement (SLA). The National Institute of Standards and Technology (NIST) defines "the cloud as a model that allows convenient on-demand network access to a common configurable resource pool of computers, such as network, storage, etc." Cloud relieves the user of the overhead of the physical installation and maintenance of their device, which automatically reduces the overall cost and enhances the system's reliability. The use of cloud-based services results in an abstract layer being added between the physical storage or servers and the users whose data or services are stored in the cloud. The current situation is such that the cloud user's data or service owner must rely entirely on the cloud service provider (CSP) for their privacy and information security. The concept of mutual trust is reached to some degree by negotiating the SLA, but a good number of cloud-specific security issues are still going to need to be addressed by either the CSP or the user itself. When it comes to IT security concerns, data occupies the top spot, regardless of the infrastructure being used. Cloud computing is no exception to this, and it focuses on extra security problems because of its distributed nature and multitenant architecture. Its generation, storage, use, delivery, and destruction constitute the data life cycle. All these stages in the data life cycle should be assisted by each CSP with sufficient protection mechanisms.

(a) Cloud computing security: One of the main driving factors behind a user's decision to switch into a cloud system or stick with the legacy system that trusts on the cloud service provider (CSP) and their services. Confidence is focused on the evaluation of whether all threats have been addressed by a supplier, including data protection areas, VM protection, as well as other government and regulatory issues. Confidentiality, honesty, and availability (CIA) are the three factors that have been considered here for the cloud system security assessment. As well as the domain is a convention commonly used by the CIA to assess the security issues of a traditional information system?

(b) Cloud computing privacy issues: Distributed computing is a growing innovation that encourages the sharing of resources, such as software and hardware and Internet servers. But there are some problems in data cloud protection and privacy that are not as reliable as opposed to conventional IT operations, protection patching in the cloud is much easier, enforcement is more difficult to show in the cloud, data loss is less in clouds, more control power would boost security. There is a profound need to securely store, supervise, exchange, and analyze enormous complex knowledge steps, to establish examples and trends that take into account the ultimate aim of enhancing the quality of human services, better protecting the country and investigating elective vitality. It is important that fogs are safe as a result of the unpredictable technique for the applications.

(c) Reliability in cloud computing: Reliability is defined as the ability of a system or component to perform its necessary functions for a specified period of time under stated conditions. There are different types of disappointments that can place pressure on a cloud administration's unwavering dominance, including excess, timeout, missing data asset, missing asset calculation, programming dissatisfaction, database annoyance, discontent with hardware, and network failure.

(d) Quality of service in cloud computing: One of the issues posed by cloud computing is the quality of service. In making cloud services appropriate to consumers, this problem plays an important role in denoting the standards of performance, reliability, and availability provided by cloud services. Many implementations have been documented by literature for in order to achieve better performance and meet the needs of producers and customers, calculate, and ensure QoS in cloud computing systems.

(e) Cloud performance management: Applications for data management implemented in IaaS cloud environments must aim to reduce costs and provide good performance at the same time. Balancing these two priorities involves difficult decision making on a variety of axes: resource provisioning, location of queries, and scheduling of queries.

(f) Scalability in cloud computing: Measuring and testing the performance of cloud-based software services is critically important in the context of rapid cloud computing growth. Scalability, elasticity, and coherence are interrelated aspects of the performance of cloud-based computing services. The performance evaluation and testing of cloud-based computing services is critically essential in order to support the service-level agreement (SLA) compliant quality of delivery of these services, particularly in the context of the rapid expansion of the amount of service delivery. Scalability is the ability of the cloud layer to increase the delivery potential of the information service by expanding the amount of information service offered. This concept focuses on the technological side of cloud-based computing services, but we note that the literature frequently uses alternate, utility-oriented (i.e., economic cost/benefit focused) approaches.

(g) Cloud interoperability and portability: An underlying evolution of cloud computing is interconnected cloud computing. The academic and industry sectors have been attracted by various advantages offered by connecting clouds. Just like everyone else does, interconnected clouds have their own set of challenges, such as protection, control, authorization and identity management, vendor lock-in, and so on. The latest evolution faces challenges. Since it is difficult to find a cloud provider that can satisfy all customer criteria, customers attempt to merge services or switch from one provider to another. But one provider's customization of services does not allow it to be done easily. It takes a great deal of effort and cost, even though it is finished. This scenario is often referred to as vendor lock-in

(h) Cloud compliance: There is an ever rising need for businesses to comply with a variety of laws, regulations, and standards in the current market environment. Companies will need to be consistent in showing that they are in compliance and this will demonstrate because of the existence of such cloud vulnerabilities. There is a strong incentive for businesses to be able to clearly show complete compliance, considering the possible severity of penalties for noncompliance.

Hence, this section discusses IoT challenges and its solutions, as well as cloud challenges and solutions for the same. Now, next section will discuss several future research gaps or possibility in (with) the respective technology in the next decade.

10 The Road Ahead with Future Technology: Future Research Directions

The future directions of these emerging technologies have the potential to completely shatter the status quo. Blockchain will be navigated toward two areas. The first will include integration with other emerging fields like IoT, autonomous vehicles, and neural interfaces like brain-to-brain interfaces (BBI) or brain-to-computer interfaces (BCI). Smart contracts and decentralized autonomous organizations have a great scope of promoting blockchain systems. The compatibility of AI with blockchain and the increased value addition will propel AI blockchain integrations. Big data security and decentralization to establish control are some possible blockchain applications with AI. This gives users the required control over their own data and can determine the access control of third-party AI. A small organization dealing with AI can utilize this decentralization to propel its operations further and break the monopoly of large corporations. Another field has a bright scope for AI blockchain integration in the field of cyber-security. With the decentralized nature of blockchain preventing central failure vulnerabilities, machine learning models can predict intrusions and threat detection in real time. This installation will provide double-layer security and resolve the lack in the transparency of AI operations. Only time will tell whether AI and blockchain dominate the future of technology as expected but there is definitely extreme potential in humans reaping both individual and combinational benefits of this technology.

Computer vision and machine learning algorithms require high-performance CPUs to enable efficient processing. Even the most efficient CPUs may not improve the performance rate of AI applications. This challenge can be solved using AI-enabled chips. Optimization of tasks can be done much more easily using the intelligence of Ai chips. Duties can be performed individually by the CPUs and function in a much faster manner. Future AI technologies will implement the use of these chips in their systems. Human sensory AI that immerses humans into a world of sight, smell, and audio simulation is viewed as the next big thing in the near future, following AR and VR. Internet of things undergoes evergrowing complexity and is the next wave of breakthroughs for humanizing devices. The convergence of IoT technology with other emerging technologies has been accomplished and will be increased exponentially moving forward. IoT is estimated to revolutionize not just consumer experiences but also promote the advent of smart cities. Cars are becoming smarter with the integration of IoT and the rise of 5G networks will only accelerate the growth of IoT. The road ahead looks intriguing and interesting for emerging technologies and only time can tell if the current expectations are met.

10.1 Advanced Analytics with Machine Learning: A Way to Forward

Our main focus is to be at the front line of giving customized arrangements dependent on joining of machine Learning strategy, programming equipment elite processing, and preparing for a wide scope of information concentrated registering, information handling, and progressed examination for logical and business applications, utilizing both open source and in house R&D. With AI we can move toward:

- Artificial intelligence (AI) for cyber-security: Intrusion detection automatically by machine and artificial intelligence: In near future, AI-based solutions may find vulnerabilities over Web and reduce the load of cyber-security professionals. Note that hackers may use AI-based solutions to perform a serious attack on cyber-physical systems or any other computing systems or networking.
- AI for Industry 4.0: AI will provide full automation in near future to industry and intelligence too. AI-based manufacturing or logistics are few examples in near future, i.e., timely, and error free delivery, increase productivity, etc. Machine intelligence in medical imaging, machine learning and AI for penetration testing and machine learning in chemical sciences are also other example of AI for Industry 4.0.
- AI for data science: AI-based data science will be helpful (in trend in near future) in retail, banking, finance, weather forecasting, or stock market prediction.
- AI—IoTs integration for other sectors: AI can be used in many other sectors like software devilment, cloud computing/fog computing. Hence, few more possibilities of AI-IoT are:
  - IoT is higher education systems
  - Impact of IoT is education now and in future
  - A learning management system enhanced with Internet of things.

Hence, this section lists various future research directions for machine learning-based IoTs—cloud applications. The readers/researchers are suggested to read work [2, 46, 47] for knowing more machine learning, deep learning, and their importance in the next decade. Note that in [47], authors provide various future research gaps and opportunities in future toward Internet of things and Internet of everything. Also, readers can find out several issues in various computing platforms (including many useful applications like Healthcare, Transportation, etc.) in [47–49].

10.2 Future Research Directions for Machine Learning Toward Internet of Things-Based Cloud Applications

Currently, a large amount of picture, audio and video and metadata data created by users, such as network and user activity information, is being transferred to the cloud. This is due to the availability of comparatively inexpensive storage of information and cloud backup. Continuous research is underway to apply machine learning to applications for speech/audio recognition, text, image, and video processing, and language translation. In view of the broad computational requirements, conventional machine learning algorithms were limited to execution on large clusters. Furthermore, in order to perform complex learning tasks without incurring large monetary costs, APIs and software libraries are now available, for example, TensorFlow and Nervana Cloud from Google. The availability in cloud environments of hardware accelerators, such as GPUs, has reduced the computation time on large quantities of data for machine learning algorithms. The industry's interest in this field is due to the ability of predictive analytics to include deep learning.

The availability in cloud environments of hardware accelerators, such as GPUs, has reduced the computation time on large quantities of data for machine learning algorithms. The industry's interest in this field is due to the potential for deep learning in predictive analytics. Cognitive computing is a closely related avenue in the sense of future clouds. Cognitive systems in this visionary model would rely on machine learning algorithms and data generated to continuously generate knowledge. The obvious advantages of using fog computing include reducing device latency and enhancing users' quality of service (QoS) and experience (QoE) while exploiting hierarchical networking and tapping into tools that are not typically used for general computing purposes. Fog computing is therefore anticipated to allow the Internet of things (IoT) vision to be realized.

11 Conclusion

With the world progressing toward an emerging technological metamorphosis, the future of technology is uncertain yet positive. The common attribution to every emerging technology is the increase in productivity and ease of usage to steer humans toward a better tomorrow. As the complexity and autonomous nature of applications increases, the human effort and manual labor-associated decreases. Of the current trends and future directions of emerging technologies, this paper has reviewed and illustrated the practical applications of the most prominent domains and societal implementations. This work discussed several serious issues like security, privacy with respect to various smart and critical applications, especially for IoT-based cloud systems. Further several critical challenges with IoT, cloud computing, and IoT-based cloud systems also have been explained. Lastly, many future research views/future directions have been listed for future researchers. Future work in any of these domains can improve upon the existing trends and aim to resolve the issues affiliated with the discussed technological applications.

Conflict of Interest The author declares that he has no conflict of interest with respect to publication of this research work.

References

1. Sampath Kumar, Y. R., & Champa, H. N. (2019). An extensive review on sensing as a service paradigm in IoT: Architecture, research challenges, lessons learned and future directions. *International Journal of Applied Engineering Research, 14*(6), 1220–1243. ISSN 0973-4562.
2. Tyagi, A. K., & Rekha, G. (2019). Machine learning with big data (March 20, 2019). In *Proceedings of International Conference on Sustainable Computing in Science, Technology and Management (SUSCOM)*, Amity University Rajasthan, Jaipur, India, February 26–28, 2019.
3. Tyagi, A. K., Rekha, G., & Aswathy, S. U. (2020). Role of Emerging Technologies in COVID 19: Analyses, Predictions, and Future Countermeasures (December 16, 2020). Available at SSRN: https://ssrn.com/abstract=3749782or http://dx.doi.org/10.2139/ssrn.3749782
4. WHO: World Health Organization. (2020). *Contact tracing in the context of COVID-19*. https://www.who.int/publications-detail/contact-tracing-in-the-context-of-covid-19
5. Albahri, O. S., Zaidan, A. A., Albahri, A. S., Zaidan, B. B., Abdulkareem, K. H., Al-Qaysi, Z. T., Alamoodi, A. H., Aleesa, A. M., M.A. Chyad, M. A., Alesa, R. M., Kem, L. C., Lakulu, M. M., Ibrahim, A. B., & Rashid, N. A. (2020). Systematic review of artificial intelligence techniques in the detection and classification of COVID-19 medical images in terms of evaluation and benchmarking: Taxonomy analysis, challenges, future solutions and methodological aspects. *Journal of Infection and Public Health, 13*(10), 1381–1396.
6. Rodrigues, J. J., Segundo, D. B. D. R., Junqueira, H. A., Sabino, M. H., Prince, R. M., Al-Muhtadi, J., & De Albuquerque, V. H. C. (2018). Enabling technologies for the internet of health things. *Ieee Access, 6*, 13129–13141.
7. Priya, R., Akshaya, M., Gomathi, S., & Lavanya, S. (2016). A smart network: Iot to monitor temperature and heartbeat of a person using rfid technology. *International Journal of Chemical Sciences, 14*, 901–905.
8. Petscharnig, S., & Schöffmann, K. (2018). Learning laparoscopic video shot classification for gynecological surgery. *Multimedia Tools and Applicatoions, 77*, 8061–8079.
9. Laguarta, J., Hueto, F., & Subirana, B. (2020). COVID-19 artificial intelligence diagnosis using only cough recordings. *IEEE Open Journal of Engineering in Medicine and Biology, 1*, 275–281. https://doi.org/10.1109/OJEMB.2020.3026928
10. Mishra, M., Parashar, V., & Shimpi, R. (2020). Development and evaluation of an AI System for early detection of Covid-19 pneumonia using X-ray (Student Consortium). In *2020 IEEE Sixth International Conference on Multimedia Big Data (BigMM)* (pp. 292–296), New Delhi, India. https://doi.org/10.1109/BigMM50055.2020.00051
11. Miner, A., Laranjo, L., Kocaballi, A. B. (2020). Chatbots in the fight against the COVID-19 pandemic. *NPJ Digital Medicine, 3*. 65. https://doi.org/10.1038/s41746-020-0280-0

12. Zeng, Z., Chen, P.-J., & Lew, A. A. (2020). From high-touch to high-tech: COVID-19 drives robotics adoption. *Tourism Geographies, 22*(3), 724–734. https://doi.org/10.1080/14616688.2020.1762118
13. Chalmers University of Technology SE–412 96 Gothenburg, Sweden, Sichitiu, M. L., & Kihl, M. (2008). Intervehicle communication systems: A survey. *IEEE Communications Surveys, 10*(2), 88–105.
14. Aloqaily, M., Otoum, S., Al Ridhawi, I., & Jararweh, Y. (2019). An intrusion detection system for connected vehicles in smart cities. *Ad Hoc Networks, 90*, 101842. ISSN 1570-8705, https://doi.org/10.1016/j.adhoc.2019.02.001
15. Zhu, H., Lu, R., Shen, X., & Lin, X. (2009). Security in service oriented vehicular networks. *IEEE Wireless Communication Magazine, 16*(4), 16–22.
16. Lee, M., & Atkison, T. (2021). Vanet applications: Past, present, and future. *Vehicular Communications, 28*, 100310. ISSN 2214-2096, https://doi.org/10.1016/j.vehcom.2020.100310
17. Yang, L., Moubayed, A., Hamieh, I., & Shami, A. (2019). Tree-based intelligent intrusion detection system in internet of vehicles. In *2019 IEEE Global Communications Conference (GLOBECOM)* (pp. 1–6), Waikoloa, HI, USA. https://doi.org/10.1109/GLOBECOM38437.2019.9013892
18. Alheeti, K. M. et al. (2015). An intrusion detection system against malicious attacks on the communication network of driverless cars. In *2015 12th Annual IEEE Consumer Communications and Networking Conference (CCNC)* (pp. 916–921).
19. Dutta, R. G., Yu, F., Zhang, T., Hu, Y., & Jin, Y. (2018). Security for safety: A path toward building trusted autonomous vehicles. In *2018 IEEE/ACM International Conference on Computer-Aided Design (ICCAD)* (pp. 1–6). San Diego, CA. https://doi.org/10.1145/3240765.3243496
20. Chaudhary, A., Tiwari, V. N., & Kumar, A. (2014). Design an anomaly based fuzzy intrusion detection system for packet dropping attack in mobile ad hoc networks. In *Souvenir 2014 IEEE International Advance Computing Conference IACC 2014* (pp. 256–261).
21. Davi, L., Hatebur, D., Heisel, M., Wirtz, R. (2019). Combining safety and security in autonomous cars using Blockchain technologies. In: A. Romanovsky, E. Troubitsyna, I. Gashi, E. Schoitsch, F. Bitsch (Eds.), *Computer safety, reliability, and security. SAFECOMP 2019. Lecture Notes in Computer Science* (vol. 11699). Springer. https://doi.org/10.1007/978-3-030-26250-1_18
22. Schmittner, C., Griessnig, G., & Ma, Z. (2018). Status of the development of ISO/SAE 21434. In *25th European Conference, EuroSPI 2018*, Bilbao, Spain, September 5–7, 2018, Proceedings. https://doi.org/10.1007/978-3-319-97925-0_43
23. Tschorsch, F., & Scheuermann, B. (2016). Bitcoin and beyond: A technical survey on decentralized digital currencies. *IEEE Communications Surveys & Tutorials, 18*(3), 2084–2123.
24. Azaria, A., et al. (2016). MedRec: Using Blockchain for medical data access and permission management. In *Proceedings of the 2nd Int'l Conference on Open and Big Data (OBD 16)* (pp. 25–30).
25. Al Omar A., Rahman M.S., Basu A., Kiyomoto S. (2017) MediBchain: A Blockchain Based Privacy Preserving Platform for Healthcare Data. In: Wang G., Atiquzzaman M., Yan Z., Choo KK. (eds) Security, Privacy, and Anonymity in Computation, Communication, and Storage. SpaCCS 2017. Lecture Notes in Computer Science, vol 10658. Springer, Cham. https://doi.org/10.1007/978-3-319-72395-2_49
26. Díaz, M., Soler, E., Llopis, L., & Trillo, J. (2020). Integrating blockchain in safety-critical systems: An application to the nuclear industry. *IEEE Access, 8*, 190605–190619. https://doi.org/10.1109/ACCESS.2020.3032322
27. Ahmad, R. W., Hasan, H., Yaqoob, I., Salah, K., Jayaraman, R., & Omar, M. (2021). Blockchain for aerospace and defense: Opportunities and open research challenges. *Computers & Industrial Engineering, 151*, 106982.https://doi.org/10.1016/j.cie.2020.106982, ISSN 0360–8352.
28. França, A. S. L., Neto, J. A., Gonçalves, R. F., & Almeida, C. M. V. B. (2020). Proposing the use of blockchain to improve the solid waste management in small municipalities. *Journal of Cleaner Production, 244*, 118529.https://doi.org/10.1016/j.jclepro.2019.118529. ISSN 0959–6526.

29. Newaz, A. I., Sikder, A. K., Rahman, M. A., & Uluagac, A. S. (2019). HealthGuard: A machine learning-based security framework for smart healthcare systems. In *2019 Sixth International Conference on Social Networks Analysis, Management and Security (SNAMS)* (pp. 389–396), Granada, Spain. https://doi.org/10.1109/SNAMS.2019.8931716
30. Javed, M. A., Hamida, E. B., Al-Fuqaha, A., & Bhargava, B. (2018). Adaptive security for intelligent transport system applications. *IEEE Intelligent Transportation Systems Magazine, 10*(2), 110–120. https://doi.org/10.1109/MITS.2018.2806636
31. Maleh, Y. (2019). *Machine learning techniques for IoT intrusions detection in aerospace cyber-physical systems*. https://doi.org/10.1007/978-3-030-20212-5.
32. Luszcz, J. (2018). Apache Struts 2: How technical and development gaps caused the Equifax Breach. *Network Security, 2018*(1), 5–8.. https://doi.org/10.1016/S1353-4858(18)30005-9. ISSN 1353–4858.
33. Fett, D., Hosseyni, P., & Küsters, R. (2019). An extensive formal security analysis of the OpenID financial-grade API. In *2019 IEEE Symposium on Security and Privacy (SP)* (pp. 453–471), San Francisco, CA, USA. https://doi.org/10.1109/SP.2019.00067
34. Rajaram, A. K., Babu, B. C., & Kishore Kumar, R. C. (2013). API based security solutions for communication among web services. In *2013 Fifth International Conference on Advanced Computing (ICoAC)* (pp. 571–575), Chennai. https://doi.org/10.1109/ICoAC.2013.6922014
35. Hussain, F., Li, W., Noye, B., Sharieh, S., & Ferworn, A. (2019). Intelligent service mesh framework for API security and management. In *2019 IEEE 10th Annual Information Technology, Electronics and Mobile Communication Conference (IEMCON)* (pp. 0735–0742), Vancouver, BC, Canada. https://doi.org/10.1109/IEMCON.2019.8936216
36. Jeong, H., & Choi, E. (2012). User authentication using profiling in mobile cloud computing. In *Aasri Conference on Power and Energy Systems* (Vol. 2, pp. 262–267).
37. Witkovski, A., Santin, A., Abreu, V., & Marynowski, J. (2015). An IdM and key-based authentication method for providing single sign-on in IoT. In *2015 IEEE Global Communications Conference (GLOBECOM)* (pp. 1–6), San Diego, CA. https://doi.org/10.1109/GLOCOM.2015.7417597
38. Zhang, L., Tang, S., & Luo, H. (2016). Elliptic curve cryptography-based authentication with identity protection for smart grids. *PLoS ONE, 11*(3), e0151253. https://doi.org/10.1371/journal.pone.0151253
39. Johnson, D., Menezes, A., & Vanstone, S. (2001). The elliptic curve digital signature algorithm (ECDSA). *IJIS, 1*, 36–63. https://doi.org/10.1007/s102070100002
40. https://www.cxotoday.com/news-analysis/iot-security-in-the-era-of-covid-19/
41. Kan, M. (2016). *IoT botnet highlights the dangers of default passwords*, InfoWorld (October 4, 2016). Available at https://www.infoworld.com/article/3127167/password-security/iot-botnet-highlights-the-dangers-of-default-passwords.html
42. Hiner, J. (2018). *New research:Most IoT devices can be hacked into botnets*. TechRepublic (March 7, 2018). Available at https://www.techrepublic.com/article/new-research-most-iot-devices-can-be-hacked-into-botnets/
43. van de Poel, I., Robaey, Z. (2017). Safe-by-design: From safety to responsibility. *NanoEthics, 11*(3), 297–306.
44. Gupta, A. et al. (2017). Scalability in internet of things: Features, techniques and research challenges. *International Journal of Computational Intelligence Research, 13*(7), 1617–1627. Research India Publications. ISSN 0973-1873.
45. Mahdavinejad, M. S. et al. (2018). Machine learning for internet of things data analysis: a survey. *Digital Communications and Networks, 4*(3).
46. Tyagi A. K., Rekha G., & Sreenath, N. (2020) Beyond the hype: Internet of things concepts, security and privacy concerns. In: S. Satapathy, K. Raju, K. Shyamala, D. Krishna, & M. Favorskaya (Eds.), *Advances in decision sciences, image processing, security and computer vision. ICETE 2019. Learning and analytics in intelligent systems* (Vol 3). Springer.
47. Tyagi, A. K., Nair, M. M., Niladhuri, S., & Abraham, A. (2020). Security, privacy research issues in various computing platforms: A survey and the road ahead. *Journal of Information Assurance & Security, 15*(1), 1–16.

48. Marwan, M., Kartit, A., & Ouahmane, H. (2018). Security enhancement in healthcare cloud using machine learning. *Procedia Computer Science, 127*, 388–397. https://doi.org/10.1016/j.procs.2018.01.136. ISSN 1877–0509.
49. Nair, M. M., Tyagi, A. K., & Goyal, R. (2019). Medical cyber physical systems and its issues. *Procedia Computer Science, 165*, 647–655. ISSN 1877-0509.

Printed by Printforce, the Netherlands